ANATOMY AT A GLANCE

Sibani Mazumdar

Professor of Anatomy
Calcutta National Medical College, Kolkata, India
IPGME & R (Institute of Postgraduate Medical Education and Research), Kolkata, India

Ex Associate Professor of Anatomy
North Bengal Medical College, Darjeeling, India

Ex Associate Professor of Anatomy
Calcutta Medical College, Kolkata, India

Ex Associate Professor of Anatomy
Nil Ratan Sarkar Medical College, Kolkata, India

D1393992

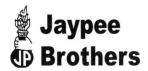

Jaypee Brothers

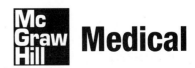

Mc Graw Hill **Medical**

© 2010, Sibani Mazumdar
First published in India in 2009 by

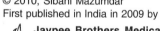

Jaypee Brothers Medical Publishers (P) Ltd.

Corporate Office
4838/24 Ansari Road, Daryaganj, **New Delhi** - 110002, India, +91-11-43574357

Registered Office
B-3 EMCA House, 23/23B Ansari Road, Daryaganj, **New Delhi** 110 002, India
Phones: +91-11-23272143, +91-11-23272703, +91-11-23282021,
+91-11-23245672, Rel: +91-11-32558559 Fax: +91-11-23276490, +91-11-23245683
e-mail: jaypee@jaypeebrothers.com, Website: www.jaypeebrothers.com

First published in USA by The McGraw-Hill Companies, 2 Penn Plaza, New York, NY 10121.
Exclusively worldwide distributor except South Asia (India, Nepal, Sri Lanka, Bhutan, Pakistan,
Bangladesh, Malaysia).

ISBN-13: 978-0-07-166720-3
ISBN-10: 0-07-166720-2

C 3776

Dedicated to

- All students (medical, dental, paramedical and nursing) —whose respect for teachers and eagerness to learn the subject, inspired me to write this book.
- My only son Avishek—whose help in processing the book inspired me.
- My husband—Dr Ardhendu Mazumdar, who unveiled me to the field of life.
- My mother—Asha Rani Biswas, whose blessings greatly inspired me.
- Professor Samar Deb—Professor and Head of the Department of Anatomy (NBMC), whose knowledge, devotion, and love for the subject gave me inspiration.
- Pupils all over the world.

MESSAGE

To my beloved students

- Though this is a small book, it is charged with energy and potential.
- This book has been written in a simple, lucid and communicative style.
- Remember "Read and Repeat" is an important step for effective learning.
- The overall objectives of this book is to develop the integrated skills of listening, speaking, reading, and writing and to develop a knowledge of Anatomy.
- Above all, now is the time to build up your character. It is that power that enables humans to win victories even after losing battles.

PREFACE

I was inspired by my students to write this book, *Anatomy at a Glance*. Every chapter includes easy-to-understand diagrams that simplify the entire learning process. The beauty of this book is that most diagrams are on the same page as the text, which facilitates retention. Most of the chapters are written in tabular form. This book will help the medical, paramedical, and nursing students. It would also be helpful to PG students for a quick review of Anatomy. It is written in simple language. In the glossary, I have included meanings of various medical terminology. At the beginning of each chapter I have given necessary terminology. In Window Dissection Chapter, students can quickly learn Anatomy point by point, as unnecessary details in Anatomy have been omitted here. In each chapter I have tried to give the *functional* anatomy. There may be unintentional errors in the writing or printing of this book. If my colleagues or students contact me I would be very appreciative. Any suggestions regarding improvement are always welcome.

Sibani Mazumdar

ACKNOWLEDGEMENTS

1. Jaypee Brothers Medical Publishers (P) Ltd.—who gave me an opportunity to publish this book.

2. All the staffs of Jaypee Brothers, Kolkata who helped me in processing the book.

3. The heads of the Departments of Anatomy Prof. Rita Roy (Calcutta National Medical College), Prof. Asis Dutta, Prof. Debabrata Kar (Institute of Postgraduate Medical Education and Research), Prof. Sumita Sarkar (KPC Medical College), Prof. Anjan Sen (Calcutta Medical College), Prof. Samar Deb (Principal of Katihar Medical College)—the trees, under which this sapling was born.

4. All the teachers and staffs in the Department of Anatomy CNMC (IPGME & R) North Bengal Medical College, Calcutta Medical College, and Nil Ratan Sarkar Medical College for their encouraging learning environment.

5. Dr Narayan Jyoti (dental surgeon), Dr Karabi Baral, Dr Viswa Prakash Das, Sandip (paramedical student), Debanjan (MBBS student), Gargi Biswas (Computer technologist) and Sudipto Das (Computer teacher), who extended their helping hands towards me.

6. The librarian and staffs of North Bengal Medical College, Calcutta Medical College (IPGME & R) and Calcutta National Medical College—whose help cannot be overstated.

7. I express my gratitude to the authors of various medical books who enriched my knowledge through their valuable writings.

8. My gratitude to Prof. P Dev (Dean of UBMES and Head of the Department of Radiology) and Dr Sohini Sengupta—Assistant Professor (Radiology IPGME & R) for incorporating radiological pictures in this book.

CONTENTS

Chapter 1

Introduction

DEFINITION OF ANATOMY

Anatomy is a science that deals with the structure and functions of the body.

Branches are:

Gross anatomy—which is visible in naked eye.

Microanatomy or histology—(which is visible with the aid of microscope).

Clinical anatomy—it is the practical application of anatomical knowledge to diagnosis and treatment.

Developmental anatomy or embryology—it is structural changes of an individual from fertilization up to full-term baby.

Radiological anatomy—study of anatomical structure by radio photo.

Surface anatomy—study of surface projection of a structure (like heart, stomach, etc).

Positioning (Body Posture) (Fig. 1.1)

Anatomical position: It is that position in which a person is standing erect, with eyes looking towards horizon, arm is by the side of the trunk, palm faces forwards.

Supine position: The subject is lying on the back with faces up.

Prone position: The subject is lying with faces down and belly, on the table.

Lateral position: Position in which, the side of the subject is adjacent to the film.

Lithotomy position: The subject is lying in supine position with flexed hip and knee. It is useful in dissection of perineum and during delivery.

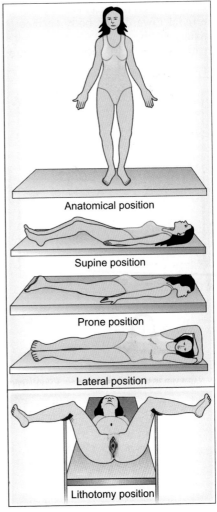

Anatomical position

Supine position

Prone position

Lateral position

Lithotomy position

Fig. 1.1: Positioning

Anatomical Terms (Figs 1.2A to D)

- Superior or cephalic towards the head or upper part of a structure, e.g. the head is superior to the neck.
- Inferior or caudal away from the head. Navel is inferior to the chest.
- Anterior or ventral towards the front part of the body.
- Posterior or dorsal towards the back part of the body.
- Towards the midline of body.
- Proximal closer to the origin (closest to the trunk).
- Distal away from the origin (away from trunk).
- Superficial towards the body surface (skin is superficial).
- Deep away from the surface (muscles are deep).

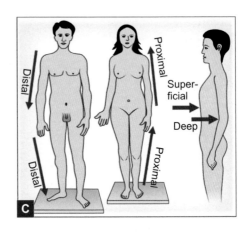

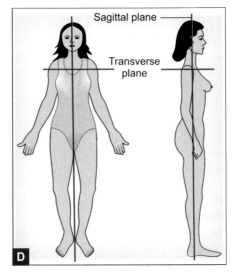

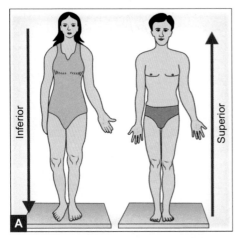

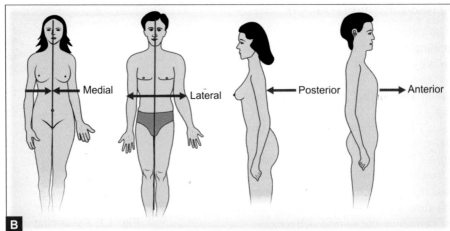

Figs 1.2A to D: Anatomical terms

Terminology Used in Description of Bones (Fig. 1.3)

Ala: Wing-like process (e.g. alar of sacrum).

Canal: A bony tunnel (e.g. vertebral canal).

Condyles: Smooth and articular projection (e.g. condyles of femur).

Crest: A ridge with certain breadth (e.g. iliac crest of hip bone).

Epicondyles: Nonarticular bony projection situated above the condyle (e.g. lateral and medial epicondyle of femur).

Facet: Small, smooth articular surface (e.g. costal facet).

Fossa: It is a depression on the surface of the bone (e.g. coronoid and olecranon fossa of lower end of humerus).

Foramen: An opening in the bone (e.g. nutrient foramen of a long bone).

Hamulus: A hook-like process (e.g. pterygoid hamulus).

Hiatus: A gap in the general outline of a bone (e.g. sacral hiatus).

Incisura: A notch in the general outline.

Lingula: A tongue-shaped projection (e.g. lingula of mandible).

Linea: A line-like elevation (e.g. linea aspara of femur).

- Lips: Elevated mergin of a crest (outer and inner lips of iliac crest).
- Meatus: A narrow passage (e.g. middle meatus of nose).
- Process: Any localized projection is known as process (e.g. olecranon process of ulna).
- Ridge: A linear elevation on surface of bone.
- Spine: A pointed bony process (e.g. spine of vertebra).
- Squama: Flat scale-like appearance of a bone (e.g. squamous part of occipital).
- Sulcus: A groove on surface of bone (e.g. intertubercular sulcus of humerus).
- Trochanters: Large nonarticular projection of varying shape and size (greater and lesser trochanters of femur).
- Trochlea: Pulley-shaped articular surface (e.g. trochlea of lower end of humerus).
- Tubercle or tuberosity: Localized rounded thickening on the surface of bone; size is smaller than trochanter (e.g. greater and lesser tubercle of humerus).

Regional Terms for Specific Body Areas (Fig. 1.4)

Anterior

- Frontal (Forehead)
- Orbital (Eye)

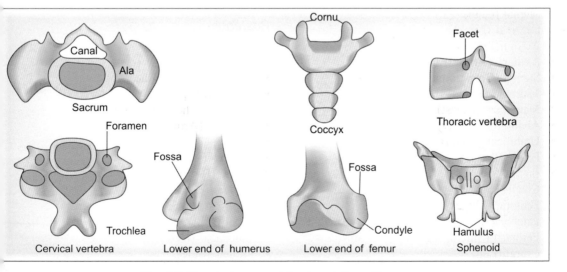

Fig. 1.3: Terminology used for description of bones

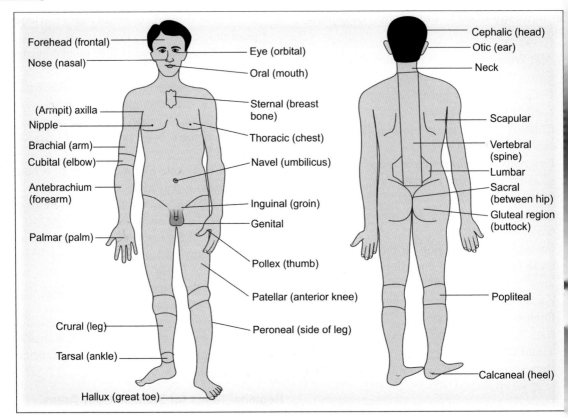

Fig. 1.4: Regions of body

- Nasal (Nose)
- Buccal (Cheek)
- Oral (Mouth)
- Mental (Chin)
- Cervical (Neck)
- Acromial (Point of shoulder)
- Axillary (Armpit)
- Sternal (Breast bone)
- Thoracic (Chest)
- Mammary (Breast)
- Abdominal (Belly)
- Umbilical (Navel)
- Pelvic (Pelvis)
- Inguinal (Groin)
- Coxal (Hip)
- Femoral (Thigh)
- Patellar (Anterior knee)
- Peroneal (Side of leg)
- Crural (Leg)
- Tarsal (Ankle)
- Digital (Toes)
- Hallux (Great toe).

Posterior

- Cephalic (Head)
- Otic (Ear)
- Occipital (Back of head)
- Vertebral (Spine)
- Scapular (Shoulder blade)
- Brachial (Arm)
- Antebrachial (Forearm)
- Lumbar (Loin)
- Sacral (Between hips)
- Gluteal (Buttock)
- Popliteal (Back of knee)
- Sural (Calf)
- Calcaneal (Heel)
- Plantar (Sole).

Skeletal System

SKELETON (FIG. 2.1)

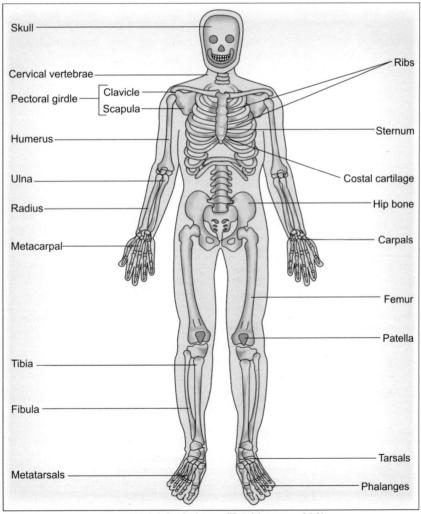

Fig. 2.1: Adult skeleton (Total bones—206)

SCLEROUS TISSUE (specialized connective tissue). It is of two types—cartilage and bones.

Difference between cartilage and bones

Cartilage	Bones
• Gives strength as well as resiliency.	• Gives strength as well as form skeletal framework of body.
• Least vascular.	• Highly vascular.
• Grows both by appositional and interstitial method.	• Grows by appositional method.
• Nonnervous.	• Has nerve supply.

Cartilage (3 types)

Hyaline cartilage (e.g. articular, costal, respiratory) (Fig. 2.2)	Elastic cartilage (e.g. epiglottis, pinna) (Fig. 2.2)	Fibrocartilage (intervertebral disk) (Fig. 2.2)
• Ground glass appearance of matrix.	• Presence of abundant elastic fibers in matrix.	• Most compressible cartilage.
• Collagen fibers present.	• More flexible than hyaline cartilage.	• Resist stretch.
• In old age, segmental degeneration of cartilage.	• No change in old age.	• In old age, intervertebral disk becomes thin.

You (students) will be surprized to know that a bone in living body is a living tissue.

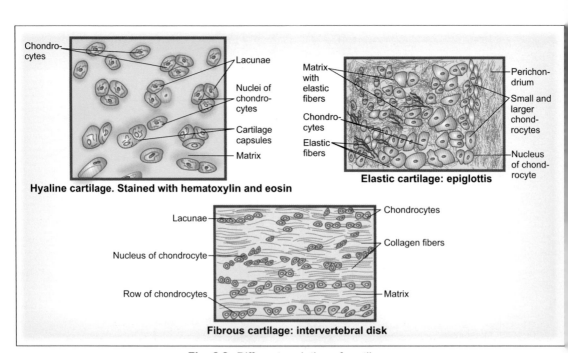

Hyaline cartilage. Stained with hematoxylin and eosin

Elastic cartilage: epiglottis

Fibrous cartilage: intervertebral disk

Fig. 2.2: Different varieties of cartilage

ssification of Bones According Shape (Fig. 2.3)

Long bone: Here length is greater than breadth. It is composed of a diaphysis and two epiphyses. The epiphysis contains spongy bone. The medullary cavity of long bone contains red

3. Flat bone: It consist of two thin plates of compact bone, enclosing a dipole (spongy bone layer), e.g. skull bone sternum. In adult, hemopoietic tissue is found within the dipole.
4. Irregular bone: Irregular in shape, e.g. hip bone, vertebrae.

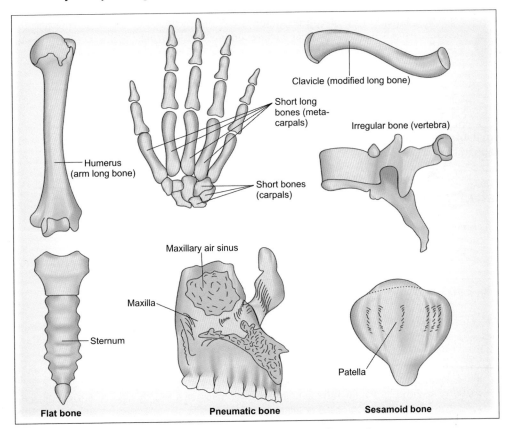

Fig. 2.3: Classification of bones according to shape

marrow for hemopoiesis; but in adults, it is replaced by yellow marrow. Periosteum covers the diaphysis. Endosteum lines the medullary cavity. Muscles are attached to periosteum (e.g. femur, tibia, humerus). Long bones continue to grow until adolescence.

Short bone: Cubical in shape. Out of six surfaces usually four surfaces are articular (e.g. carpal and tarsal bone).

5. Sesamoid bone: Seed-like. Develops within a tendon of muscle, having no periosteum and harvesian system (e.g. patella in a quadriceps femoris and pisiform in flexor carpi ulnaris tendon).
6. Pneumatic bone: Pneuma means air. A bone contains air-filled cavity, e.g. maxilla.
7. Accessory bone: Extra-bone particularly seen in seventh cervical and first lumbar vertebra. It is due to separation of costal element from transverse process.

Bones of Superior Extremity

Names	Comments	Important features	Anatomical position

Clavicle (Collar bone) (Figs 2.4A and B)	Modified long bone; horizontally placed, shape like 'f'.	Two ends: 1. **Sternal**: Quadrangular
		        2. **Acromial**: Flat
		Shaft:
		1. Medial 2/3rd (convex in front) has 4 surfaces:
		  a. **Anterior surface**: origin of calvicular head of **pectoralis major**.
		  b. **Posterior surface**: origin of **sternohyoid**.
		  c. **Superior surface**: near sternal end few fibers of **sternocleidomastoid**.
		  d. **Inferior surface**:
		    i. A rough area medially.
		    ii. A subclavian groove laterally gives attachment to **clavipectoral fascia** (in anterior and posterior margins) insertion of **subclavius** muscle.
		2. Lateral 1/3rd (concave in front) has
		  a. Two borders:
		    i. Anterior—concave, gives attachment of **deltoid**.
		    ii. Posterior—rough, convex gives attachment of **trapezius**.
		  b. Two surfaces:
		    i. Superior, subcutaneous (palpable).
		    ii. Inferior, present conoid tubercle and trapezoid ridge.
			• Place medial 2/3r convexity in fron Subclavian groove o inferior surface.
			• Sternal end lies more i anterior plane.

Scapula (shoulder blade) (Fig. 2.5)	Flat triangular; lies in back opposite second to seventh rib.	Two surfaces:
		a. **Ventral**—hollow out **subscapularis** is attached
		b. **Dorsal**—marked by spine which divides the surface —two fossae:
		  i. Supraspinous—supraspinatus attached.
		  ii. Infraspinous—infraspinatus attached. It has head or glenoid, neck and body.
		Three borders:
		a. **Superior**—shortest; marked medially by suprascapular notch.
		b. **Medial or vertebral**—largest; in the: **ventral aspect**—gives attachment of serratus anterior.
		dorsal aspect—from above downwards: gives attachment to levator scapulae, rhomboidus minor and major.
		c. **Lateral or axillary**—thickest border, in the:
		  i. **ventral aspect**—gives attachment of subscapularis.
		  ii. **dorsal aspect**—from above downwards: Teres major and minor.
			• Superior border with suprascapular notch above.
			• Spine in on dorsa surface.
			• Tip of the coracoid process directed forwards and slightly laterally.
			• Glenoid looks laterally and upwards.

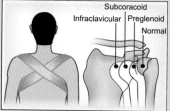

Fig. 2.4A: Figure of 8 bandage in fracture clavicle

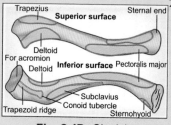

Fig. 2.4B: Clavicle

Contd...

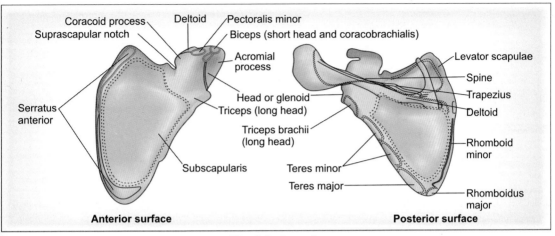

Fig. 2.5: Scapula

Names	Comments	Important features	Anatomical positions
		Three angles: a. **Superior**—meeting of superior and medial borders—obscured by muscle. b. **Inferior angle**—meeting of lateral and medial borders—over lies seventh rib. c. **Lateral angle or glenoid**—provide a shallow-socket for head of humerus—forming gleno-humeral or shoulder joint—synovial ball and socket joint. Three processes: a. **Spinous process**—dorsal border or crest of spine—deltoid is attached at lower lip, trapezius is attached at upper lip. b. **Coracoid process**—it is atavistic type of epiphysis—gives attachment of pectoralis minor, short head of biceps, coracobrachialis and coracoclavicular ligament. c. **Acromial process**—projecting forwards from spine.Acromian angle (junction of lateral and inferior border) gives attachment of deltoid—lateral border. attachment of trapezius—medial border. It has **upper end, lower end** and **shaft**.	
Humerus (arm bone) (Figs 2.6A and B)	Longest and largest bone of upper limb.	**Upper end presents** *Head*—globular, articular, forms shoulder joint. It is directed upwards, medially, and slightly backwards. *Neck-anatomical*—constriction adjoining head, capsular ligament is attached here. *Morphological*—junction between epiphysis and diaphysis (epiphyseal line).	• Place globular head above. • Place bicipital grooves coronoid and radial fossa in front.

Contd...

Names	Comments	Important features	Anatomical positions

Surgical—it is the most constricted portion, in the upper part of shaft - vulnerable to trauma.

Tubercles—greater–lies in lateral part; covered by deltoid, produces rounded contour of shoulder. There are three impressions for attachment of supraspinatus, infraspinatus and teres minor muscles.

Lesser—separated from greater tubercle by bicipital groove; gives attachment to subscapularis.

Shaft

Three borders—anterior, medial and lateral lower part of lateral and medial border is prominent and known as lateral supracondylar line.

Three surfaces

a. Anteromedial surface: marked by bicipital groove. It presents two lips:
   i. Pectoralis major—is attached in lateral lip,
   ii. teres major—at medial lip. In floor lies latissimus dorsi.
b. Anterolateral surface: in the middle rough impression—deltoid tuberosity. Deltoid is inserted.
c. Posterior surface: in the middle third. There is shallow spiral groove (lodges radial nerve and arteria profunda brachii.

Lower 1/3rd is flat. Gives origin to medial head of triceps, linear origin of lateral head of triceps above spiral groove.

Lower end

Articular part—Pulley-shaped articular surface medially (trochlea), rounded articular surface laterally (capitulum).

Nonarticular part—coronoid fossa, radial fossa in front and olecranon fossa behind capsular ligament of elbow joint attached at the margin of articular area and it includes three fossae.

i. Medial epicondyle gives common origin of flexor muscle.
ii. Ulnar nerve lies behind the medial condyle and behind lateral epicondyle common extensor of forearm arises.

• Place greater tubercle on lateral aspect.

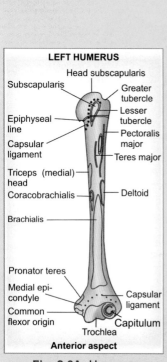

Fig. 2.6A: Humerus

Abbreviation

FDH–Flexon digtorum superficialis
FPL–Flexor pollicis longus
FDS–Flexor digitorum superficialis
EPL–Extensor pollicis longus
EPB–Extensor pollicis brevis

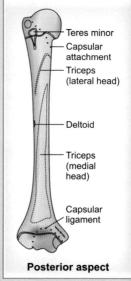

Fig. 2.6B: Humerus

Names	Comments	Important features	Anatomical positions
Radius (Figs 2.6C and D)	Lateral bone of forearm. It has upper end, shaft and lower end. Forms elbow joint, wrist joint, superior, middle, and inferior radioulnar joint.	**Upper end** Head—cup-shaped upper surface forms joint with capitulum of humerus—forms part of elbow joint. Neck—constricts part below head. Tuberosity—rough projection below and medial side of neck—gives attachment to biceps brachii. **Shaft**—three borders: a. Anterior border—upper part form anterior oblique line. Flexon digitorum superficialils is attached.	• Place dorsal tubercle posteriorly. • Disk like head should be placed above. • Styloid process should be on lateral aspect.

Contd...

Names	Comments	Important features	Anatomical positions

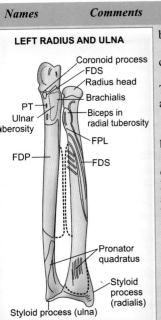

LEFT RADIUS AND ULNA

Coronoid process
FDS
Radius head
Brachialis
PT
Ulnar
tuberosity
Biceps in radial tuberosity
FPL
FDP
FDS
Pronator quadrata
Styloid process (radialis)
Styloid process (ulna)

Anterior aspect

Fig. 2.6C: Radius and ulna

Abbreviations

DH–Flexure digotorum super-cialis FPL–Flexor pollicis ngus, FDS–Flexor digitorum uperficialis, EPL–Extensor ollicis longus, EPB–Extensor ollicis brevis, EI–Extensor dicis

b. Posterior border—upper part form posterior oblique line.
c. Interosseous border—sharp; starts from radial tuberosity. Interosseous membrane is attached
Three surfaces:
a. Anterior—hollow out in upper part-flexor pollicis longus, pronator quadratus is attached (in the lower part).
b. Posterior—supinator, abductor pollicis longus, extensor pollicis brevis is attached.
c. Lateral—pronator teres, supinator is inserted.
Lower end—enlarged; presents five surfaces:
a. Anterior surfaces—concave.
b. Posterior surfaces—marked by ridges and grooves; dorsal tubercle is present. From lateral to medial-abductor pollicis longus, extensor pollicis brevis, extensor carpii radialis longus and brevis, extensor digitorum is related.
c. Medial surfaces—there is a notch present.
d. Lateral surfaces—forms styloid process-insertion of brachioradialis.
e. Inferior surfaces—articular; lateral triangular impression articulate with scaphoid, medial one to lunate.

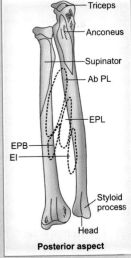

Triceps
Anconeus
Supinator
Ab PL
EPL
EPB
EI
Styloid process
Head

Posterior aspect

Fig. 2.6D: Radius and ulna

| Ulna | Medial bone of forearm. Forms elbow joint; superior, middle and inferior radioulnar joint. | **Upper end**—hook-like—two processes:
a. Coronoid process—lateral surface present radial notch. Anterior surface present rough ulnar tuberosity gives—attachment to brachialis.
b. Olecranon process—superior surface gives—attachment of triceps, capsular ligament.
Shaft—three borders—
a. Anterior
b. Posterior—palpable; common aponeurotic origin of flexor and extensor carpi ulnaris.
c. Interosseous—attachment of interosseous membrane.
Three surfaces:
a. Anteriors—nutrient foramen present here. Gives attachment to flexor digitorum profundus, pronator quadratus and supinator.
b. Posterior—divided into:
  i. Upper oval area—anconeus is inserted.
  ii. Lower large area—origin of abductor pollicis longus, extensor pollicis longus and extensor indicis. | • Place more expanded end with olecranon process and coronoid process above.
• Head with styloid process below.
• Place trochlear notch anteriorly. Sharp interosseous border is lateral. |

Classification of Bones in General

A. According to Shape
1. Long bones—three types
   a. Long long bone, e.g. Humerus
   b. Short long bone, e.g. Metacarpal
   c. Modified long bone, e.g. Clavicle
2. Short bones (Cubical in shape), e.g. Carpals and tarsals
3. Flat bones: Sternum
4. Irregular bones: Hip bone
5. Sessamoid bones: Patella
6. Pneumatic bones: Maxilla
7. Accessory bones: Cervical ribs

B. According to Development
1. Membranous: Parietal bone
2. Cartilaginous: Femur bone
3. Membrano-cartilaginous: Clavicle

C. According to Position
1. Axial bones : Skull 29
   Vertebral 26
   Ribs and sternum 25
2. Appendicular bones:
   Bones of upper limb 64
   Bones of lower limb 62

Articulated Skeleton of Hand (Fig. 2.7)

It comprises of 8 marble size short bones of carp closely united by ligaments, 5 metacarp (numbered from thumb to little finger as 1 to and phalanges (comprising of 14 bones), 3 in e (2 to 5 finger) except first (consists of 2 phalange Gliding movements occur between the car bones. So it is flexible (can be assessed dur wearing of short bangles inside the hand). T carpal bones are arranged into two rows:

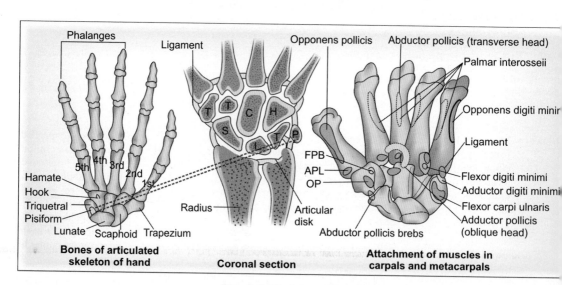

Bones of articulated skeleton of hand   Coronal section   Attachment of muscles in carpals and metacarpals

Fig. 2.7: Skeleton of hand

oximal row (from lateral to medial side)—
phoid (boat shaped), lunate (crescentic moon
e), triquetral (triangular), pisiform (pea seed
e).

stal row (from lateral to medial side)—
pezium (distal articular surface saddle shaped),

trapezoid (boot shaped), capitate (longest carpal
bone with a head), hammate (hammer-like with
hook).

Applied Anatomy of Bones (In General)

FRACTURE—break in the normal outline of bone
(Fig. 2.8).

Fracture type	Description	Comments
Simple	Bone break clearly but does not penetrate the skin.	Sometimes called closed fracture.
Compound	Broken end of bone protrudes through soft tissue and skin.	More serious than simple fracture.
Comminuted	Broken fragments into many pieces.	Common in aged whose bones are more brittle.
Green stick	Bones break incompletely, much like green twigs break.	Common in children whose bones are more flexible.
Derpessed	Broken bone portions are pressed inward.	Typical in skull fracture.

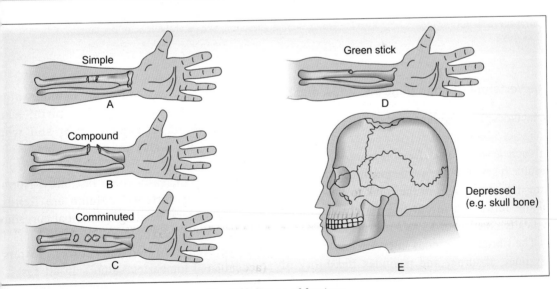

Fig. 2.8: Types of fracture

Osteoporosis: A diminution of bone mass; particularly in elderly fellow.

Injury of upper limb bone

Bone involved	Comments
Fracture of clavicle	It is common, particularly in children and young adults, due to fall of outstretched hand. Fracture is usually in mid-shaft region in children.
Fracture of scapula	Fracture in the body of scapula is due to direct blow. Fracture in the neck of scapula is due to fall on shoulder.
Fracture of surgical neck of humerus	It can occur with a fall on, the outstretched hand, particularly in the elderly woman.
Fracture of shaft of humerus	It is produced when a fall is accompanied by twisting injury. It may involve the radial nerve and there is wrist drop.
Supracondylar fracture	It is common injury to children and adolescents due to fall on the outstretched hand. The structures at risk are brachial artery and median nerve.
Forearm fracture	These fractures interfere with pronation and supination.
Colles' fracture	Fracture in the lower end of the radius with or without 'dinner fork' deformity due to fall on the outstretched hand.
Scaphoid fracture	Above 70% of carpal fractures, only the scaphoid is broken, due to fall on the outstretched hand. Palpation of anatomical snuffbox is more painful. High rate of non-union and avascular necrosis (in proximal part) is common.
First metacarpal Fracture	Also known as Bennet's fracture, occurs at the base of the thumb.

The Vertebral Column (Figs 2.9, 2.10A and B)

It includes 26 irregular vertebrae (7 cervical, 12 thoracic, 5 lumbar, sacrum and coccyx) connected in such a way that a flexible curved structure results. It supports the axial structure of trunk and transmits the weight of the trunk to lower limb. In the fetus and infant the vertebral column typically consists of 33 separate pieces of bone.

The fibrocartilaginous intervertebral disk acts as shock absorber and provides flexibility of vertebral column. When somebody views the vertebral column from side; four curvatures are seen. The primary curvature (curvature present during developing fetus) are thoracic, and sacral; the secondary curvatures or compensatory curvatures (that develop after birth, when baby can hold its head upright and when start to sit and walk) are cervical and lumbar curvatures.

Curvature increases spine flexibility. Normal movement of vertebral column are flexion, extension, lateral bending. Abnormal curvatures are scoliosis (lateral bending), kyphosis (dorsal exaggerated thoracic curvature), lordosis (accentuated lumbar curvature). In all cases of abnormal curvatures back pain is common.

In old age, the height of the vertebral column diminishes due to diminished thickness of intervertebral disk mainly.

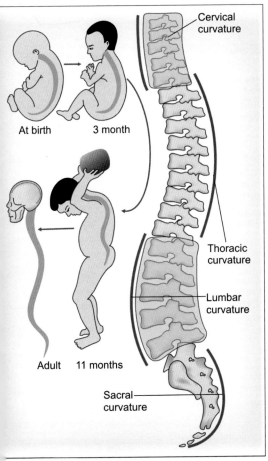

Fig. 2.9: The vertebral column add-its different curvatures (in children adult)

Cervical curvature

Thoracic curvature

Lumbar curvature

Sacral curvature

At birth

3 month

Adult   11 months

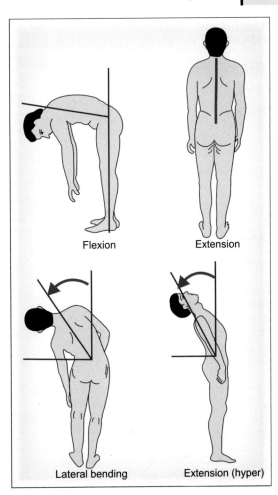

Flexion

Extension

Lateral bending

Extension (hyper)

Fig. 2.10A: Movements of vertebral column

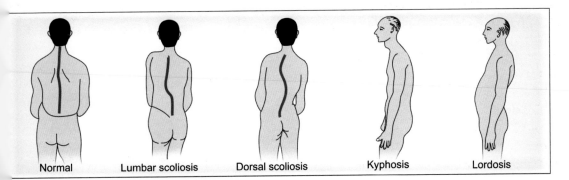

Normal

Lumbar scoliosis

Dorsal scoliosis

Kyphosis

Lordosis

Fig. 2.10B: Abnormal vertebral curvatures (comparing with normal)

Regional Characteristics of Cervical, Thoracic and Lumbar Vertebrae (Typical) (Fig. 2.11)

Characteristic	Typical cervical (3—6)	Typical thoracic (2,3 to 9th)	Typical lumbar (1—4)
Body	Small, wide side to side. Transverse diameter > antero-posterior diameter.	Larger than cervical, heart-shaped. Transverse and antero-posterior diameters are equal	Massive, kidney shaped (i.e., indentation on posterior part of body). Transverse > Antero-posterior diameter.
Spinous process	Short, bifid, projects directly backwards.	Long, sharp, projects downwards.	Short, project horizontal backwards.
Vertebral forearm	Triangular in shape.	Circular in shape.	Triangular in shape.
Transverse process.	Contain foramina (foramina transversarium).	Club shaped bear facets for ribs.	Thin. Slender and close to tip bears a vertical ridge for attachment of lumbar fascia.
Superior and inferior articular process	Fused to form articular pillar.	Thin articular process superior facet looks, backward and interior facet looks forward.	Superior articular process has concave facet directed postero-medially. Interior articular process has vertical convex articular facets facing posteromedially.
Movements allowed	Flexion, extension, lateral bending and rotation. This vertebral region has greatest range of movement.	Rotation, lateral flexion possible but limited by ribs. Flexion and extension prevented.	Flexion and extension some lateral flexion, rotation prevented

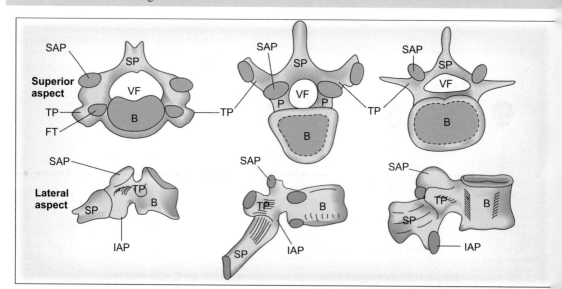

Fig. 2.11: Movements of vertebral column

Abbreviations: SAP—Superior articular process, SP—Spinous process, VF—Vertebral foramen, TP—Transverse process, B—Body, IAP—Interior articular process

ATYPICAL CERVICAL VERTEBRAE (Fig. 2.12A)

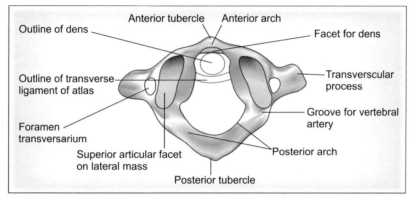

Fig. 2.12A: Atypical cervical vertebrae (Atlas)

Names	*Comments*	*Important features*	*Anatomical positions*
Atlas (First cervical)	Support globe of head; ring like. Forms atlanto-occipital and atlanto-axial joint.	(1) No body (2) No lamina and spine (3) Presents anterior and posterior arches and two lateral masses (4) Tip of the transverse process is palpable between angle of mandible and mastoid temporal bone (5) Superior articular process has kidney-shaped facet (6) Inferior articular process has oval facet.	• Anterior arch which has a circular face on posterior aspect place in front.
Axis (Second cervical)	Allow rotation of head and atlas around the dens. Named so because of prominent adontoid process.	(1) Odontoid (dens) process projects from upper part of the body—Apical ligament and alar (cheek) ligament is attached. (2) Lamina is thick. (3) Spine is thick and bifid. (4) Transverse process is small and no costo-transverse bar.	• Groove presents on the upper surface of posterior arch, should be placed above. • Odontoid process marked by oval facet in front should be placed anteriorly.
Vertebra prominence (Seventh cervical)		(1) Spine—not bifid, long and horizontal. (2) No facet in body by which one can separate it from first thoracic. (3) Absence of costotransverse bar in transverse process.	• Convex superior articular facet should be placed superiorly • Place body with neurocentral lip upwards. • Strong horizontal spinous process should be placed backward

ATYPICAL THORACIC VERTEBRAE (Fig. 2.12B)

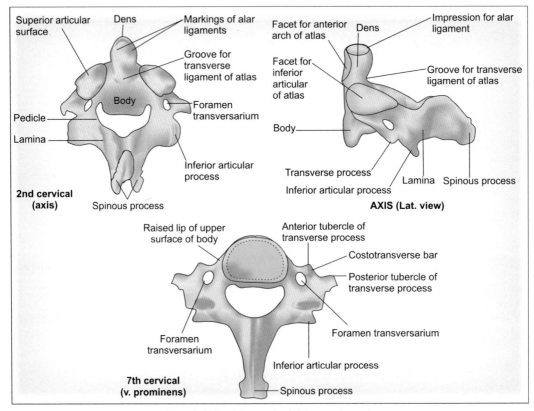

Fig. 2.12B: 7th cervical (V. prominens)

Names	*Comments*	*Important features*	*Anatomical positions*
First thoracic	All thoracic vertebrae except tenth, eleventh and twelfth vertebrae h ave upper and lower facet. Upper one articulates with numerically corresponding rib and lower one with upper facet of rib below.	(1) Body cervical, type, i.e. transverse diameter is greater than anteroposterior diameter. (2) Upper facet is circular for first rib. (3) Lower half facet (demifacet)—for upper facet of second ribs. (4) Spine directed horizontal like cervical.	• Place body anteriorly and superior articular facet above.
Tenth thoracic	Same as first thoracic, but body is gradually larger and attains lumbar shape (kidney shape). Body is lumbar type. Thoracic aorta becomes abdominal at the lower border of T12.	(1) Body is larger, only superior semilunar facet if present for tenth rib. (2) Inferior demifacet is absent. (3) The transverse process may or may not present facet for tenth rib tubercle. (4) Obliquity of spine diminishes.	• Place semilunar costal facet in the upper part. • Place body anteriorly

Contd...

Names	Comments	Important features	Anatomical positions
Eleventh thoracic	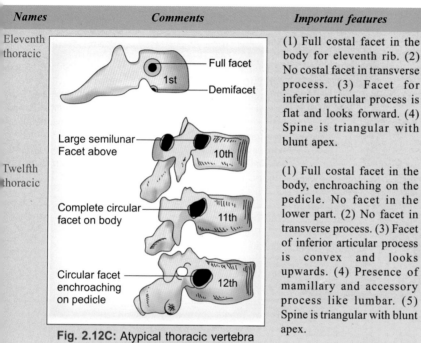	(1) Full costal facet in the body for eleventh rib. (2) No costal facet in transverse process. (3) Facet for inferior articular process is flat and looks forward. (4) Spine is triangular with blunt apex.	• Place body anteriorly with single facet above. • Place body anteriorly with single facet above.
Twelfth thoracic		(1) Full costal facet in the body, enchroaching on the pedicle. No facet in the lower part. (2) No facet in transverse process. (3) Facet of inferior articular process is convex and looks upwards. (4) Presence of mamillary and accessory process like lumbar. (5) Spine is triangular with blunt apex.	• Shaft (Inner surface) should be directed upwards and laterally

Fig. 2.12C: Atypical thoracic vertebra

ther Atypical Vertebrae

Names	Comments	Important features	Anatomical positions
Fifth lumbar Figs 2.12C and D)	Inferior vena cava is formed in front and right side of body.	Massive body—(1) Anterior part of the body is more thicker. (2) Short and thick transverse process projects from the pedicle. (3) Distance between the two superior articular process is equal or less than the distance between the two inferior articular process. (4) Spine quadrilateral and down turned.	• Place body with thickened anterior part in front and spine in behind.

Fig. 2.12D: Atypical lumbar vertebra

Contd...

Names	Comments	Important features	Anatomical positions
Sacrum (wedge shaped bone) (Figs 2.13A and B)	Formed by fusion of fifth sacral vertebra.	**Ventral surface**: It is marked by four transverse ridges. Lateral to it lies four ventral foramina; sympathetic trunk descends medial to ventral sacral foramina ventral surface; gives E-shaped origin of pyriformis muscle. **Dorsal surface**: (1) Marked by medial sacral crest (formed by fusion of spinous process), intermediate (fusion of articular process) and lateral sacral crest (fusion of transverse process). (2) Presence of four dorsal sacral foramina—transmit dorsal rami of sacral nerves. (3) Sacral hiatus (U shaped)—transmit S5, coccygeal nerve and filam terminale. **Base**—broad; formed by first sacral vertebra. Lower part of body projecting downwards and forwards—sacral promontory (anteroposterior diameter of inlet of pelvis is measured). Sympathetic trunk, lumbosacral trunk, obturator nerve lies in front alar (wing-like) process. **Apex**—lower part of sacrum, articular with coccyx. **Lateral surface—Upper part**—presence of ear-like articular surface–form sacro-illiac joint with hip bone. **Lower part**—gluteus maximus is attached.	• Broad base is directed upwards. • Tapered apex directed downwards. • Pelvic surface is directed forwards and tilted downwards as if sacrum is pickling something from ground. • Dorsal surface is recognized by sacral crests.

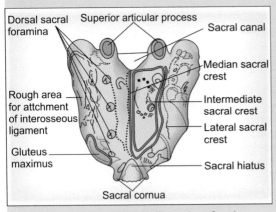

Fig. 2.13A: Sacrum (Dorsal surface)

Labels: Dorsal sacral foramina; Superior articular process; Sacral canal; Median sacral crest; Intermediate sacral crest; Lateral sacral crest; Rough area for attchment of interosseous ligament; Gluteus maximus; Sacral hiatus; Sacral cornua

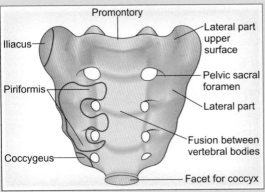

Fig. 2.13B: Sacrum (Ventral surface)

Labels: Promontory; Iliacus; Piriformis; Coccygeus; Lateral part upper surface; Pelvic sacral foramen; Lateral part; Fusion between vertebral bodies; Facet for coccyx

| Coccyx (triangular small bone) (Fig. 2.13C) | Formed by fusion of four rudimentary coccygeal vertebrae | **Base**—formed by first coccygeal vertebra. From its postero-superior aspect coccygeal cornua project. **Apex**—Formed by fourth coccygeal vertebra. **Pelvic surface**—attachment of coccygeus and levator ani. **Dorsal surface**—attachment of filum terminale (second piece)—gives origin to gluteus maximus, external anal sphincter (last piece). | • Base identified by oval facet directed upwards. • Dorsal surfaces will be identified by coccygeal cornu. |

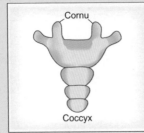

Fig. 2.13C: Coccyx

Labels: Cornu; Coccyx

plied Anatomy (Vertebrae)

ondylosis (misnomer spondylitis): It is a generated condition, characterized by eneration of intervertebral disks, and formation osteophytes (bony overgrowth).

ondylolisthesis: It is congenital (present from :h) the vertebral body and arch are not fused. All the diseases describe above produces pain he spine (vertebral column).

berculosis: Most common source of vertebral :ection; the infection begins at the anterior margin of the vertebral body near the intervertebral disk. Abscess (pus) formation is common and can form paraspinal abscess. It may track down through the psoas sheath producing psoas abscess.

Coccydynia: It refers to any painful condition in the region of coccyx.

Prolapsed disk: It means a herniated disk; mainly nucleus pulposus herniated out, through annulus pulposus. It is also known as slipped disk. It is most commonly seen in lower lumbar region.

s and Sternum

Names	Comments	Important features	Anatomical positions

ternum oreast bone) Fig. 2.14)	Flat bone: consists of two compact bone layers and spongy bone in between.	Three parts:
		1. Manubrium (cranial part)
		2. Body (middle part)
		3. Xiphoid process (caudal part).
		MANUBRIUM
		1. Concavo-convex anterior surface—sternocleidomastoid (in upper part) and pectoralis major (in lower part) are attached.
		2. Concave posterior surface—gives attachment to sterno-hyoid above and sterothyroid below. It is related with arch of aorta with three branches.
		  a. Superior border—in the center lies jugular notch, gives attachment to two layers of deep cervical fascia enclosing space of Burn.
		  b. Lateral border—has two costal facet for cartilage (cartilaginous joint), of first rib and second rib (synovial joint).
		  c. Inferior border—oval area; articulate with upper part of body forming manubrio-sternal joint, also known as sternal angle (important for surface marking and counting of ribs).
		BODY: Two surfaces, two borders.
		1. Anterior surface—it is marked by promi-nent transverse ridge (three in number)—indicate fusion of four sternebrae, on either side of midline—pectoralis major is attached.
			• If three parts are joined together, then place triangular manubrium above.
			• Anterior surface is very rough and convex.
			• If only body is present, then, upper and lower end is identified by distance between articular facets. Upper part distance is more and lower part distance is less.
			• Lower end of the bone should be placed forwards and upper end backwards.

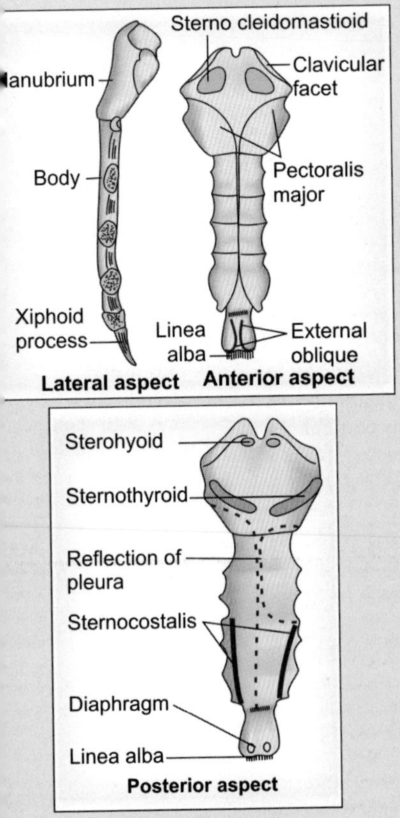

Sterno cleidomastioid
Clavicular facet
Manubrium
Pectoralis major
Body
Xiphoid process
Linea alba
External oblique
Lateral aspect   Anterior aspect

Sterohyoid
Sternothyroid
Reflection of pleura
Sternocostalis
Diaphragm
Linea alba
Posterior aspect

Fig. 2.14: Sternum

Contd...

Names	Comments	Important features	Anatomical positions
	It contains red bone marrow throughout life, and forms anterior boundary of superior and inferior medias-tinum.	**2. Posterior surface**—it is flat, faint transverse ridges; related to anterior border of two lungs with pleura. The left part of lower, two pieces of sternebrae are direct contact with heart and pericardium. **Lower end**—joins with xiphoid, which unites at 40 years of age. Lateral border—has six facets on either side—first and last are half facet. The distance between the two adjacent central facets are gradually diminishing from above downwards. **XIPHOID PROCESS**—small part. Its size and shape vary. At the tip, linea alba is attached. 1. On **anterior surface**—external oblique apo-neurosis and rectus abdominis is attached. **2. Posterior surface**—Gives transverse attachment abdominis and gives attachment of diaphragm.	

Ribs

12 pairs, classified into typical and atypical ribs

Typical Ribs

Names	Comments	Important features	Anatomical positions
Typical Rib (third to ninth) (Fig. 2.15)	Elastic arches of bone, present anterior end and posterior end and body or shaft.	**Anterior end**—cup-shaped depression for costal cartilage. **Posterior end**—present head, neck and tubercle. 1. **Head**—present two facets; lower large facet articulates with the same number of thoracic vertebra. Upper facet articulates with the lower facet of vertebra above. 2. **Neck**—it has elevated upper border is known as crest of neck. 3. **Tubercle**—lateral nonarticular part present a medial facet of articulation with facet of transverse process of same number of vertebrae. **Shaft or body**—has thick **upper border** gives insertion of external intercostals, internal intercostals and intercostalis intimus. **Sharp lower border**—gives origin to external intercostals. **Costal groove** (which is faint in anterior aspect) gives origin to internal intercostals. Ridge above the groove gives origin to intercostalis intimi.	• It should place in pen holding fashion with cup-shaped anterior end lies below the posterior end. • Posterior end above. • Thick and rounded superior border is above. • Sharp inferior border below. • Costal groove should be on internal surface.

Contd...

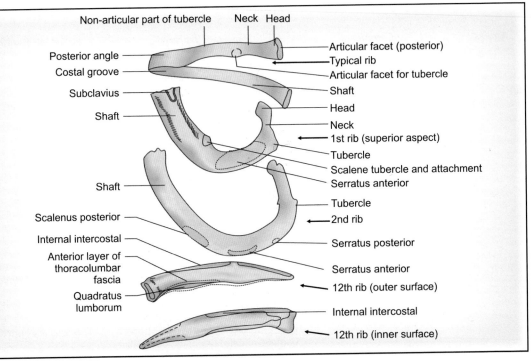

Fig. 2.15: Typical and atypical ribs

Atypical Ribs

Names	Comments	Important features	Anatomical positions
First Rib (Vertebrosternal)	Brodest, shortest, most curved rib; form lateral boundary of inlet of thorax.	Single facet at head. Inspite of external and internal surface (as in other ribs) it has rough superior surface marked by two grooves. The anterior groove lodges subclavian vein. The posterior groove lodges subclavian artery. Inferior surface—smooth. Inner border—it has a tubercle in the middle (scalene tubercle)—scalenus anterior muscle is attached. Whole border gives attachment to suprapleural membrane. Outer border—convex; thick behind and thin in front.	• It should be placed obliquely so that anterior end is nearly 4 cm below the posterior end. • Rough superior surface with two prominent grooves should be above.
Second Rib (Vertebrosternal)	Twice the length of first. Shaft is not twisted like first. So when it is placed on a plane surface, both the ends touch the surface.	Double facet at head. The shaft is flat with external rough surface looking upwards; and internal smooth surface downwards and inwards, external surface gives attachment to first external intercostals, serratus anterior	• It should be placed in pen holding fashion with cup-shaped anterior end below and posterior end above. • Thick and rounded superior border is above.

Contd...

Atypical Ribs

Names	Comments	Important features	Anatomical positions
		(first and second digitations). Internal surface gives origin to second external intercostals near its outer border and related to second posterior intercostals nerve, artery, and vein.	• Sharp inferior border below. • Costal groove should be on internal surface.
Tenth Rib	Vertebrochondral rib.	Single facet in head. Facet present in tubercle. Other features like typical ribs.	• Same as typical.
Eleventh Rib	Vertebral.	Single facet in head. No facet in tubercle. Slight angle, slight tubercle, shallow central groove.	• Place in horizontally, i.e. anterior end and posterior end in the same line.
Twelfth Rib	Vertebral (very short ribs)	Single facet in head. No angle, no tubercle, no costal groove. Lower border is sharper than upper border. Upper border is slopping downwards, towards the tip—gives attachment to last external intercostals. Lower border—middle layer of thoracolumbar fascia is attached. Anterior surface— quadratus lumborum muscle is attached.	• Horizontal in position with the head directed medially. • Tip directed laterally • Anterior surface looks forwards and upwards.

Applied Anatomy

Single rib fracture: due to compression force. Pain is experienced at the site of fracture during respiration.

Frail chest: As a result of crushing injury (motor vehicle accident) produces comminuted (multiple) fracture of a number of ribs The frail segment (a number of fractured ribs) sucked in, during inspiration and driving out during expiration (paradoxical respiration).

Cervical rib: When the costal element in the seventh cervical vertebra grows and separates out it is called cervical rib. Common anomaly— presses the brachial plexus and sometime subclavian artery producing symptoms

Bones of Inferior Extremity

Names	Comments	Important features	Anatomical positions
Hip bone (coxal bone) (Figs 2.16A and B)	Irregular bone formed by fusion of ILIUM, ISCHIUM and PUBIS, and cup-like acetabulum occurs at the point of fusion. Form symphyseal joint with opposite hip	**THREE PARTS** 1. **ILIUM (superior portion of hip bone)—It has three borders** a. **Superior border**–It is also known as **Iliac crest** gives attachment to fascia lata, external oblique, transversus abdominis and gluteus maximus muscles (near its posterior part).	• Place elevated iliac crest above and anterior superior iliac spine and pubic tubercle in same vertical plane. • Posterior superior iliac spine lies above 5 cm away from midline.

Contd...

Names	*Comments*	*Important features*	*Anatomical positions*
	bone, sacroiliac joint with sacrum.	b. **Anterior border**—It has two spines and a notch: • **Anterior Superior Iliac Spine**—palpable attachment of inguinal ligament and sartorius muscle. • **Anterior Inferior Iliac Spine**—stem of iliac femoral ligament and rectus femoris muscle (straight head) is attached. c. **Posterior border**—Presents two spine and a notch: • posterior superior iliac spine—represents in the living body by a dimple in the buttock—gives attachment to sacrotuberous ligament (also attached at • posteroinferior iliac spine) • presence of greater sciatic notch. d. **Medial border**—forms iliac part of arcuate line.	• Acetabulum is on lateral aspect.

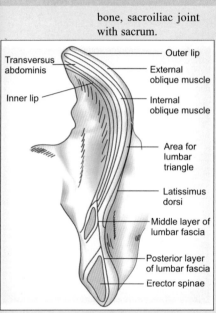

Fig. 2.16A: Iliac crest (viewed from above)

Contd...

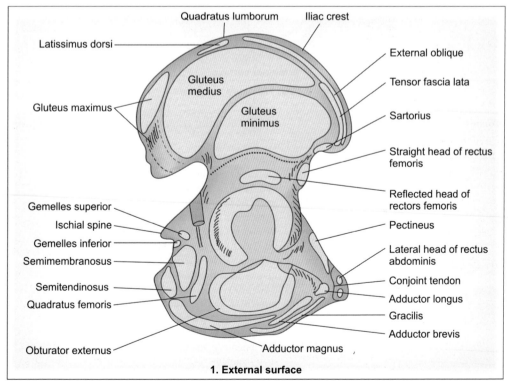

1. External surface

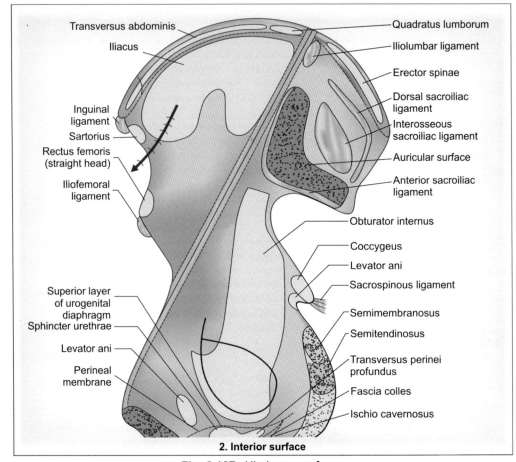

Transversus abdominis

Iliacus

Inguinal ligament

Sartorius

Rectus femoris (straight head)

Iliofemoral ligament

Superior layer of urogenital diaphragm
Sphincter urethrae

Levator ani

Perineal membrane

Quadratus lumborum

Iliolumbar ligament

Erector spinae

Dorsal sacroiliac ligament

Interosseous sacroiliac ligament

Auricular surface

Anterior sacroiliac ligament

Obturator internus

Coccygeus

Levator ani

Sacrospinous ligament

Semimembranosus

Semitendinosus

Transversus perinei profundus

Fascia colles

Ischio cavernosus

2. Interior surface

Fig. 2.16B: Hip bone, surfaces

Names	Comments	Important features	Anatomical positions
		Three Surfaces: 1. **Gluteal Surface**—Presents three gluteal lines—anterior, posterior, and inferior. Area behind the posterior gluteal lines gives attachment to gluteus maximus. Between posterior and anterior gluteal lines gluteus medius is attached; below inferior gluteal line gluteus minimus is attached. 2. **Sacropelvic Surface**—it has **auricular impression**, articulate with auricular surface of sacrum; **rough iliac tuberosity** gives attachment to interosseous sacro-iliac ligament.	

Contd...

| ames | *Comments* | | *Important features* | *Anatomical positions* |

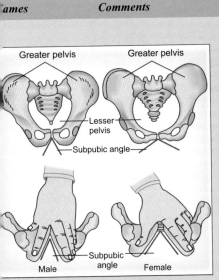

Fig. 2.17: Comparision between male and female pelvis

omparison between male and female pelvis
ig. 2.17)

	Male	Female
ıb pubic ıgle	Narrower	wider
esser pelvis	Less spaceous	More spaceous
ony rominence	More marked	Less marked
reauricular ılcus	Not prominent	Prominent
cetabula	Larger, closer	Smaller and further apart

3. **Pelvic surface** is smooth, marked by preauricular sulcus (more prominent in female).

   a. **Iliac Fossa**—gives origin of iliacus muscle; right fossa lodges caecum with appendix. Left fossa lodges part of desending colon.

ISCHIUM—It has a ramus and a body. Body presents three surfaces:

i. **Femoral Surface**—Quadratus femoris is attached.

ii. **Dorsal Surface**—Lower part form ischial tuberosity (we sit on it) gives attachment to hamstring muscles (semitendinosus, semi-membranesus, adductor magnus, long head of biceps).

iii. **Pelvic Surface**—lies pudendal canal, with internal pudendal vessels and pudendal nerve.

RAMUS—presents external surface and internal surface.

PUBIS—V-shaped bone; articulates with opposite pubis. It has a both form symphyseal joint .

BODY

1. **Anterior Surface**—Presence of pubic crest. Lateral end of pubic crest is known as Pubic tubercle

   a. where medial end of inguinal ligament is attached;

   b. guide for identifying inguinal and femoral hernia.

   c. gives attachment to adductor longus muscle .

2. **Posterior Surface**—Smooth, related to urinary bladder. Gives attachment of levator ani and obturator internus along the obturator foramen.

Superior Ramus—Run upwards and laterally. (1) Gives attachment to pectineus muscle (2) Vas deferens is in relation (in male).

Inferior Ramus—Unite at 8 years with ramus of ischium, forms common ischiopubic rami. It gives attachment

Contd...

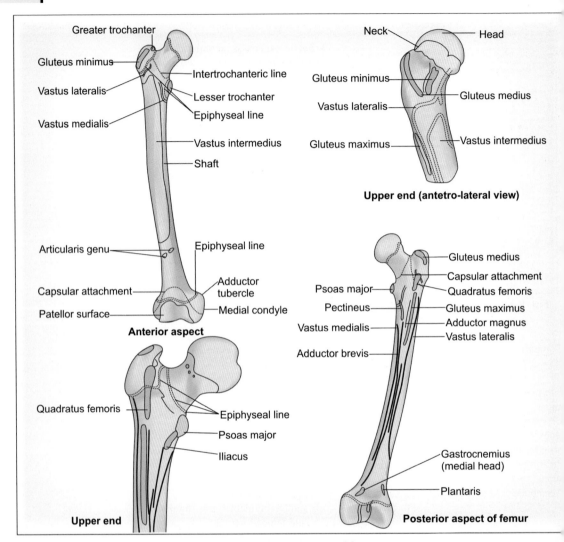

Fig. 2.18: Different views of femur

Names	Comments	Important features	Anatomical positions
Femur (Thigh bone) (Fig. 2.18)	Largest, longest and strongest bone in the body. Its length is roughly 1/8th of a person's height. It has an upper end, shaft and lower end. It takes part in formation of hip joint and knee joint.	to obturator externus, adductor magnus, adductor brevis, gracilis muscle on the external surface and perineal muscle on internal surface. **UPPER END** 1. **Head**—Globular, directed upwards and medially; articulate with acetabulum forming hip joint. A pit in the head-fovea capitis-ligamentum teres femoris is attached.	• Globular head above. • Linea aspara and condyles are behind. • Greater trochanter is behind.

Contd...

Names	*Comments*	*Important features*	*Anatomical positions*
Femur (Contd...)		2. **Neck**—long and constricted on the middle.	

2. **Neck**—long and constricted on the middle.
   Anterior surface—of the neck marked by a rough line **inter-trochanteric** line; capsular ligament of hip joint is attached here.
   Posterior surface—near its junction with shaft, an elevated ridge is present known as **intertrochanteric crest**—in the middle of which, quadratus femoris muscle is attached. 1 cm above the crest, the capsular ligament fits as tight collar.
3. **Greater Trochanter**—Quadrilateral eminence; pyriformis, gluteus medius, gluteus minimus and, obturator internus is attached.
4. **Lesser Trochanter**—Iliacus and psoas muscle are inserted.

SHAFT
Three Borders
1. Lateral
2. Medial border which is rounded.
3. Posterior border (linea aspara) vastus medialis, medial intermuscular septum, adductor brevis above, adductor longus below; and adductor magnus is attached to it.

Three Surfaces
1. Anterior,
2. Medial and
3. Lateral surface.
Anterior surface—origin of vastus intermedius, vastus medialis and vastus lateralis.

LOWER END
Two Condyles:
1. **Medial Condyle**—convex medial surface easily palpable. Presence of adductor tubercle;gives insertion to adductor magnus.
2. **Lateral Condyle**—lateral surface is flat and less prominent. Presence of oblong groove for attachment of popliteus. Presence of epicondyle (Lateral). Lateral collateral ligament is attached.
3. **Intercondyler Fossa**—separates two condyle behind.

Contd...

Names	Comments	Important features	Anatomical positions
		4. **Intercondylar Line**—attachment of capsular ligament of knee joint. Attachment of anterior cruciate ligament at the posterior part of medial surface of lateral condyle. Posterior cruciate ligament is attached at the anterior part of the medial surface of lateral condyle.	• Broader upper end should placed above. • Tibial tuberosity and shin facing forwards. • Medial malleolus should be situated on medial aspect.
Tibia (Fig. 2.19A)	Larger medial bone of leg; consists of upper end, shaft and lower end. It forms knee joint, superior, middle and inferior tibio fibular joint.	**UPPER END** **Two Condyles** 1. **Medial**—larger than lateral; in its posterior aspect groove for semimem-branous present. 2. **Lateral condyle**—oval facet in front; for attachment of iliotibial tract. In posterior aspect a facet for articulation with head of fibula. **A tuberosity**—palpable tibial tuberosity. Upper smooth part gives attachment to ligamentum patellae. **SHAFT** **Three Borders** 1. **Medial border**—attachment of medial collateral ligament. Soleus is attached in middle 1/3rd of medial border. 2. **Lateral border** (interosseous border)—interosseous membrane is attached. 3. **Anterior border (shin)**—palpable; gives attach-ment to deep fasca of leg and superior extensor retinaculum (in lower part). **Three Surfaces** 1. **Medial surface**—Subcutaneous, except in upper part. Upper part gives insertion to sartorius, gracilis and semitendinosus. 2. **Lateral surface**—in its proximal 3/4th it is transversely concave. Gives attachment to tibialis anterior muscle. 3. **Posterior surface**—divided by oblique soleal line into upper popliteal surface and lower surface, (which is again divided by vertical ridge into medial and lateral part). It gives attachment of popliteus, soleus, flexor digitorum longus.	

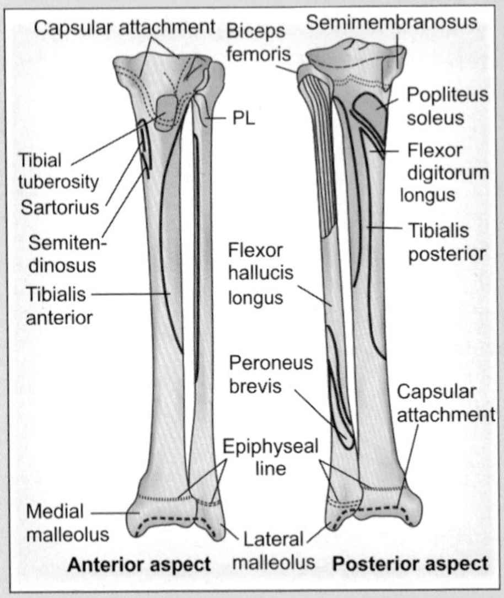

Fig. 2.19A: Tibia and fibula with attachments

Labels (Anterior aspect): Capsular attachment, Biceps femoris, Tibial tuberosity, Sartorius, Semitendinosus, Tibialis anterior, Medial malleolus, Lateral malleolus

Labels (Posterior aspect): Semimembranosus, PL, Popliteus soleus, Flexor digitorum longus, Tibialis posterior, Flexor hallucis longus, Peroneus brevis, Capsular attachment, Epiphyseal line

Contd..

Names	Comments	Important features	Anatomical positions
		LOWER END—projected medial part is known as medial malleolus—gives attachment to deltoid ligament. It has anterior, posterior, medial, lateral and inferior surfaces. 1. **Lateral surface**—lower part forms fibular notch, articulates with lower end of fibula. 2. **Anterior surface**—structure in relation (from medial to lateral)—Tendons of tibialis anterior, extensor hallucis longus, anterior tibial vessels, extensor digitorum longus. 3. **Posterior surface**—related with tendon of tibialis posterior, flexor digitorum longus, posterior tibial vessels, tibial nerve and flexor hallucis longus. 4. **Inferior surface**—articulates with superior, medial, and inferior surface of talus.	
Fibula (Lateral bone of leg) (Fig. 2.19B)	Stick like; has upper end, shaft and lower end.It forms superior, middle and inferior tibiofibular joint and ankle joint.	**UPPER END**—prominent head lies 2 cm below knee joint. Present articular facet at upper end for articulation with tibia.Junction between head and shaft is known as neck. **Shaft: Three Borders** 1. **Anterior border**—begins from below, from the apex of a subcutaneous triangular area the lateral surface and ends is neck. 2. **Posterior border**—prominent in lower part, ascends upwards from posterior groove of lateral malleolus and fades upwards. The interosseous border is medial to anterior border and in the upper part it is placed in close proximity with this border. **Three Surfaces** 1. **Lateral surface** (peroneal)—between anterior and posterior border—gives attachment to peroneus longus above and peroneus brevis below. 2. **Medial (extensor) surface**—between anterior and interosseous	• Hold the bone by pressing the thumb at malleoler fossa so that fossa lies below and behind.

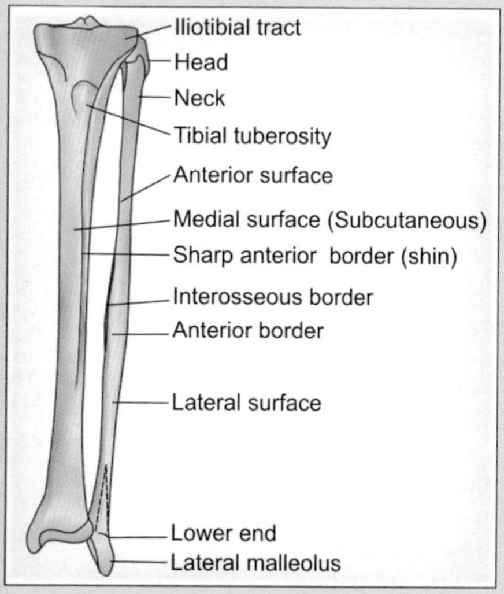

Iliotibial tract
Head
Neck
Tibial tuberosity
Anterior surface
Medial surface (Subcutaneous)
Sharp anterior border (shin)
Interosseous border
Anterior border
Lateral surface
Lower end
Lateral malleolus

Fig. 2.19B: General feature of tibia and fibula

Contd...

Names	Comments	Important features	Anatomical position
		border—extensor digitorum longus, extensor hallucis longus and peroneus tetrius arises from the surfaces. 3. **Posterior (flexor) surface**—between posterior and interosseous border—soleus and flexor hallucis longus and tibialis posterior is attached to it.	
Patella (Fig. 2.20)	Largest sessamoid bone having no periosteum and haversian system.	**LOWER END**—it is known as lateral malleolus—subcutaneous bony projection; in it, medial aspect there is a facet in front and a groove behind (malleolar fossa). It has broad base, (directed above), pointed apex (directed below). Rough anterior surface in front and upper part of the posterior surface is occupied by articular smooth area. It has medial border and lateral border. Base gives attachment of quadratus femories, apex ligamentum patellae.	• Place rough anteri⟨ surface in front. • Place articular area posterior surfac⟨ above medial bord⟨ present a vertic⟨ facet behind.

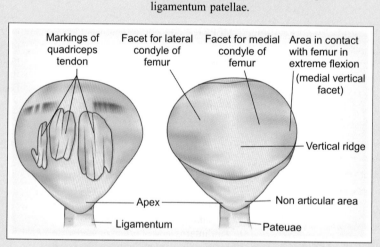

Fig. 2.20: The patella (Anterior and posterior aspects)

Talus (Ankle bone) (Fig. 2.21)	Important tarsal bone that overrides calcaneum and it is depressed during transmission of body weight in standing position. Talocalcaneal, talocalcaneonavicular joint are contributed by this bone.	Presents globular head, constricted neck and body. **HEAD**—articulates with navicular. **NECK**—gives attachment to capsular ligament. Long axis make angle of long axis of body—about 140°. In infant the angle is larger. In its plantar aspect deep groove is present known as sulcus tali.	• Head is directe⟨ forwards. • Trochlear surface o⟨ body is above. • Place complete trian gular facet on latera⟨ aspect.

Contd.

Names	*Comments*	*Important features*	*Anatomical positions*

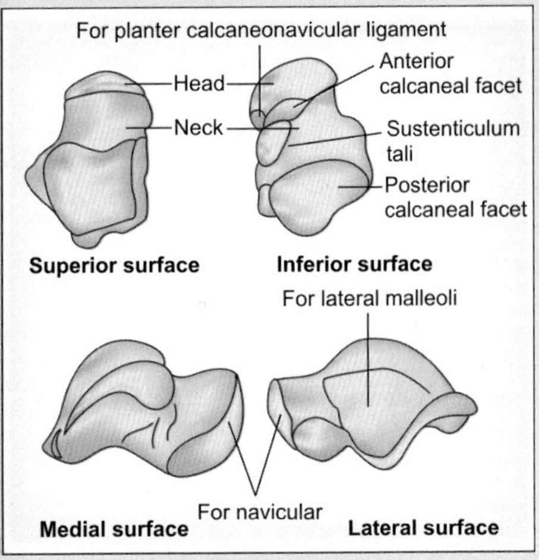

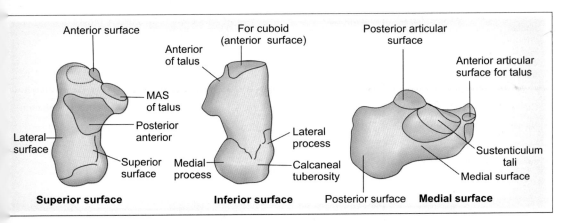

For planter calcaneonavicular ligament
Head
Neck
Superior surface

Anterior calcaneal facet
Sustenticulum tali
Posterior calcaneal facet
Inferior surface

For lateral malleoli

For navicular
Medial surface   **Lateral surface**

Fig. 2.21: Talus

BODY
Presents five surfaces.
1. **Superior or dorsal surface—** articular, pully-like surface articulate with **inferior articular surface—**of tibia and fibula, forming ankle joint.
2. **Inferior or plantar surface—** marked by oval facet—articulate with calcan-eum forming subtalar joint.
3. **Medial surface**
   a. **Upper part—**occupied by comma-shaped facet articulate with medial malleolus of tibia.
   b. **Lower non-articular part—** rough for deltoid ligament (deep part).
4. **Lateral surface—**occupied by triangular facet—articulates with facet on medial aspect of lateral malleolus.
5. **Posterior surface—**marked by medial and lateral tubercle (posterior tubercle) at the lower part.

| CALCANEUM (heal bone) (Fig. 2.22) | Largest tarsal bone, forming heel having six surfaces. | **Superior surface (dorsal)—**Presence of an articular facet in front— articulates with a facet in the undersurface of head of talus. A deep groove—sulcus calcanei, form sinus tarsi with sulcus tali. A big middle | • Facet for cuboid should lie in front. The sulcus calcanei are above. |

Contd...

Anterior surface
Anterior of talus
MAS of talus
Posterior anterior
Lateral surface
Superior surface
Superior surface

For cuboid (anterior surface)
Lateral process
Medial process
Calcaneal tuberosity
Inferior surface   Posterior surface

Posterior articular surface
Anterior articular surface for talus
Sustenticulum tali
Medial surface
Medial surface

Fig. 2.22: Calcaneum (largest tarsal bone)

Names	Comments	Important features	Anatomical positions
		calcaneal facet articulates with facet in inferior surface of talus. **Inferior surface (planter)**—Rough and marked by calcaneal tuberosity in posterior part. **Anterior surface**—Occupied by concavo-convex articular facet; articulates with cuboid, forms calcano-cuboid joint. **Medial surface**—Presence of shelf-like projection—sustenticulum tali produces which is a palpable bony marking. **Lateral surface**—Rough, marked by a tubercle (peroneal tubercle) in the middle.	• Sustenticulum tali should place medially. • Anterior part is in higher position than posterior part.

Articulated Skeleton of Foot (Figs 2.23 and 2.24)

It includes tarsal bone (seven in number), matatarsals (five numbered from great toe to little toe as 1st–5th) and the phalanges (same as hand). Tarsal bones form the posterior half of the foot. Body weight is carried primarily by two largest and most posterior tarsal bones—the talus calcaneum. The intermediate row comprising of navicular, on medial aspect (boat-shaped bone wit a tuberosity on plantar aspect) and cuboid (cub like, with a crest and groove on plantar surface on the lateral aspect. Medial (largest of thre cuneiform); Intermediate (shortest of three, dist: surface is occupied by a triangular facet which doe not cover this surface wholely) and lateral (dist: surface occupied by a triangular facet whic completely occupies that surface) cuneiform bone

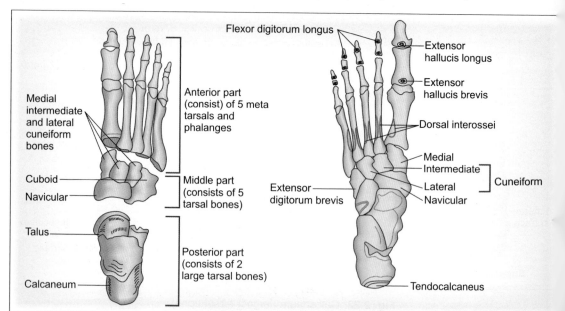

Fig. 2.23: Skeleton of foot

Difference between Metatarsal and Metacarpal

Metacarpals	Metatarsal
• Head is larger than base, except first metacarpal. • Dorsal surface has flat triangular area. • First metacarpal has a shaddle-shaped facet at the base to articulate with trapezium.	• Base is larger than head, except first metatarsal. • No such marking. • First metatarsal has kidney-shaped facet at the base.

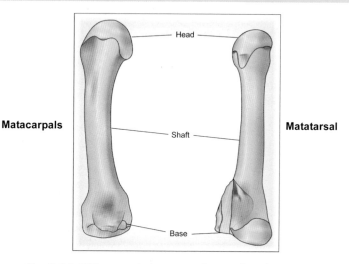

Fig. 2.24: Difference between metacarpal and metatarsal

Differences between Pectoral Girdle and Pelvic Girdle (Figs 2.25 and 2.26)

Pectoral girdle	Pelvic girdle
• Two components—clavicle and scapula which remains separate. • Comparatively lightly built for mobility.	• Three components—ilium, ischium and pubis which fuse at the age of 25 to becomes a single hip bone. • Strong and heavily built for resistance to stress.

Contd...

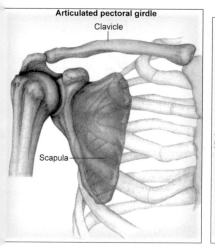

Fig. 2.25: Pectoral girdle

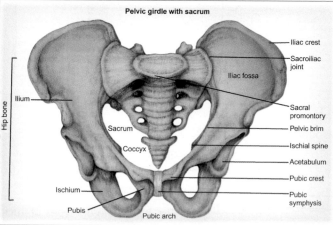

Fig. 2.26: Pelvic girdle

Pectoral girdle	*Pelvic girdle*
• No articulation with vertebral column. • No direct ventral articulation (clavicles are connected by interclavicular ligament). • Articulations of clavicle with axial skeleton are relatively small (Manubrium sterni) mobile and ventral. • Shallow joint with limbs which allows free mobility. • Stability is less.	• Articulates with sacrum (auricular articular surface). • Direct ventral articulation at symphysis pubis. • Articulation of hip bone with axial skeleton (sacrum) are relatively large, less mobile and dorsal. • Deep joint with limb with limited range of movement. • More stable.

Injury of Lower Limb Bones (Figs 2.27 and 2.28)

Bone involved (Fig. 2.22)	*Comment*
• Fractured neck of femur are of two types—intracapsular and extracapsular	Intracapsular fracture, may interfere with the blood supply of head, due to damage of retinacular blood vessels–avascular necrosis of head occurs. Extracapsular fracture occur outside the capsules and damage of blood supply is little. So satisfactory union is there.
• Supracondylar fracture of femur	Accompanied by pain, swelling and inability to make the movement of leg (occur due to direct trauma).
• Patellar fractures	May be transverse or stellate. Transverse fracture is due to indirect violence of quadriceps and stellate fracture is due to direct blow over patella.
• Fracture of tibial condyles	Are relatively common and may be articular or nonarticular. The lateral condyle is most frequently involved.
• Combined fracture of tibia and fibula (in shaft region)	It is a common injury to men due to accident.

Contd...

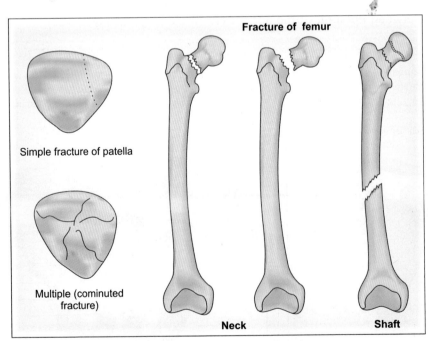

Fracture of femur

Simple fracture of patella

Multiple (cominuted fracture)

Neck

Shaft

Fig. 2.27: Different types of fractures (femur)

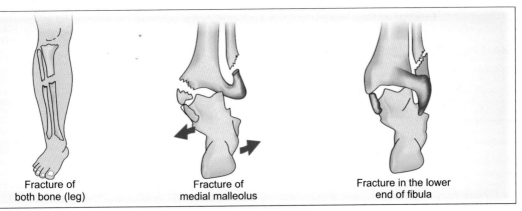

| Fracture of both bone (leg) | Fracture of medial malleolus | Fracture in the lower end of fibula |

Fig. 2.28: Different types of fracture of leg bones

Bone involved (Fig. 2.22)	Comment
March fracture	It is also known as stress fracture of metatarsal. Traditionally seen in military recruits. It is a fatigue fracture occurring with the repetitive stress after prolonged period of rest. Pain felt during palpation of the metatarsal which is involved.

...ial Bones

Bones	Comments	Important marking	Anatomical positions

...ntal ...g. 2.29)	Forms forehead, roof of orbit and anterior cranial fossa. It contains two unequal fron-tal air sinuses.	• It has squamous part and orbital part.
		• Presence of nasal notch and ethmoidal notch > nasal notch (articular from medial to lateral) nasal bone, frontal process of maxilla and lacrimal bone is articulated.
		• It has supraorbital foramina (or notch) which allows the supraorbital vessels and nerve to pass.
		• Squamous part—it has
		  (a) **External surface**—convex
		  (b) **Internal surface**—concave.
		• **External surface** present Glabella—meeting point of two superciliary arches. Supercilary arch—it is formed due to the projection of frontal air sinus. Eyebrows lies super-ficial to it. Frontal tuberosity—bulge over each orbit.
		• Supraorbital margin—arched ridge just below the eyebrows.
			• Orbital surface will face downwards
			• Orbital plate will be horizontal.
			• Concave cerebral surface of squama facing posteriorly.

...rietal ...gs 2.30A ...d B)	Form most of superior and lateral aspect of the skull.	• Presence of **four angles—arterosuperior** Occupied by unossified membrane (fontanellae) at the time of birth. Antero inferior angle pointed and inferiorly.	• Inferior border is bevelled on the middle at the expense of external surface

Contd...

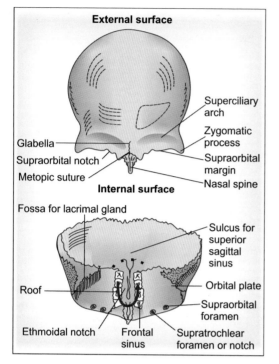

Fig. 2.29: Frontal bone

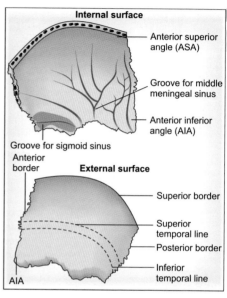

Fig. 2.30A: Parietal bone

Bones	Comments	Important marking	Anatomical position
	During birth un-obssibial memb-rane present which helps in moulding of foetal head.	placed. Postero superior angle (lambda), porture inferior angle (marked an internal surface by sigmoid sulcus). • **Four borders** 1. Anterior 2. Posterior 3. Superior 4. Inferior border articulates with, (from before backward) sphenoid (greater wing) squamous and mastoid part of temporal bone. **Two surfaces** 1. External surface marked by superior and inferior temporal lines—inferior temporal line gives attachment to temporails muscle. 2. Internal surface marked by grooves and sulcus—criddle meningeal groove, sagittal sulcus and sigmoid sulcus (on postero inferior angle). • Parietal eminence: Most prominent part; biparietal diameter is measured here. Ossification centre starts from here.	• Pointed anteri inferior angle (mark internally by groc for middle mening vessels) placed dow wards and anterior • Smooth convex ext nal surface with par tal tuberosity shou be placed laterally.

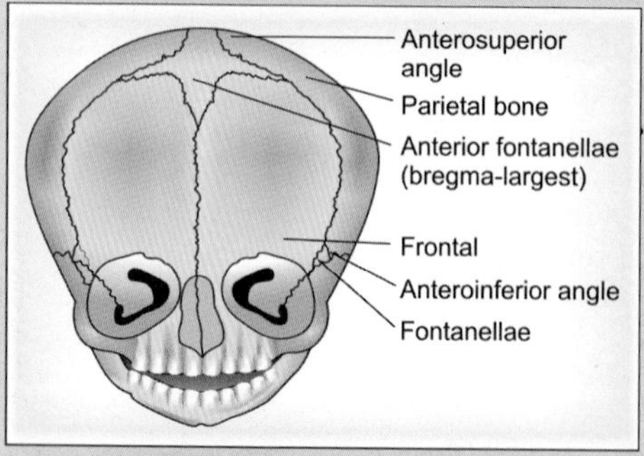

Fig. 2.30B: Fontanellae

Conte

Names	Comments	Important features	Anatomical positions
Occipital (Fig. 2.31)	Forms posterior aspect and most of the base of the skull It has squamous, condylar, and basilar part.	• **External surface of squamous part** presents prominent tubercle known as external occipital protuberance (convex) and three nuchal lines (a) highest, (b) superior, (c) inferior. Superior nuchal line gives attachment to trapezius, sternocloidomastoid, (d) inferior nuchal lines. • External occipital crest—ligamentum nuche is attached. • **Internal surface**—concave; marked by four fossae and three sulcus. (1) Upper fossae—lodges occipital poles—of brain. (2) Lower fossae—lodges cerebellar hemisphere. Sulcuses are—(1) Superior sagittal sulcus—from internal occipital protruberance to superior angle. (2) Two transverse sulci—on either side of internal occipital protrubance. • Foramen magnum—(1) gives passage to lower part of medulla with meninges, two vertebral arteries, sympathetic nerve and venous plexus. (2) Spinal root of accessory nerve and one anterior and two posterior spinal arteries. • Hypoglossal canal: Allow passage of hypoglossal nerve (twelfth cranial nerve). • Occipital condyles: Articulates with superior articular process of atlas forming atlanto-occipital joint. movements of this joint are Flexion, Extension, Lateral bending.	• Foramen magnum must be horizontal. • Apex of squamous part face upwards, occipital condyle face downwards. • Basilar part directed upwards and forwards.
Temporal (Fig. 2.32)	Forms inferolateral aspects of skull and contributes to the middle cranial fossa. It has squamous, mastoid, tympanic and petrous part. Important foramina of this bone are stylomastoid F, internal acoustic meatus.	Temporal bone has three processes—zygomatic, mastoid, and styloid process· • **Zygomatic process**—helps to form the zygomatic arch which forms the prominence of cheek. • **Styloid process**—Deeply situated, gives attachment to stylohyoid ligament, styloglossus, stylopharyngeous and stylohyoid muscles. • **Mastoid process**—Palpable behind the auricle; gives attachment to sternocleidomastoid, posterior belly of digastric and other neck muscles.	• Squamous part directed upwards and styloid process pointed downwards.) • Apex of petrous part looks forward and medially. • Zygomatic process directed forwards and medially. • External auditory meatus lies on the lateral aspect.

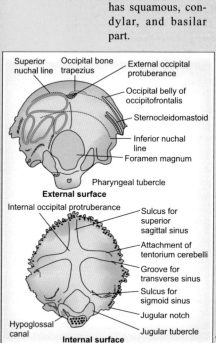

External surface labels: Superior nuchal line, Occipital bone, trapezius, External occipital protuberance, Occipital belly of occipitofrontalis, Sternocleidomastoid, Inferior nuchal line, Foramen magnum, Pharyngeal tubercle — **External surface**

Internal surface labels: Internal occipital protruberance, Sulcus for superior sagittal sinus, Attachment of tentorium cerebelli, Groove for transverse sinus, Sulcus for sigmoid sinus, Jugular notch, Hypoglossal canal, Jugular tubercle — **Internal surface**

Fig. 2.31: Occipital bone

Contd...

Names	*Comments*	*Important features*	*Anatomical positions*

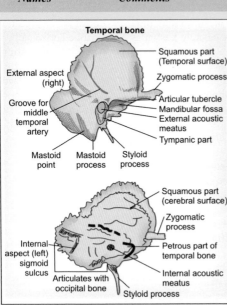

Fig. 2.32: Temporal bone

Stylomastoid foramen—allows facial nerve (seventh cranial) to pass. Jugular foramen–allows passage to internal jugular vein, nineth, tenth, eleventh, cranial nerves. Internal acoustic meatus—allows passage of seventh and eighth cranial nerves and auditory vessels. Carotid canal—S-shaped channel in petrous part, transmits internal carotid artery.

Mandibular fossa—oval shaped depression, anterior to external auditory meatus, form socket for head of mandible forming temporo-mandibular junction. **Squamous part**—in scale like has smooth external surface, form temporal fossa and rough internal surface. **Petrous part**—wedge-shaped, it houses middle and internal ear. **Mastoid part**— It lies posterior to external auditory meatus. Rough lower projected part produce mastoid process; contains mastoid air cells. At the junction of mastoid and squamous part lies external auditary meatus. Triangular area above the meatus is known as suprameatal triangle; deep to which lies mastoid antrum.

- Basilar part (basiocciput)—fuses with basi sphenoid and form clivus (slope). It lodges brain stem.
- **Condylar part**—It has articular and non-articular arm.

Sphenoid (bird like with wings stretched outwards) (Figs 2.33A to C)	Single bone, situated in the middle of base of skull.It has two wings— 1. Lesser wing· Greater wing—has two surfaces: lateral, cerebral. 2. A body with six sufaces— a. Superior b. Inferior c. Anterior d. Posterior	1. Sella turcica (hypophyseal fossa)—present in superior surface; lodges pituitary gland 2. Optic foramen—gives passage to second (optic) cranial nerve and ophthalmic artery. 3. Super-ior orbital fissure—allows passage to cranial nerves—third, fourth, sixth and ophthalmic division of fifth cranial nerve. 4. Foramen rotandum—gives passage to maxillary division of trigeminal nerve. 5. Foramen ovale—it transmits sensory part of mandibular nerve, motor root of trigeminal nerve, anterior division of middle meningeal sinus, lesser superficial petrosal nerve.	• Pterygoid looks downwards. • Jugum sphenolae and sphenodal air sinus facing forwards.

Contd...

Names	Comments	Important features	Anatomical positions
	Two lateral. Two ptery-goid process • Two air filled cavi-ties in the center part of body (sphenoidal air sinus).	6. Foramen spinosum–middle menin-geal artery and posterior division of middle meningeal sinus. 7. Foramen lacerum—Opening at the junction of the sphenoid, temporal and occipital bone. It transmits a branch of ascending pharyngeal artery.	

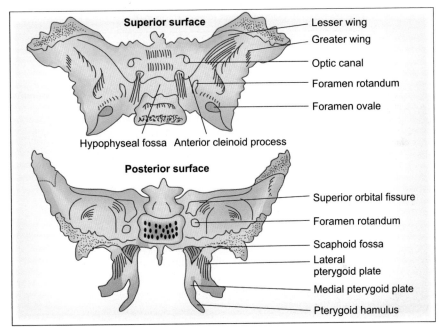

Fig. 2.33A: Sphenoid

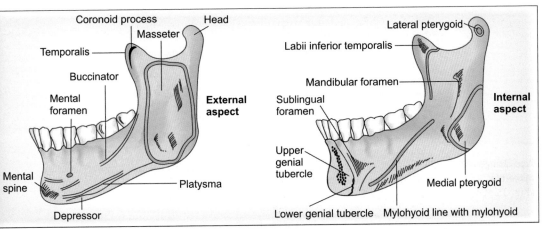

Fig. 2.33B: Mandible

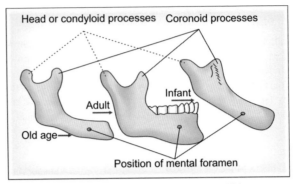

Head or condyloid processes Coronoid processes

Infant

Adult

Old age→

Position of mental foramen

Fig. 2.33C: Age changes of mandible

Mandible

Names	Important features	Anatomical positions
Mandible Parts (Fig. 2.33B)	Forms lower jaw (immovable). It is the strongest and largest bone of the face.Mandible has (1) C-shaped body, (2) two rami (right and left); (3) three processes—(a) pointed coronoid process, (2) rounded condyloid process (also known as head) and (3) alveolar process contains socket for teeth.	• Place the mandible in such a way that the coronoid, condyloid process, and alveolar process should be looked upwards.
a. External surface	**1. Body**: It has two surfaces, convex external and concave internal.External surface near the midline lies a ridge known as symphysis menti indicates the mandible develops in two halves. In the lower part on either side of symphysis menti is mental tubercles. On each side a faint ridge extends upwards and backwards from mental tubercle (oblique line). Main muscles arise from external surface, they are buccinator (opposite three molar teeth). From the lower border (also known as base); anterior belly of digastic arises.	• Convex external surface should be placed outwards.
b. Internal surface	Presence of mylohyoid line in internal (extends from third molar tooth to symphysis menti) and this line demarcates two fossa upper sublingual; lower submandibular fossa lodging the salivary glands. Behind the symphysis menti lies two pairs of tubercle. Upper genial tubercle gives the attachment to genioglossus lower one to geniohyoid. **2. Ramus**: It has outer and inner surface. At outer surface masseter is attached. Internal surface near the angle of mandible medial pterygoid is attached.Neck gives the attachment to lateral pterygoid. **3. Coronoid process**: Sharp coronoid process gives insertion of temporalis. **4. Condyloid process**: Also known as head. Articulates with atricular fossa of mandible forming a temporomandibular (synovial) joint.	
Age changes of mandible (Fig. 2.33C)	At birth the bone presents two halves. 1 year after birth it becomes a single bone. The coronoid process projects at a higher level than condyloid process. The mental foramen is at the lower border of the body (Fig. 2.33C). In adult— 1. Teeth (sixteen in number) have errupted.	

Contd..

Names	Important funcitons	Anatomical positions
	2. Condyloid process is higher than coronoid process.	
	3. Mental foramen is situated at midposition of the body.	
	In old age—	
	1. Absorption of the alveolar process.	
	2. Mental foramen is close to alveolar process	
Applied	Fracture (#) of mandible single or multiple, is common. Forward dislocation of mandible even during yawning displaces the TM joint.	

axilla

Bones	Comments	Important features	Anatomical positions
Maxilla (Fig. 2.34)	Second largest bone of face forming upper jaw, part of hard palate, orbits and nasal cavity. It is a pneumatic, quadrangular bone. From cheek and part of orbit.	**Body**—(pyramidal shape) contains maxillary air sinus. **Four surfaces** presents— 1. **Anterior surface,** 2. **Infratemporal or posterior surface**, 3. **Orbital surface,** 4. **Nasal surface** (medial) it presents maxillary hiatus). **Processes**— 1. **Frontal**—articulates with frontal bone, 2. **Zygomatic**— articulates with zygomatic bone, 3. **Alveolar**—contains sixteen teeth in adult,	• Frontal process should be directed upwards from body. • Alveolar process directed downward. • Zygomatic process projects laterally. • Palatine process directed postero-medially. • Like posterosuperior border placed posterior superiorly. • Temporal process project backward.

Contd...

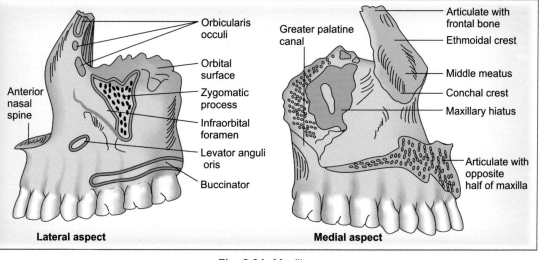

Fig. 2.34: Maxilla

Names	*Comments*	*Important features*	*Anatomical positions*

4. **Palatine**—forms anterior 2/3rd of hard palate.

Anterior surfaces of body have:
1. Incisive fossa,
2. Canine eminence,
3. Infraorbital foramen (just below the orbital margin—infraorbital vessels and nerve come out),
4. Nasal notch—separates the anterior surfaces from medial surface.

Infratemporal surface (posterior surfaces)—lateral part forms infratemporal fossa. Medial part forms pterygopalatine fossa. Maxillary tuberosity lies at the lower and posterior part of this surface. Sometimes this tuberisity is damaged during removal of upper 3rd molar teeth.

Orbital surface—forms the floor of orbit. Posterior border forms anterior boundary of inferior orbital fissure (greater wings of sphenoid forms posterior border). It transmits maxillary nerve and its zygomatic branch, inferior ophthalmic vein and sympathetic nerve.

Nasal (medial) surface—identified by large maxillary hiatus which is partially reduced in size by processes from inferior nasal chonchae, palatine and lacrimal bones.

Zygomatic
(or Japonicum)
(Fig. 2.35)

Three surfaces—
1. lateral, 2. temporal 3. orbital
Five borders—
1. anterosuperior,
2. anteroinferior,
3. posterosuperior,
4. postero-inferior,
5. posteromedial.
Three processes—
1. frontal, 2. temporal, 3. maxillary. At the upper part of the body— thyrohyoid membrane, hyoepiglottic ligament and genioglossus is attached. At the anterior surface of the body geniohyoid, hyoglossus, mylohyoid, sternohyoid and omohyoid is attached.

- Lateral surface convex with zygomatic facial foramen
- Convex anterior surface place anteriorly. Lesser cornu directed upwards. Tip of greater cornu directed backwards.

Contd.

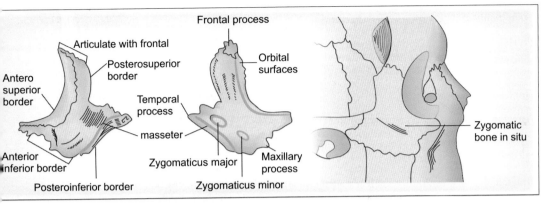

Fig. 2.35: Zygomatic bone

Names	Comments	Important features	Anatomical positions
Hyoid (Fig. 2.36)	Lies in front of neck; U-shaped bone.	At greater cornu—origin of middle constri-ctor. Attachment of thyrohyoid membrane. Lesser cornu—origin of middle constrictor and stylohyoid ligament.	

Important Landmarks in Cranium (Figs 2.37 and 2.38)

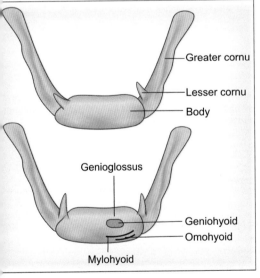

Fig. 2.36: Hyoid bone

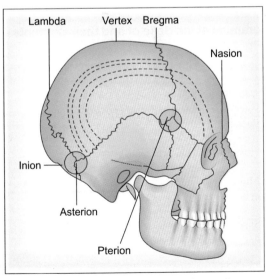

Fig. 2.37: Important landmarks in cranium

Bony landmarks	Location	Importance
Pterion (Fig. 2.37)	Junction of greater wing of sphenoid, squamous temporal, frontal and anteroinferior angle of parietal bone.	(1) Position of anterior division of middle meninge artery and sinus. (2) Position of stem of lateral sulcus of brain. (3) Insula lies deep to it. (4) Broca's area of speech is situated here.
Asterion	Meeting point of three bones— posteroinferior angle of parietal, squamous part of occipital and mastoid part of temporal.	Position of sigmoid sinus.
Bregma	Point of calvaria at the junction of coronal and sagittal suture.	Occupied by anterior fontanelle (unossifie membrane) at the time of birth. It ossifies at eighte months of age.
Lambda	Point on calvaria (skull cap) at the junction of sagittal and lamboid sutures.	Occupied by posterior fontanelle which ossify s months after the birth of the baby.
Nasion (L.nose)	Junction of nasal and frontal bones.	Length of the skull is measured from here.
Inion (Situated at back of head)	Most prominent point of external occipital protuberance.	Length of the skull is measured from here.
Vertex (L.whorl)	Superior point of neurocranium in the midline, in anatomical plane.	Used for measurement of height.

Foramina at the Base of and their Contents (Fig. 2.38)

Foramina	Contents (structures come through)
Anterior cranial fossa Foramen caecum, anterior and posterior ethmoidal foramina	Nasal emissary vein connecting superior sagittal sinus wit veins of nose. Anterior and posterior ethmoidal vessels an nerve.
Foramina in cribriform plate of ethmoid	Rootlets of olfactory nerve.
Middle cranial fossa optic canals	Optic nerve and ophthalmic arteries.
Superior orbital fissure	Inferior ophthalmic vein, ophthalmic nerve and occulomoto troclear, abducent nerve and sympathetic nerve fibers.
Foramen rotandum	Maxillary nerve.
Foramen ovale	Mandibular division of trigeminal nerve and accessor meningeal artery and lessser superficial petrosal nerve.

Contd.

...mina in Cranial Fossa and their Contents (Fig. 2.38)

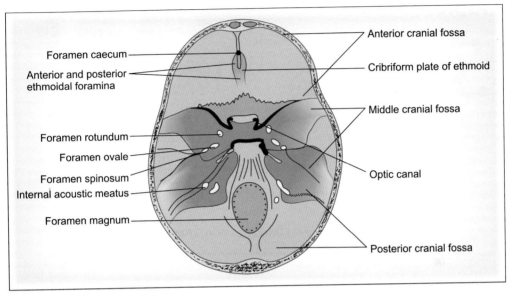

Fig. 2.38: Base of skull

Foramina	Contents (structures come through)
...ramen spinosum	Middle meningeal artery and vein and a branch of mandibular nerve.
...ramen lacerum	Structure actually lies across, are, internal carotid artery and its accompanying sympathetic and venous plexuses.
...osterior cranial fossa ...ramen magnum(magna—large)	Medulla with its covering meninges, vertebral arteries, spinal root of accessory, anterior and posterior spinal arteries several dural veins.
...gular foramen	Glossopharyngeal (IX), Vagus (X), Accessory (XI) nerves, sigmoid sinus continued as superior bulb of internal jugular vein, inferior petrosal sinus and meningeal branch of ascending pharyngeal artery.
...ypoglossal canal	Hypoglossal nerve.
...ternal auditors meatus	Passes seventh and eighth cranial nerve.

Chapter

3

Joints

Joints—Joints are the junction between two or more bones, bones with cartilage or cartilage with cartilage.

JOINTS [Functional Classification] (Figs 3.1 to 3.3)

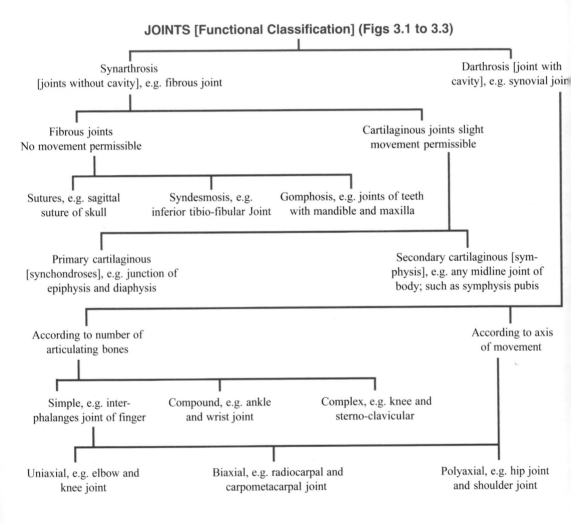

Synarthrosis [joints without cavity], e.g. fibrous joint

Darthrosis [joint with cavity], e.g. synovial joint

Fibrous joints No movement permissible

Cartilaginous joints slight movement permissible

Sutures, e.g. sagittal suture of skull

Syndesmosis, e.g. inferior tibio-fibular Joint

Gomphosis, e.g. joints of teeth with mandible and maxilla

Primary cartilaginous [synchondroses], e.g. junction of epiphysis and diaphysis

Secondary cartilaginous [symphysis], e.g. any midline joint of body; such as symphysis pubis

According to number of articulating bones

According to axis of movement

Simple, e.g. inter-phalanges joint of finger

Compound, e.g. ankle and wrist joint

Complex, e.g. knee and sterno-clavicular

Uniaxial, e.g. elbow and knee joint

Biaxial, e.g. radiocarpal and carpometacarpal joint

Polyaxial, e.g. hip joint and shoulder joint

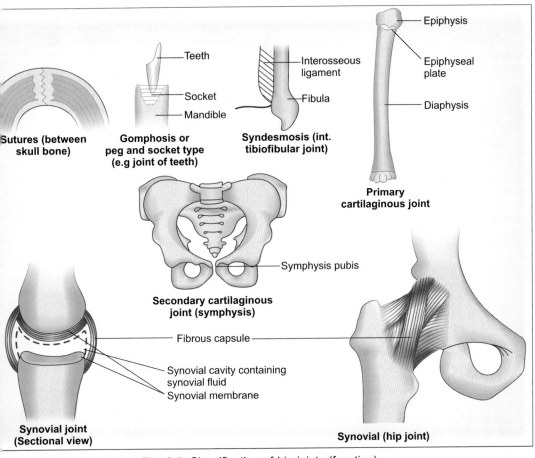

Fig. 3.1: Classification of hip joints (function)

...ortant Joints of Whole Body at a Glance (Skip it in Case of Beginner)

Joints	Articulating bones	Structural type	Movements allowed
...mporo-mandibular ...nt	Mandibular fossa of temporal bone and condyles of mandible.	Type – synovial Subtype – condyloid	Elevation, depression, protraction, retraction and slight lateral movement.
...anto-occipital	Condylar process of occipital with superior kidney shaped articular process of atlas.	Type – synovial Subtype – condyloid	Flexion, extention, lateral bending and circum-duction.
...anto-axial	Atlas (c-1) with axis (c-2)	Type – synovial Subtype – pivot	Uniaxial joint. Rotation of head.
...ervertebral	Between adjacent vertebral bodies	Type – secondary cartilaginous Subtype – symphysis	Gliding movement

Contd...

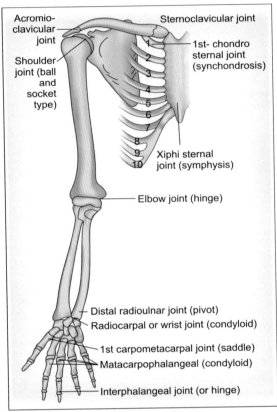

Acromio-clavicular joint

Shoulder joint (ball and socket type)

Sternoclavicular joint

1st- chondro sternal joint (synchondrosis)

Xiphi sternal joint (symphysis)

Elbow joint (hinge)

Distal radioulnar joint (pivot)

Radiocarpal or wrist joint (condyloid)

1st carpometacarpal joint (saddle)

Matacarpophalangeal (condyloid)

Interphalangeal joint (or hinge)

Fig. 3.2: Joints of upper limb and sternum

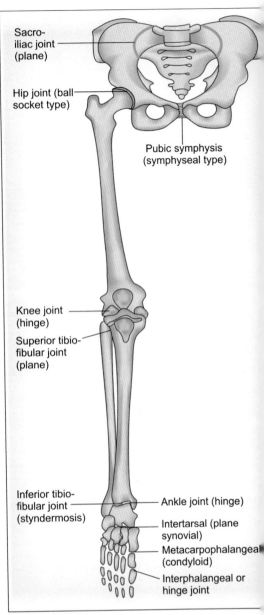

Sacro-iliac joint (plane)

Hip joint (ball-socket type)

Pubic symphysis (symphyseal type)

Knee joint (hinge)

Superior tibio-fibular joint (plane)

Inferior tibio-fibular joint (styndermosis)

Ankle joint (hinge)

Intertarsal (plane synovial)

Metacarpophalangeal (condyloid)

Interphalangeal or hinge joint

Fig. 3.3: Joints of lower limb

Name	*Comment*	*Important features*	*Anatomical position*
Costo-vertebral joint	Vertebrae and ribs	Type—synovial Sub type—plain	Gliding movement
Sterno-clavicular joint	Sternum and clavicle	Type—synovial Sub type—saddle	Gliding movement
Sterno-costal joint	Sternum and first rib	Synchondrosis (primary cartilaginous joint)	No movement
Other sterno-costal joint	Sternum and second to seventh rib	Type—synovial Subtype—double plane	Gliding movement
Acromioclavicular joint	Acromion of scapula and lateral end of clavicle	Type—synovial Subtype—plane	Gliding, elevation, depression, protraction and retractions
Shoulder joint	Glenoid cavity of scapula with head of humerus	Type—synovial Subtype—ball and socket joint	Multiaxial joint. Movements are—flexion, extension, abduction, adduction, circumduction and rotation.
Elbow joint	Lower end of humerus with upper end of ulna and radius	Type—synovial Subtype—hinge	Uniaxial joint. Movements are—flexion and extension.
Radioulnar joint (proximal and distal, both)	Radius and ulna	Type—synovial Subtype—pivot	Uniaxial, rotation.
Wrist joint (radio-carpal)	Lower end of radius with proximal carpals, i.e. scaphoid and lunate.	Type—synovial Subtype—condyloid	Biaxial joint. Movements are—flexion, extension, abduction, aduction and circumduction.
Sacroiliac joint	Articular surface of sacrum and articular surface of hip bone	Type—synovial Subtype—plane	Slight gliding possible
Hip joint (coxal joint)	Acetabulum of hip bone and head of femur	Type—synovial Subtype—ball and socket type	Multiaxial joint. Movements are—flexion, extension, abduction, adduction and some degree of rotation.
Tibio-fibular joint Proximal	Proximal part of tibia and fibula	Type—synovial Subtype—plane	Gliding
Distal	Distal end of tibia and fibula.	Type—fibrous Subtype—syndesmosis	Slight movement during dorsiflexion of foot.
Ankle joint	Articular surface of lower end of tibia and fibula with superior, medial and lateral articular surface of talus	Type—synovial Subtype—hinge	Dorsiflexion (extention) Planter flexion of foot
Subtalar joint	Inferior articular surface of body of talus with superior surface of calcaneum.	Type—plane	Inversion and eversion of foot.
Talo-calcanonavicular joint	Head of talus articulate with calcaneum and navicular	Talonavicular part—ball and socket type	Gliding and rotarory movement
Calcanocuboid joint	Anterior articular surface of calcaneum	Type—plane	Inversion and eversion of foot.

Important Joints of Superior Extremity

Name of joints and bones concerned	Important ligaments	Movements	Muscle involved	Nerve supply	Stability	Closed packed position	Loose packed position
Shoulder joint or Glenohumeral (polyaxial, ball and socket type) bones concerned – • Glenoid fossa of scapula • Articular surface of head of humerus (Figs 3.4A and B)	Capsular ligaments Glenohumeral ligaments (thickening part of capsule)	1. Flexion (bending) 2. Extension (straightening) 3. Abduction (move away from midline) 4. Adduction (move towards the mid line) 5. Lateral rotation 6. Medial rotation Circumduction (combination of all movements in sequence)	1(a) Deltoid (anterior fibers), Pectoralis major (clavicular part) (b) Biceps brachi (long and short head) (c) Coraco-brachialis 2. Posterior fibers of deltoid, latissimus dorsi and teres major. 3. Middle fibers of deltoid, supraspinatus. 4. Supraspinatus, pectoralis major (sternal part) latissimus dorsi. Infraspinators, teres major, deltoid (posterior fibfer). Subscapulares, latissimus dorsi, teres major.	• Axillary • Supras-capular • Lateral pectoral	Unstable joint. Stability is maintained by – rotator cuff muscles (e.g. supraspinatus, infraspinatus, subscapularis) and teres minor	Abduction and lateral rotation	Semi-abduction. In loose packed position. All movements are free.

Contd...

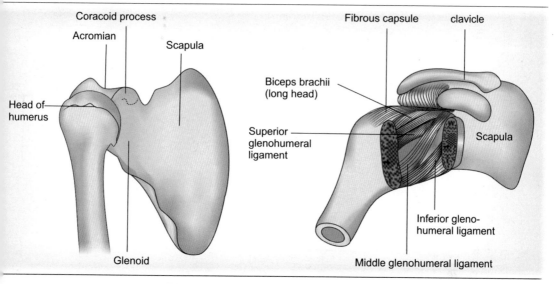

Fig. 3.4A: Shoulder joint and its interior

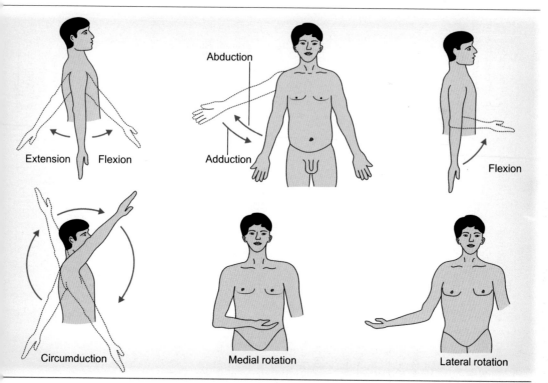

Fig. 3.4B: Movements of shoulder joint

Name of joints and bones concerned	Important ligaments	Movements	Muscle involved	Nerve supply	Stability	Closed packed position	Loose packed position
Elbow joint (hinge, uniaxial variety) (Figs 3.5A and B) Bones concerned: Articular surface of lower end of humerus (i.e. trochle and capitulum)	• Capsular ligament • Radial co-lateral ligament • Ulnar co-lateral ligament	1) Flexion 2) Extension	1a) Brachialis 1b) Biceps-brachii 1c) Brachioradialis 1d) Pronator teres 2a) Triceps brachii 2b) Anconeus	• Musculocutaneous, via its branch to brachialis. • Radial, via nerve to anconeus. • Ulnar nerve • Median nerve	Stable joint. Stability is maintained by – bony configuration and ligaments.	Extension and semipronation.	Semiflexion and supination.
Wrist joint (biaxial condylar variety) (Fig. 3.6) Bones concerned: Articular surface of lower end of radius, scaphoid and lunate.	• Fibrous capsule. • Palmar radio-carpal ligament • Dorsal radio-carpal ligament • Radial co-lateral ligament • Ulnar co-lateral ligament	1) Flexion 2) Extension	• Prime-mover: • Flexor carpi ulnaris • Flexor carpi radialis **Assisted by:** • Flexor digitorum superficialis, • Flexor digitorum profulus, • Flexor pollicis longus, and Abductor pollicis longus. a) Extensor carpi radialis, longus and brevis. b) Extensor carpi ulnaris. c) Extensor digitorum. d) Extensor indicis.	• Anterior interosseous nerve- branch of median nerve. • Posterior interosseous nerve – branch of radial nerve. • Deep terminal branch of ulnar nerve.	Maintained by configuration and ligaments.	Dorsiflexion	Semiflexion

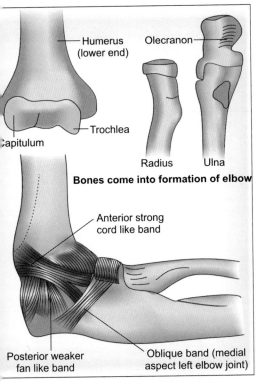

Bones come into formation of elbow

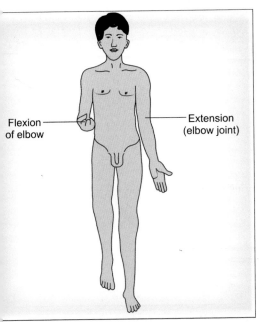

Fig. 3.5A: Elbow joint and ligaments

Fig. 3.5B: Movements of elbow joint

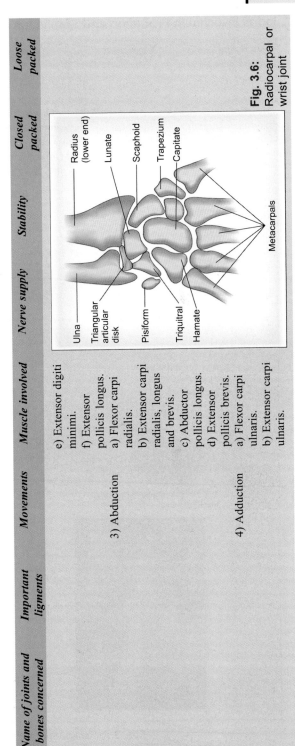

Fig. 3.6: Radiocarpal or wrist joint

Name of joints and bones concerned	Important ligments	Movements	Nerve supply	Stability	Closed packed	Loose packed	Muscle involved
							e) Extensor digiti minimi. f) Extensor pollicis longus.
		3) Abduction					a) Flexor carpi radialis. b) Extensor carpi radialis, longus and brevis. c) Abductor pollicis longus. d) Extensor pollicis brevis.
		4) Adduction					a) Flexor carpi ulnaris. b) Extensor carpi ulnaris.

Joints Involved in Pronation and Supination

Name and bones concerned	Ligaments	Movements	Muscles producing the movement	Nerve supply	Stability
Superior (synovial, uniaxial, pivot type) and inferior radio-radio ulnar joint. Superior – articular area of head of radius with articular area of ulna. Inferior radio-ulnar joint – head of ulna with ulnar notch of radius (Fig. 3.7).	• Capsular • Annular • Capsular ligament • Palmar ligament • Dorsal ligament • Lateral ligament	Pronation and supination in a vertical axis; the axis passes through the center of head of radius, and through the ulnar attachment of articular disk (lower).	Pronation – Giving something (king pronate) – done chiefly by pronator quadratus. Assisted by pronator teres (when the movement is rapid and against resistance). Supination—[more powerful, antigravity movement (begger supinate)] i.e. taking something • Supinator • Biceps brachii.	• Musculo cutaneous • Median • Radial nerves	Maintained by strong ligament

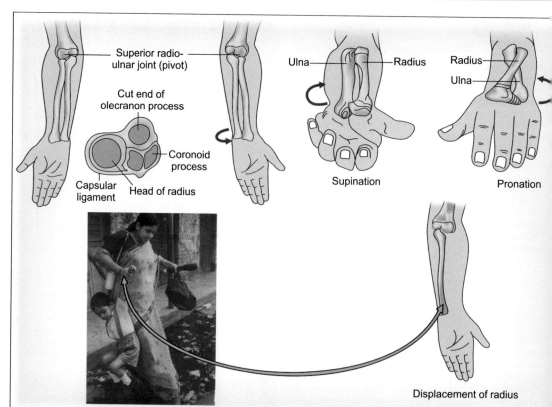

Fig. 3.7: Radio-ulnar joints, movements and applied

concerned	Ligments	Movements	Muscle involved	Nerve supply	Stability	Closed packed	Loose packed
First carpometa-carpal joint (poly - axial, saddle shaped)	• Capsular ligament	1. Flexion	a. Flexor pollicis brevis b. Opponens pollicis and assisted by flexor pollicis longus.	Digital branch of median nerve going to thumb.	Stable joint	Full oppo-sition	Neutral position of thumb
Distal articular surface of trapezium.	• Palmar ligament	2. Extension	a. Extensor pollicis-longus and brevis.				
	• Dorsal ligament	3. Abduction	a. Abductor pollicis longus. b. Abductor pollicis longus and abductor pollicis brevis.				
	• Lateral ligament	4. Opposition	Assisted by – extensor pollicis brevis. a. Flexor pollicis brevis. b. Assisted by – adductor pollicis.				
Proximal saddle-shaped articular surface of first metacarpal. (Fig. 3.8)		5. Circumduction	All movements (in a sequence)				
		6. Adduction	Adductor pollicis				

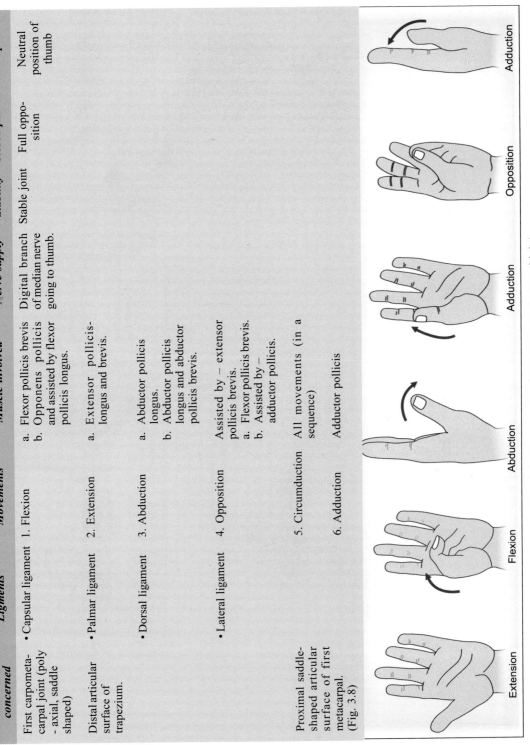

Fig. 3.8: Movements of 1st carpo metacarpal joint

Extension   Flexion   Abduction   Adduction   Opposition   Adduction

Joints of Inferior Extremity

Name and bones concerned	Ligments	Movements	Muscle involved	Nerve supply	Stability	Closed packed position	Loose packed position
Hip Joint (poly-axial, ball and socket joint) Articular surface of acetabulum of hip bone. Articular surface of head of femur. (Figs 3.9A and B)	A. Capsular ligament (three parts) 1. Iliofemoral ligament. 2. Pubofemoral ligament 3. Ischiofemoral ligament B. Ligamentum teres femoris. C. Acetabular labrum.	1. Flexion (bending) 2. Extension (straightening) 3. Abduction 4. Lateral rotation (external rotation)	a. Iliacus b. Psoas c. Rectus femoris d. Sartorius a. Gluteus maximus b. Biceps femoris c. Semitendinous d. Adductor magnus (ischial fibres) a. Adductor longus b. Adductor brevis c. Adductor magnus d. Gracilis e. Pectineus a. Pyriformis b. Obturator internus and externus.	By branches from – lumbar plexus via – 1. Obturator nerve 2. Nerve to rectus femoris 3. Accessory obturator nerve.	Stable due to bony configuration and ligaments.	Extension and medial rotation	Semiflexion

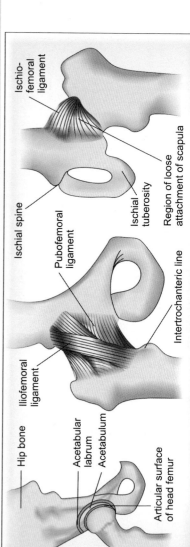

Hip bone — Iliofemoral ligament

Acetabular labrum

Acetabulum

Articular surface of head femur

Intertrochanteric line

Pubofemoral ligament

Ischial spine

Ischio-femoral ligament

Ischial tuberosity

Region of loose attachment of scapula

Contd...

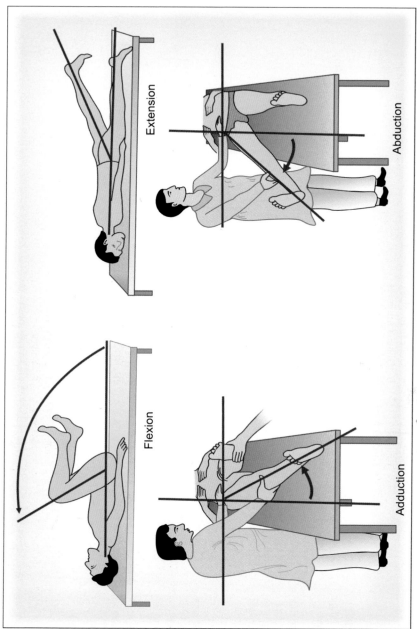

Fig. 3.9B: Movement of hip joint

Joints of Inferior Extremity

Name and bones concerned	Ligments	Movements	Muscle involved	Nerve supply	Stability	Closed packed position	Loose packed position
	D. Transverse acetabular ligament.		c. Two-gamelii d. Quadratus femoris e. Gluteus maximus				
		5. Medial rotation 6. Circumduction	a. Gluteus medius b. Gluteus minimus c. Tensor fasciae latae				Semiflexion
KNEE JOINT (modified hinge joint) Bones concerned— 1. Articular area of lower end of femur. 2. Articular area on posterior surface of patella. 3. Articular area of upper end of tibia (Figs 3.10A and B)	• Capsular ligament. • Tibial (medial) collateral ligament. • Fibular (lateral) collateral ligament. • Oblique popliteal ligament. • Cruciate ligament, medial and lateral menisci.	1. Flexion 2. Extension 3. Medial rotation 4. Lateral rotation	Combination of all movements in sequence. a. Biceps femoris b. Semitendinous c. eminembranous d. Gastrocnemius Quadriceps femoris Satorius, gracilis. Biceps femoris	Obturator nerve (posterior division) Genicular branches of tibial and common peroneal.	Maintained mainly by ligaments and partially by muscles.	Full extension	
ANKLE JOINT (hinge; uniaxial) (Fig. 3.11)	Capsular ligament Deltoid (medial) Lateral ligament	1. Dorsiflexion (flexion) 2. Plantar flexion (extension)	a. Tibialis anterior b. Extensor hallucis longus. c. Extensor digitorum longus. d. Peroneus tertius. a. Gastrocnemius. b. Soleus c. Tibialis posterior d. Flexor digitorum longus e. Flexor hallucis	Deep peroneal	Bony configuration	Dorsiflexion	Neutral position

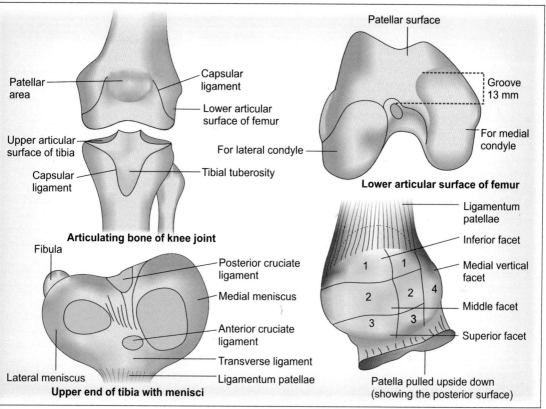

Articulating bone of knee joint

Patellar area

Capsular ligament

Lower articular surface of femur

Upper articular surface of tibia

Capsular ligament

For lateral condyle

Tibial tuberosity

Patellar surface

Groove 13 mm

For medial condyle

Lower articular surface of femur

Fibula

Posterior cruciate ligament

Medial meniscus

Anterior cruciate ligament

Transverse ligament

Lateral meniscus

Ligamentum patellae

Upper end of tibia with menisci

Ligamentum patellae

Inferior facet

Medial vertical facet

Middle facet

Superior facet

Patella pulled upside down (showing the posterior surface)

Fig. 3.10A: Knee joint

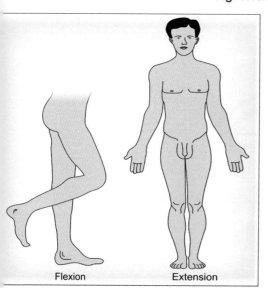

Flexion

Extension

Fig. 3.10B: Movement of knee joint

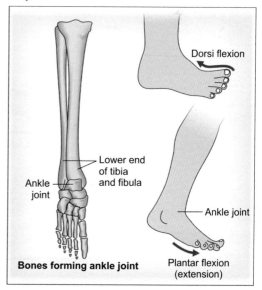

Dorsi flexion

Lower end of tibia and fibula

Ankle joint

Ankle joint

Bones forming ankle joint

Plantar flexion (extension)

Fig. 3.11: Ankle joint and its movements

Arches of Foot

Comments	Factors maintaining the arch	Applied
• It acts as an elastic platform which helps to carry body weight efficiently and economically. • It helps in propagation, in plane or uneven surface, due to segmental nature. • Foot has three arches, which are also present at birth. The arches are: 1. Medial longitudinal arch – bones are: calcaneum, talus, navicular, three cuneiform bones, first three metatarsals. 2. Lateral longitudinal arch – bones are calcaneum, cuboid, fourth and fifth metatarsal bones. 3. Transverse arch. Bones are: bones of all metatarsals and cuboid and three cuneiform. (Figs 3.12A to D)	1. SHAPE OF BONES – Bones are faceted and shaped in such a way that they fit with each other. 2. INTERSEGMENTAL TIERS – They are the binders of bones (ligaments). Important tiers (ligaments) of medial arch are – SPRING LIGAMENT (plantar calcanonavicular ligament). For lateral arch – Long Plantar Ligament Short Plantar Ligament for Transverse Arch – Deep Transverse Ligament. 3. BOW STRING OR TIE — BEAM ARRANGEMENT – two ends of the arch connected by muscles or ligaments. FOR MEDIAL ARCH – Medial part of plantar aponeurosis. Abductor hallucis (muscle of sole). FOR LATERAL ARCH – lateral part of plantar aponeurosis and abductor digiti minimi (intrinsic muscle of sole). FOR TRANSVERSE ARCH – Peroneus longus tendon and tibialis posterior 4. SLING ARRANGEMENT – Suspends arch from above. FOR MEDIAL ARCH – Suspended by flexure hallucis longus. FOR LATERAL ARCH – Peroneus longus et brevis. FOR TRANSVERSE ARCH – peroneus longus.	• Flat foot (pes planus) – It can be congenital or acquired (due to over-weight) and prolong standing. • High arch (pes cavus) – Height of arch is more. • Talipes equinus – Heal raised; person walks on toes. • Talipes calcaneus – Person walks on heel. • Talipes varus – Person walks on lateral border of foot. • Talipes valgus – Person walks on medial border of foot. • Talipes equinovarus – Most common combination. It is also called clubfoot. • Above all deformities produce impairment of movements and pain.

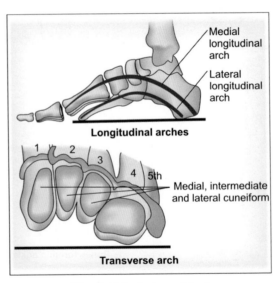

Fig. 3.12A: Arches of foot

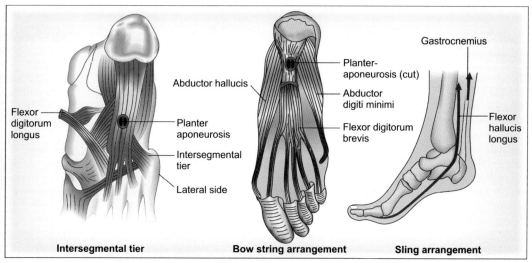

Fig. 3.12B: Maintenance of arches

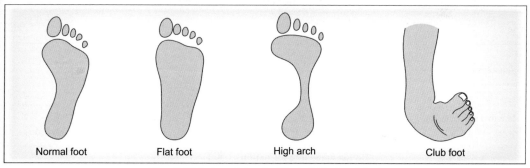

Fig. 3.12C: Imprints of different kinds of feet

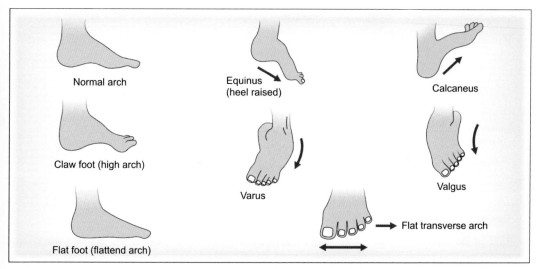

Fig. 3.12D: Different deformities of foot

Joints of Head and Neck

Name and bones concerned	Ligaments	Movements	Muscle concerned	Nerve suppl
Temporo mandibular joint (TM Joint) • Articular area of head of mandible. • Articular area of mandibular fossa of temporal bone and its articular tubercle (Fig. 3.13).	1. Capsular ligament. 2. Lateral temporo-mandibular ligament. 3. Stylomandi-bular ligament.	1. Protrusion 2. Retraction 3. Elevation 4. Depression 5. Side-to-side chewing movement.	1. Lateral and medial pterygoid muscle. 2. Temporalis (posterior fibre), assisted by – Masseter, Digastric, Geniohyoid. 3. Temporalis Masseter. 4. Medial pterygoid. Lateral pterygoid. Digastric. Geniohyoid. Mylohyoid. 5. Medial and lateral pterygoid of each side, acting alternately.	Auriculotempe – from posteri division of mandibular Masseteric branch – from anterior divisi of mandibular.

Cont

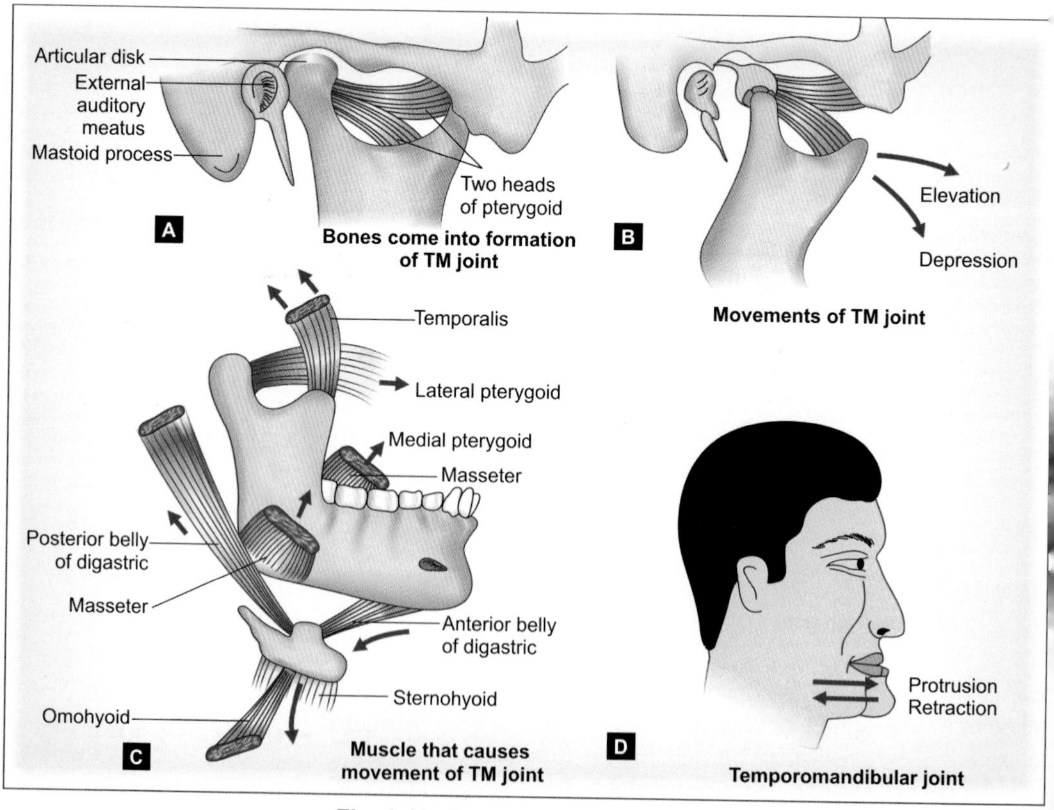

Articular disk
External auditory meatus
Mastoid process
Two heads of pterygoid

A **Bones come into formation of TM joint**

B

Elevation
Depression

Movements of TM joint

Temporalis
Lateral pterygoid
Medial pterygoid
Masseter
Posterior belly of digastric
Masseter
Anterior belly of digastric
Sternohyoid
Omohyoid

C **Muscle that causes movement of TM joint**

D

Protrusion
Retraction

Temporomandibular joint

Fig. 3.13: Tenporo mandibular joint

Name and bones concerned	Ligaments	Movements	Muscle concerned	Nerve supply
nio-vertebral Joints unto-occipital Joint novial) Bones cerned: ndyles of occipital e and reciprocally ved superior cular surface of first vical vertebra. las) (Fig. 3.14).	Fibrous capsule. Anterior atlanto-occipital membrane. Posterior atlanto-occipital membrane.	Flexion (main) with a little lateral flexion and rotation.	Longus capitis. Rectus capitis anterior.	First cervical nerve.
LANTO-AXIAL NT [synovial, axial, pivot type] NE CONCERNED: as and axis forms ee synovial nts – Lateral Medial	1. Atlantoaxial ligament. 2. Apical. 3. Alar ligament 4. Transverse ligament. 5. Cruciform ligament. 6. Membrana tectoria.	Simultaneous of all three joints. Rotation of axis which are checked by alar ligament.	Oblicus capitis inferior. Rectus capitis posterior major. Splenius capitis. Contralateral (opposite side). Sternomastoid	Second cervicle

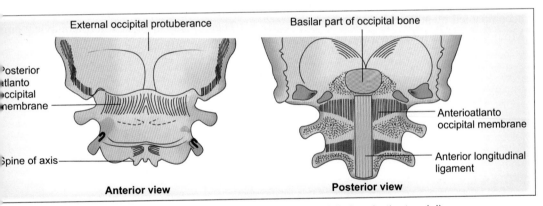

External occipital protuberance

Basilar part of occipital bone

Posterior atlanto occipital membrane

Spine of axis

Anterioatlanto occipital membrane

Anterior longitudinal ligament

Anterior view

Posterior view

Fig. 3.14: Craniovertebral joints (atlanto to occipital and atlantoaxial)

plied Anatomy [Joints]

mmon Joint Injuries

ain: The ligaments reinforcing a joint are tched or torn. The lumbar region, the knee and le are common sites of sprain. RICE; R – for ; I – for ice, C – for compression and E – for vation, are the standard treatment for pulled scle, stretched tendons or ligaments.

Cartilage Injuries

- It is common in knee joint, particularly in case of sportsman.
- The avascular cartilage [medial menisci] is unable to repair itself.
- The patient is unable to fully extend the knee and there is true locking.

Dislocation

- It involves displacement of articular surfaces of bones.
- It is usually accompanied by sprains, inflammation, and joint immobilization, like fracture, dislocation must be reduced [go back to original position]. Shoulder joints, finger joints, thumb, patella and temporo-mandibular joint is commonly dislocated.
- *Sublaxation* is the partial dislocation of a joint. Shoulder joint is commonly sublaxated due to loose capsule on inferomedial aspect.
- Temperomandibular joint is also dislocated due to loose capsule; even a large yawning produce dislocation.

Inflammation and degenerative disease of joint
[includes bursitis, tendinitis and various forms of arthritis]

- *Osteoarthritis:*
  Most common degenerative joint disease accompanied by stiffness and pain.
  Most common in aged [above 40 years]

particularly in women.
Weight bearing joints are mostly affected.

- *Rheumatoid arthritis:*
  Occurs in any age group [three times mo female].
  It is most crippling arthritis [due to a immune disease] involving severe inflamm of joints.
  Small joint like joint of finger, wrist, a and feet are affected in the same time [sides are involved].

- *Frozen shoulder:*
  It is a syndrome [combination of severe s and symptoms] characterized by a gl restriction of glenonumeral movement, pai muscle wasting. Commonly affects the mi aged and elderly persons.
  Spontaneous recovery occurs.

- *Tennis elbow [lateral epicondylitis]:*
  This is a common over used condi [repeatitive rotation at the elbow].
  There is pain in the lateral epicondyle [com extensor origin].

Chapter 4

Muscular System

INTRODUCTION

Muscle (mouse-like appearance) tissue has the special property of contractility due to presence of abundant actin and myocin protein filament. Muscle cells are known as myocytes. In man, muscle tissue constitutes 40 to 50% of body mass. There are three types of muscles.

Feature	Skeletal (Fig. 4.1A)	Cardiac (Fig. 4.1C)	Smooth (Fig. 4.1B)
Fibers-shape	• The fibers are cylindrical.	Fibers are cylindrical and branched (intercalated disc present at the junction).	Fibers are fusiform or spindle shaped.
Position of nuclei	• Peripherally situated multiple nuclei.	Single central nucleus.	Single central nucleus.
Cross striations	• Numerous prominent cross striation showing light and dark band.	Cross striation may or may not be present (when it is faintly stained).	No such features.
Situation	• They are usually attached to body skeleton.	Present in heart musculature.	Muscle of organs like gastrointestinal tract, urinary tract, etc.
Function	• Voluntary in function.	Involuntary in function.	Involuntary in function.

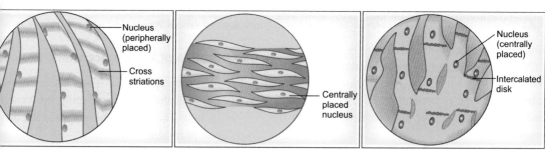

Fig. 4.1A: Skeletal muscle   **Fig. 4.1B:** Smooth muscle   **Fig. 4.1C:** Cardiac muscle

(Terminology) Associated with Muscle (Fig. 4.2)

- Origin: The attachment that moves least.
- Insertion: The attachment that moves more.
- Tendon: The end of a muscle is connected to cartilage by strong, rounded fibrous tissue are known as tendon, e.g. tendoachills.
- Aponeurosis: The flated muscles are attached by a thin strong sheet of fibrous tissue kn as aponeurosis, e.g. External oblique aporosis.
- Raphae: A raphae is interdigitation of tendi ends of fibers of flat muscle, e.g. Myloh raphae.
- Retinaculum: Condensation of white fib tissue (deep fascia) around the joint. It stabi the long tendons during movement of a joi

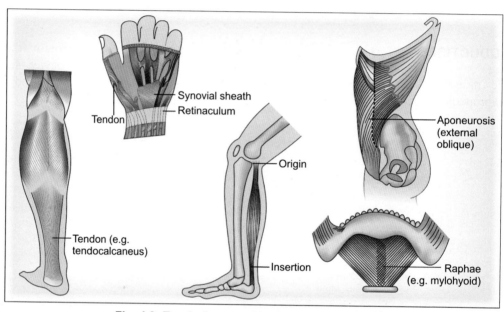

Synovial sheath
Retinaculum
Tendon
Aponeurosis (external oblique)
Origin
Tendon (e.g. tendocalcaneus)
Insertion
Raphae (e.g. mylohyoid)

Fig. 4.2: Terminology used in description of muscle

CLASSIFICATION OF VOLUNTARY MUSCLE

The individual fiber of a voluntary muscle are arranged either parallel or oblique to the long axis of a muscle. According to their arrangement of fibers, they are classified below (Fig. 4.3).

While resting, every skeletal muscle is in a partial state of contraction. This is known as muscle tone. In paralysis of skeletal muscle, tone is absent, and flabby. In the long run, there is wasting of muscles.

There are three types of voluntary muscles fibers–*fast (glycolytic)*–Tire quickly or white type (pale)–Used in powerful movement.

Slow, oxidative (fatigue resistance) – muscle: Used in maintaining posture.

Intermediate fast oxidative (fatigue resistanc Used during walking. Most muscles contai mixture of fibers types.

Classification of Muscle According to Acti

- *Prime movers (agonists):* The muscles bear chief responsibility for producing movemen
- *Antagonist:* The muscle that opposes the acti of another muscle.
- *Synergists:* Helps the prime movers by effecti the same action (by stabilizing joint preventing undesirable movements).

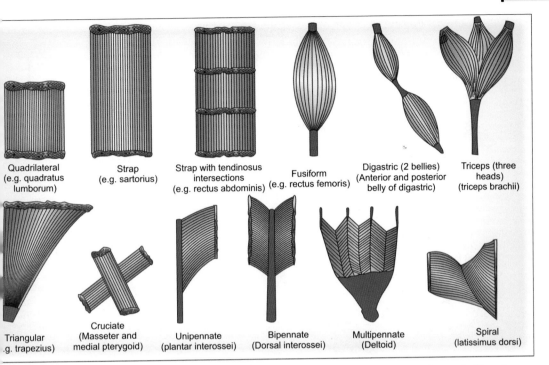

Quadrilateral (e.g. quadratus lumborum) · Strap (e.g. sartorius) · Strap with tendinosus intersections (e.g. rectus abdominis) · Fusiform (e.g. rectus femoris) · Digastric (2 bellies) (Anterior and posterior belly of digastric) · Triceps (three heads) (triceps brachii)

Triangular (e.g. trapezius) · Cruciate (Masseter and medial pterygoid) · Unipennate (plantar interossei) · Bipennate (Dorsal interossei) · Multipennate (Deltoid) · Spiral (latissimus dorsi)

Fig. 4.3: Classification of voluntary muscle (according to shape and direction of muscle fibers)

Fixator: Its function is to immobilize a bone or muscle from origin to allow the desirable movement.

...es and Muscles as Body Lever System

...ver is a bar that moves on fulcrum. When an ...rt is applied to the lever, a load is moved. In ...body bones are the levers, joints are the fulcrum ...the effort is exerted by skeletal muscle.

...st class levers (effort – fulcrum – load) ...y operate at a mechanical advantage or ...dvantage, e.g. humero ulnar and part of elbow ...t (Fig. 4.4A).

...ond class lever (fulcrum – load – effort) all ...rate at a mechanical advantage, e.g. ankle joint ...;. 4.4B).

...rd class lever (fulcrum – effort – load) always ...rate at a mechanical disadvantage, e.g. elbow ...t (Fig. 4.4C).

Naming of Muscle

According to Shape

- Deltoid=(triangular), e.g. deltoid muscle of arm.
- Quadratus = (square), e.g. quadratus lumborum of abdomen.
- Rhomboid = (diamond shaped), e.g. rhomboids major muscle of back.
- Teres = (round), e.g. teres major of upper limb.
- Gracilis = (slender), e.g. gracilis muscle in thigh.
- Rectus = (straight), e.g. rectus abdominis of abdomen.
- Lumbrical = (worm like), e.g. lumbricals of hand and feet.

According to Size

- Major = big, e.g. pectoralis major (muscle of thorax).
- Minor = small, e.g. pectoralis minor (muscle of thorax).

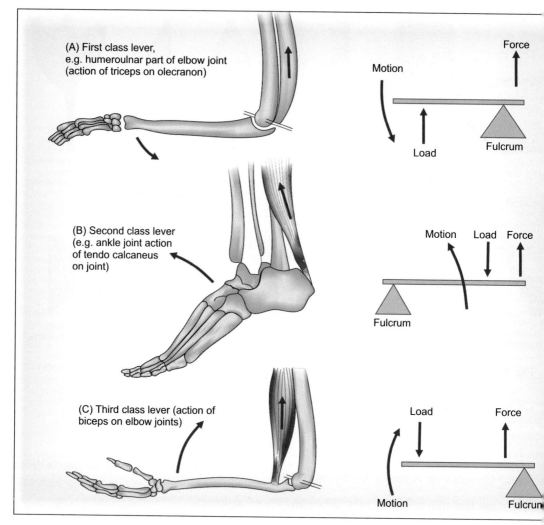

Fig. 4.4: Lever system

- Longus = long, e.g. adductor longus (of thigh).

- Brevis = short, e.g. adductor brevis (of thigh).

- Magnus = large, e.g. adductor magnus (of thigh).

- Latissimus = broadest, e.g. latissimus dorsi (back muscle).

- Maximus = largest, e.g. gluteus maximus (hip muscle).

- Minimus = smallest, e.g. gluteus minimus (another hip muscle).

According to Number of Heads of Origin

- Biceps = Bi – two; ceps – head – e.g. bi
  brachii (front muscle of arm).
- Triceps = Tri – three; Triceps brachii (bac
  arm).
- Quadriceps = Quadri – four; Quadriceps fem
  (muscle of front thigh).
  Often several criteria are combined in nan
  of a muscle = For example, Extensor c
  radialis brevis – tells us, extensor (musc
  action), carpi (of wrist), radialis (of radial s
  i.e. on lateral side), brevis (short).

lied

fect of exercise on muscles

Regular aerobic exercise results in increase efficiency endurance (tolerance), strength, and resistant to fatigue of skeletal muscles. Resistance exercise causes skeletal muscle hypertrophy (increase in size) and gains in skeletal muscle strength.

ramp: Sustained spasm of an entire muscle asts for a few seconds to several hours) causing e muscle to become tough and painful; ommon in calf, thigh and hip muscle.

oasm: A sudden involuntary muscle twitch ange from mere irritation to very painful) due chemical imbalance; common in eyelid, facial uscle.

uscle strain: Excessive stretching and rceable tearing (due to overuse and abuse) – e injured muscle is painful and inflammed. uadriceps and hamstring muscle strain is very ommon in athlets.

5. *Muscle injury:* Very common; formation of hematoma (blood accumulated swelling) within the muscle, e.g. hamstring, gastrocne-mius hematoma.
6. *Wasting:* Wasting due to disuse, and confinement in bed due to peripheral nerve injury.
7. *Rotator cuff weakness:* Supraspinatus, infraspinatus teres minor, subcapularis form the rotator cuff. Most problems arise due to tear (complete or partial) of supraspinatus. The abduction is impaired and arm drop.
8. *Biceps and triceps tendinitis (tendon inflammation):* Biceptial tendinitis causes pain in the anterior aspect of elbow or in upper arm as a result of overuse or strain.
   Tricepital tendinitis causes posterior elbow pain and tenderness in the triceps insertion.
9. *Quadriceps weakness:* It occurs due to constant use of high heel or tear of few fibers of muscles (due to over work) and due to prolonged immobilization. The patient gets tired early when walks on a staircase.

cle Connecting Upper Limb to Thoracic Wall (Fig. 4.5)

Muscle	Origin	Insertion	Description	Nerve supply	Action
toralis major ctus – chest or – large)	Clavicle, sternum and upper six postal cartilages.	Lateral lip of bicipital groove of humerus.	Large, fan shaped muscle, covering upper portion of chest, forms anterior axillary fold.	Medial and lateral pectoral nerves from brachial plexus.	Adductus arm and rotate it medially. *Laterally* Clavicular fiber also flex arm.
toralis minor nor – small)	Third, fourth and fifth ribs.	Coracoid process of scapula.	Flat, thin muscle lies under cover of pectoralis major.	Medial pectoral nerve.	Depress point of shoulder, when the scapula is fixed. It elevates the ribs from insertion.
clavius (sub – eath, clav – vicle)	First rib cartilage	Clavicle	Small, cylindrical muscle extending from first rib to clavicle.	Nerve to subclavius from upper trunk of brachial plexus.	Depresses the clavicle. Steadies clavicle during movement of shoulder girdle.
ratus anterior rratus – saw th like xer muscle)	Upper eight ribs.	Entire anterior surface of medial border and inferior angle of scapula.	Lies deep to scapula, forms medial wall of axilla, origins has saw tooth like appearance.	Long thoracic nerve.	Move scapula forward around the thoracic wall; rotates scapula and raises the point of shoulder.

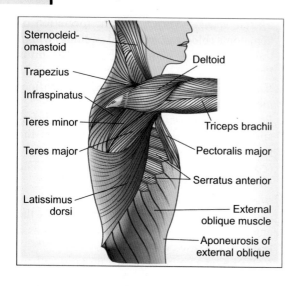

◀◀

Fig. 4.5: Muscle connecting the upper limb to thoracic wall

Muscle Connecting Upper Limb to Vertebral Column (Fig. 4.6)

Muscle	Origin	Insertion	Description	Nerve supply	Action
Trapezius	Occipital bone, ligamentum nuchae. Muscle arises also from spines of C7 and all thoracic spines.	A continuous insertion along the acromin and spine of scapula (upper border) and lateral third of clavicle.	Most superficial muscle of back. Flat triangular in shape. Upper fibers run downwards, middle fibers run horizontally and lower fibers pass upwards.	Spinal part of accessory nerve (eleventh cranial nerve)	Stabilize and rota scapula, upper fib elevates the scapu middle fibers pull the spinel mediall and lower fibers p the medial border of scap downwards.
Latissimus dorsi (Latissimus – widest dorsi – on dorsal aspect)	From iliac crest, lumbar fascia, spines of lower six thoracic vertebrae, lower three or four ribs and inferior angle of scapula.	It winds around the teres major to insert in the floor of bicipital groove of humerus.	Broad, flat triangular muscle of lumbar region, forms posterior wall of axilla.	Thoracodorsal nerve	Extends, adduct a medially rotates t arm. It is promine during hammering rowing and swimming.
Rhomboid major (Rhomboid –diamond shaped)	Second to fifth thoracic spine.	Medial border of scapula.	Rectangular muscle lying deep to trapezius.	Dorsal scapular nerve	Raises medial bor of scapula upward and medially.
Rhomboid minor	Ligamentum nuchae, spines of C7 and T1.	Medial border of scapula.	Rectangular muscle lying deep to trapezius and inferior to levator scapulae.	Dorsal scapular nerve	Raises medial bor of scapula and stabilizes scapula.

Cont

uscle	Origin	Insertion	Description	Nerve supply	Action
s major tator cuff cle]	Lower 3rd of lateral border of scapula.	Medial lip of bicipital groove of humerus.	Thick muscle, located inferior to teres minor, helps to form the posterior border of axilla.	Lower subscapular nerve from post cord of brachial plexus	Medially rotate and adduct arm and stabilizes shoulder joint.
es minor tator cuff cle)	Upper 2/3rd of lateral border of scapula.	Greater tuberosity of humerus (lower impression).	Small elongates muscle lies inferior to infraspinatus and may be inseparated from the muscle.	Axillary nerve	Laterally rotate the arm and stabilizez shoulder joint.
scapularis o-under) ator cuff scle	Subscapular fossa.	Lesser tuberosity of humerus.	Forms part of posterior of axilla. Tendon passes infront of shoulder joint.	Upper and lower sub-scapular nerve of post cord of brachial plexus	Chief medial rotator of arm and stabilize shoulder joint.

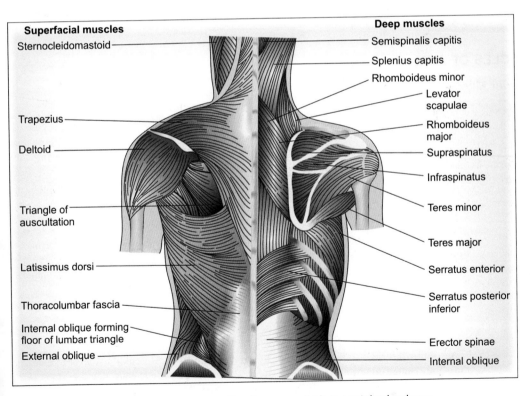

Fig. 4.6: Muscle connecting the upper limb to vertebral column

Muscles Connecting the Scapula to Humerus (Fig. 4.6)

Muscle	Origin	Insertion	Description	Nerve supply	Action
Deltoid (Delta – triangular muscle)	Lateral one third of clavicle, acromian, spine of scapula.	In deltoid tuberosity in middle of lateral surface of shaft of humerus.	Thick, multipennete muscle, forming the roundness of shoulder. A site commonly used for intramuscular injection.	Axillary nerve.	Abducts arm. Ant fibers flex and med rotate the arm. Post fiber extends laterally rotate the Action in antagoni pectoralis major latissimus dorsi.
Supraspinatus (supra – above a muscle lies above the spine) [Rotate cuff muscle].	Supraspinous fossa of scapula.	Greater tuberosity of humerus, shoulder joint.	Lies deep to trapezius and it is a rotator cuff muscle.	Supra - scapular nerve.	Abducts and stabil shoulder joint. Pre downward disloca of shoulder w carries a heavy suitc
Infraspinatus (Infra –below– so a muscle below the spine of scapula) [Rotator cuff muscle].	Infraspinous fossa of scapula.	Greater tuberosity of humerus, shoulder joint.	Partially covered by deltoid and trapezius.	Supra scapular nerve.	Laterally rotates arm and stabil shoulder joint.

MUSCLES OF ARM

Anterior Muscles (Fig. 4.7A)

Muscle	Origin	Insertion	Description	Nerve supply	Action
Biceps Brachii (Biceps – two head)	Long head – from supraglenoid tubercle of scapula. Short head – Coracoid process of scapula.	Tuberosity of radius and bicepital aponeurosis.	Fusiform muscle. Two head unite near about the middle of arm.	Musculocutaneous nerve.	Flexes elbow joint supinate the forea Long head stabil shoulder joint.
Coraco-brachialis (Coraco-coracoid process brachium-arm)	Coracoid process of scapula.	Medial aspect of shaft of humerus.	Small cylindrical muscle.	Musculocutaneous nerve.	Flexes arm; we adductor synergist pectoralis major.
Brachialis	From anterolateral and anteromedial surface of lower end of humerus.	Coronoid process of ulna.	Strong muscle. Lies deep to biceps brachii on distal humerus.	Musculocutaneous nerve.	Flexor of elbow join

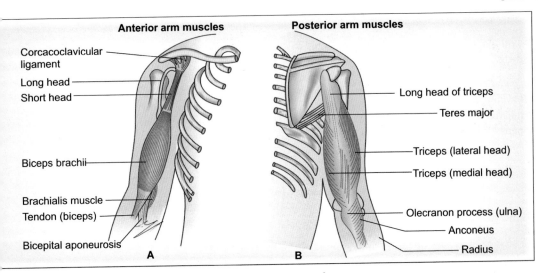

Anterior arm muscles

- Corcacoclavicular ligament
- Long head
- Short head
- Biceps brachii
- Brachialis muscle
- Tendon (biceps)
- Bicepital aponeurosis

A

Posterior arm muscles

- Long head of triceps
- Teres major
- Triceps (lateral head)
- Triceps (medial head)
- Olecranon process (ulna)
- Anconeus
- Radius

B

Figs 4.7A and B: Muscles of arm

...terior Muscles (Fig. 4.7B)

Muscle	Origin	Insertion	Description	Nerve supply	Action
...ceps bra-...i (Tri—...ee ...s—head ...ee ...ded ...scle)	Long head—Infraglenoid tubercle of scapula. Lateral head – upper half of posterior humerus. Medial head – Lower half of posterior humerus, below the radial groove.	Superior surface of olecranon process of ulna.	Large fleshy belly, and only muscle of posterior compartment of arm. Long and lateral head lie superficial to me-dial head	Radial nerve.	Extensor of elbow joint.

...scles of Forearm (Figs 4.8A and B)

...ht muscle arranged in lateral to medial aspect

Muscle	Origin	Insertion	Description	Nerve supply	Action
...onator ...es (Pro-...tion—...sition of ...rearm to ...ve some-...ing to ...mebody).	Humeral head – Medial epicondyle of humerus. Ulcer head – Medial border of coronoid process of ulna.	Lateral aspect of shaft of radius.	Two headed superficial muscle located between brachioradialis on its lateral aspect and flexor carpi radialis on its medial aspect. Form medial boundary of cubital fossa.	Median nerve.	Pronation and flexon of forearm.

Contd...

Muscle	Origin	Insertion	Description	Nerve supply	Action
Flexor carpi radialis	Anterior surface of medial epicondyle of humerus.	Bases of second and third metacarpal.	Runs obliquely across the forearm. It has chord like tendon at the region of wrist.	Median nerve.	Flexes and abdu... hand at wrist jo...
Palmaris longus	Anterior surface of medial epicondyle of humerus.	Flexor retinaculum and palmar aponeurosis.	Small muscle with a long tendon; often absent.	Median nerve.	Weak wrist flex...
Flexor carpi ulnaris	Humeral head – Anterior surface of medial epicondyle of humerus. Ulnar head – Medial aspect of olecranon process and posterior border of ulna.	Pisiform, hook of hammate and base of fifth metacarpal bone.	Medial most muscle of flexor group. Two headed ulnar nerve lies lateral to its tendon.	Ulnar nerve.	Flexes and addu... the arm at wrist joint.
Flexor digitorum superficialis (digitorum – concerned with finger) or toe superficial – close to surface.	Humero-ulnar head – Anterior surface of medial epicondyle of humerus; medial border of coronoid process of ulna. Radial head – from anterior oblique line of shaft of radius.	By four tendon into middle phalanges of two to five fingers.	Intermediate group of muscle, visible at the distal part of forearm. Median nerve is plastered behind this muscles	Median nerve.	Flexer mid... phalanx of fing... and assist in flex... proximal phal-... and head.

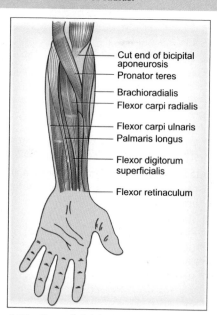

Fig. 4.8A: Superficial flexor muscles of forearm

Cut end of bicipital aponeurosis
Pronator teres
Brachioradialis
Flexor carpi radialis
Flexor carpi ulnaris
Palmaris longus
Flexor digitorum superficialis
Flexor retinaculum

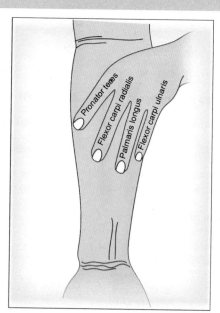

Fig. 4.8B: Arrangement of superficial flexors o... forearm (like 4 fingers in hand)

ep Muscles

uscle	Origin	Insertion	Description	Nerve supply	Action
xor licis gus lax – mb. long xor of mb.	Anterior surface of shaft of radius.	Distal phalanx of thumb.	Lies side by side with flexor digitorum. Profundus.	Anterior interosseous branch of median nerve.	Flexes distal phalanx of thumb.
exor gitorum ofundus rofunda– ep)	Anteromedial surface of shaft of ulna.	Distal phalax of medial 4 fingers.	Extensive origin covered by flexor digitorum superficialis.	Medial half by ulnar and lateral half by median.	Only muscle that can flex distal interphalangeal joint.
onator aadratus uodrate– uare ape).	Pronator ridge on the anterior surface of lower end of ulna.	Anterior surface of lower end of shaft of radius.	Deepest muscle of distal forearm. Only muscle that arise solely from ulna and inserted solely in radius.	Anterior interosseous branch of median nerve.	Pronates forearm along with pronator teres.

scles of Posterior Compartment of Forearm
perficial (Lateral to Medial) (Fig. 4.9)

Muscle	Origin	Insertion	Description	Nerve supply	Action
achio- dialis	Lateral supracondylar ridge of humerus	Base of styloid process of radius.	Form lateral boundary of cubital fossa.	Radial nerve.	Rotates fore-arm to the mid prone position.
tensor rpi radialis ngus ongus-long)	Lateral supracondylar ridge of humerus.	Posterior surface of base of second metacarpal bone.	Parallel to brachio-radialis on lateral forearm and may blend with it.	Radial nerve.	Extends and abducts hand at wrist joint.
xtensor rpi dialis evis (brevis short)	Lateral epicondyle of humerus.	Posterior surface of base of third metacarpal bone.	Shorter than extensor carpi radialis longus and lies deep to it.	Deep branch of radial nerve.	Extends and abducts hand at wrist joint.
xtensor gitorum	Lateral epicondyle of humerus.	Middle and distal phalanx of medial four fingers.	Lies medial to extensor carpi ralialis brevis. Four tendons at the wrist passes deep to extensor retinaculum.	Deep branch of radial nerve.	Extends little fingers and hand.

Contd...

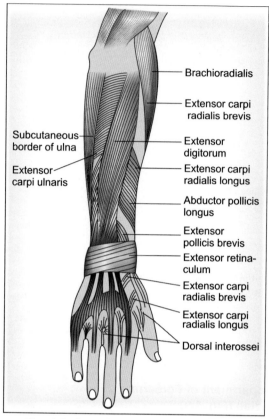

Fig. 4.9: Superficial extensors of forearm

Muscle	Origin	Insertion	Description	Nerve supply	Action
Extensor digiti minimi	Posterior surface of lateral epicondyle of humerus	Extensor expansion of little finger.	It is the detached portion of extesor digitorum.	Deep branch of radial nerve (posterior interosseous).	Extends metacarpo-phalangeal joint of little finger.
Extensor carpi ulnaris	Posterior surface of lateral epicondyle of humerus.	Base of fifth metacarpal.	Medial most muscle of superficial compartment. It is long and slender in shape.	Deep branch of radial	Extends and adduct hand at wrist joint
Anconeus	Posterior surface of lateral epicondyle of humerus.	Lateral surface of olecranon in a fan shaped manner	Small, triangular muscle behind the cubital joint. It is partially blended with triceps.	(Posterior interosseous). Radial nerve.	Extends and abduct ulna during pronation

p Group

uscle	Origin	Insertion	Description	Nerve supply	Action
inator rning m eriorly)	Lateral epicondyle of humerus, annular ligament.	Neck and shaft of radius.	Deep muscles at posterior aspect of elbow largely concealed by superficial muscle.	Posterior interosseous nerve (deep branch of radial).	Supination of forearm.
ductor licis gus	Posterior surface of shaft of radius.	Base of first metacarpal bone.	It lies lateral and parallel to extensor pollicis longus.	Posterior interosseous nerve.	Abducts and extends thumb.
tensor licis vis and gus.	Posterior surface of shaft of radius.	Brevis – base of proximal phalanx of thumb. Longus – base of distal phalanx of thumb.	Deep muscle pair with a common origin and action.	Posterior interosseous nerve.	Brevis extends metacarpo-phalangeal joint of thumb and longus – extends distal phalanx.
tensor licis	Posterior surface of shaft of ulna.	Extensor expansion of index finger.	Tiny muscle arising close to wrist.	Posterior interosseous nerve.	Extends metacarpo-phalangeal joint of index finger.

scles of Inferior Extremity (Fig. 4.10)

scle of Anterior Compartment (extensor group)

thigh (seven muscles)

Muscle	Origin	Insertion	Description	Nerve supply	Action
rtorius artor eans tailor. ilor's uscle)	Anterior superior iliac spine.	Inverted hockey stick like insertion in the upper medial surface of shaft of tibia.	Long, slender, superficial strap muscle, descends downwards and medially, crosses both hip and knee joint. It forms lateral boundary of femoral triangle.	Femoral (anterior division)	Flexes, and laterally rotates thigh. Weak flexor of knee. This position is usually seen in tailor which uses their both legs on the machine.
iacus	Iliac fossa of hip bone.	With psoas into lesser trochanter of femur.	Large, fan-shaped muscle, fibers covering downwards and passes below the inguinal ligament toward insertion.	Femoral nerve.	Flexes hip. Flexes trunk and thigh as in sitting posture.

Contd...

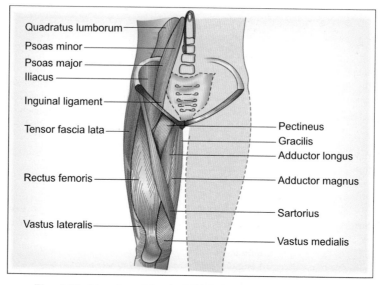

Fig. 4.10: Muscles of front of thigh (extensor compartment)

Muscle	Origin	Insertion	Description	Nerve supply	Action
Poas major	By fleshy slips from transverse processes, bodies (upper and lower border) and disc of all lumbar vertebrae and T12.	With iliac (together known as ilio-psoas) into lesser trochanter of femur.	Longer, thicker, more medial muscle of the ilio-psoas pair; descends along the pelvic brim, below the inguinal ligament and in front of hip joint, towards insertion.	Ventral rami of L1-L3.	• Prime mo of hip jo (flexion). • Flexes trun on the thig • Important postural muscle.
Pectenius	Pecten pubis	Upper end of linea-aspara of shaft of femur.	Short, flat quadrilateral muscle. It lies over adductor brevis on proximal thigh.	1. Nerve to pectenius (branch of femoral nerve). 2. From obturater.	Flexes and adducts thigh
Rectus femoris (rectus – straight)	Straight head – arises from anterior inferior iliac spine. Reflected head – from ilium above acetabulum.	Through patella inserted to tibial tuberosity via ligamentum patellae.	Superficial muscle of extensor compartment of thigh. Runs straight down in thigh. This is the only muscle of extensor group which crosses the hip joint.	Femoral (posterior division)	Extends kn and flexes thi at hip joint.
Vastus lateralis	Greater trochanter, intert-rochanteric line, linea	Through patella inserted to tibial	Largest, bulky compo-nent of quadriceps	Femoral (posterior division)	Extends knee.

Cont.

uscle	Origin	Insertion	Description	Nerve supply	Action
	aspara and lateral lip of gluteal tuberosity of femur.	tuberosity via ligamentum pate-llae.	femoris. It is a site for intramuscular injection particularly in infant.		
stus dialis	Linea aspara, medial aspect of inter trochanteric line medial supracon-dylar line.	Through patella inserted to tibial tuberosity via ligamentum patellae.	Forms inferomedial aspect of thigh. Fibers pass downward and medially towards medial border of patella.	Femoral (posterior division)	• Extends knee. • Stabilizes patella.
stus inter edialis	From anterolateral and anteromedial surface of upper 2/3rd of femur.	Through patella inserted to tibial tuberosity via ligamentum patellae.	Obscured by rectus femoris, intermediate in position on anterior thigh. It appears to be inseparable from vastus medialis.	Femoral nerve	• Extends knee

scles of Medial Compartment of Thigh
dductor Group–Five Muscles)

luscle	Origin	Insertion	Description	Nerve supply	Action
racilis lender)	• By thin aponeurosis from body of pubis. • From ischiopubic rami.	Upper part of medial surface of shaft of tibia posterior to sartorius.	Long, thin, superficial muscle broad above and narrow below.	Obturator nerve (Anterior division)	Adduct thigh, flexes knee and rotate it medially.
dductor ongus ongus – ng)	Body of pubis as a C shaped tendon.	Linea aspara in the middle of 1/3rd of femur.	Large, fan shaped muscle. Most anterior muscle among three adductors.	Obturator nerve (anterior division).	• Adducts thigh. • Flexes medially rotate thigh.
dductor revis revis – hort)	Body and inferior ramus of pubis.	Linea aspara between pectineous and adductor longus.	Largely concealed by adductor longus and pectineus. It is some what triangular muscle lies in contact with obturator externus.	Obturator nerve (anterior division) sometimes posterior division.	• Adducts thigh.
dductor nagnus Magna – arge)	• From ischiopubic rami. • Inferolateral aspect of ischial tuberosity.	From medial margin of gluteal tuberosity upto adductor tubercle of lower end of femur.	A hybrid, triangular, massive muscle with a broad insertion. The linear attachment of muscle is interrupted by a series of openings (for four perforating arteries)	Adductor portion. Posterior division of obturator nerve. Hamastring portion by sciatic nerve.	• Adducts thigh. • Hamstring portion extends hip.

Muscles of Posterior Compartment of Thigh (Flexor Group) (Fig. 4.11A)

They are called hamstring.
Group of muscle four in number.

Muscle	Origin	Insertion	Description	Nerve supply	Action
Biceps femoris (Bi – two ceps two headed), e.g. two headed muscle	Long head – ischial tuberosity. Short head – linea aspera, lateral supracon-dylar line of shaft of femur.	Head of fibula.	Most lateral muscles of hamstring group. In the lower part it forms the lateral boundary of popliteal fossa and common peroneal nerve lies in its medial aspect.	Long head – tibial portion of sciatic nerve. Short head – common pero-neal part of sciatic nerve	Extends and flxes kn
Semiten-dinosus (semi-half, i.e. lower half of it is transformed onto tendon)	Ischial tuberosity(upper area).	Medial aspect of upper tibial shaft.	It is quite fleshy and lies medial to biceps in upper part. Lower third of thigh it is replaced by a long tendon.	Tibial portion of sciatic nerve	Extends and flxes kn
Semimemb-ranosus. (nearly half of the muscle flattened form, i.e. me-mbrane like)	Ischial tuberosity (upper part)	Medial condyle of tibia in a tubercle for semimem-branosus.	Deep semitendinosus and posteromedial aspect of thigh.	Tibial portion of sciatic nerve	Extends and flxes kn

Adductor magnus – Discussed in muscles of medial compartment of thigh.

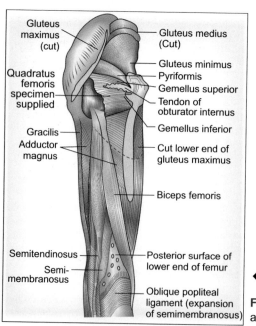

Fig. 4.11A: Muscles of gluteal region and posterior compartment of thigh

Muscles of Leg (Fig. 4.12A)

Anterior Compartment (Five in Number)

All muscles of anterior compartment are dorsiflexor of ankle and have a common innervation by deep peroneal nerve.

Muscle	Origin	Insertion	Description	Nerve supply	Action
Tibialis anterior	Lateral surface of shaft of tibia (upper 2/3rd) and from lateral condyle of tibia.	Inferior surface of medial cuneiform and base of first metatarsal bone.	Superficial muscle of anterior leg, readily palpable, lateral to tibia. In the lower 1/3rd of leg the muscle belly is replaced by tendon.	Deep peroneal nerve.	Dorsiflexion of ankle and invert foot. Maintain medial long-itudinal arch.
Extensor digitorum longus	• Lateral condyle of tibia. • Proximal 3/4th of extensor surface of fibula. • Interosseous membrane.	Inserted into distal phalanx of 2-5 toes through dorsal digital expansion.	Lies lateral to tibialis anterior muscle. In upper 1/3rd of leg anterior tibial vessel and deep peroneal nerve lies between it, and tibialis anterior.	Deep peroneal nerve.	Dorsiflexor of foot and prime mover in toes extension.
Peroneus tertius ('Perone – fibula tertius – third)	• Lower 1/4th of extensor surface of fibula. • Interosseous membrane.	Inserted on dorsum of fifth metatarsal, passing anterior to lateral malleolus.	Small muscle, usually continuous and fused with distal part of extensor digitirum longus. Not always present.	Deep peroneal nerve.	Dorsiflexes and evert foot.
Extensor hallucis longus (hallux – great toe)	Arises from middle half of anterior surface of fibula.	Inserted on distal phalanx of great toe.	It lies deep to extensor digitorum longus and tibialis anterior. It has narrow origin.	Deep peroneal nerve	Dorsiflexes foot and extends great toe.

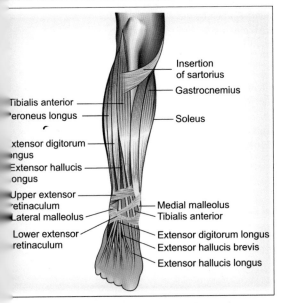
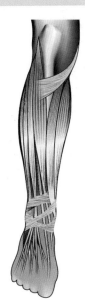

Tibialis anterior
Peroneus longus

Extensor digitorum longus
Extensor hallucis longus
Upper extensor retinaculum
Lateral malleolus
Lower extensor retinaculum

Insertion of sartorius
Gastrocnemius
Soleus

Medial malleolus
Tibialis anterior
Extensor digitorum longus
Extensor hallucis brevis
Extensor hallucis longus

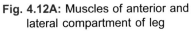

Fig. 4.12A: Muscles of anterior and lateral compartment of leg

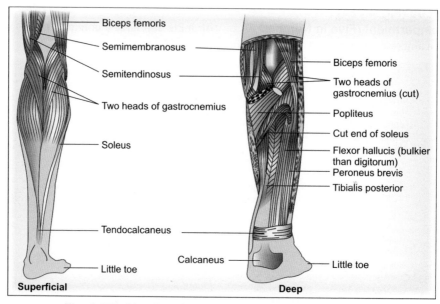

Fig. 4.12B: Muscles of back and lateral compartment of leg

Muscles of Lateral Compartment of Leg (Fig. 4.12B)

Muscle	Origin	Insertion	Description	Nerve supply	Action
Peroneous longus (longus– long).	Arises from head and proximal 2/3rd of lateral surface of shaft of fibula.	By a long tendon which crosses the sole obliquely and inserted into base of first metatarsal and medial cunei-form.	More superficial muscle of the two. In the lower 1/3rd it ends in tendon which passes behind the lateral mallesus and enter into sole.	Superficial peroneal nerve.	Plantar flexo and evertor o foot.
Peroneus brevis (brevis – short)	Distal 2/3rd of lateral surface of fibula.	Dorsal surface of base of fifth metatarsal lateral to peroneus tertius.	Smaller than longus and lies deep to it. It ends in a tendon which lies behind the lateral malleolus (brevis is deep).	Superficial peroneal nerve.	Plantar flexo and evertor c foot.

cles of Posterior Compartment (Back) of Leg

plied by Tibial Nerve) (Fig. 4.12B)

erficial Group

scle	Origin	Insertion	Description	Nerve supply	Action
rocnemius st rficial)	Medial, larger head arises from a depression behind adductor tubercle. Lateral head from lateral surface of femur.	Via tendo-calcaneus (largest tendon in the body- 15 cm in length). It is inserted into middle part of posterior surface of calcaneum.	Paired superficial muscle. Prominent bellies that form prominence of calf. Along with soleus it is known as triceps surae.	Tibial nerve.	Plantar flexor of foot at ankle joint and flexes knee joint.
taris	Lower part of lateral supracondylar line of femur.	Posterior surface of calcaneum.	Generally very small and feeble, but varies in size and extent, may be absent.	Tibial nerve.	Plantar flexor of foot at ankle joint and flexes knee joint.
eus	Soleal line middle 1/ 3rd of medial border of shaft of tibia, upper 1/4th of fibula	Via tendo achills into posterior surface of calcaneum.	Lies deep to gastroc-nemius; is a broad flat muscle. Within it venous plexuses lies which pump venous blood upwards by muscle action. So soleus is known as peripheral heart.	Tibial nerve.	Plantar flexor foot

p Group

uscle	Origin	Insertion	Description	Nerve supply	Action
liteus	·Intracapsular but extra–synovial, originates from groove on lateral surface of lateral condyle of femur.	Posterior surface of shaft of tibia above soleal line.	Thin, triangular muscle at posterior knees; passes downwards and medially in a fan shaped manner. It forms floor of popliteal fossa.	Tibial nerve.	Flexes knee. Un-lock knee joint by lateral rotation of femur on tibia and loose the ligaments.
xor itorum gus	Posterior surface of shaft of tibia below soleal line and medial to vertical ridge.	Bases of distal phalanges of lateral four toes.	It is thin and pointed proximally; runs medial to tibialis posterior and partly overlies posterior on it. It is long and nar-row muscle.	Tibial nerve.	• Weak plantar flexor. • Flexes toes and helps foot "to grip" the ground. • Support medial and lateral longitudinal arch.

Contd...

Muscle	Origin	Insertion	Description	Nerve supply	Action
Flexor hallucis longus	Posterior surface of distal 2/3rd of fibula.	Base of distal phalanx of hallux (great toe).	Bipennate muscle. Bulckier than flexor digitorum longus, and laterally placed	Tibial nerve.	• Flexes distal phalanx of big • Weak plantar flexor of ankl • Support medi longitudinal a
Tibialis posterior	Posterior surface of shaft of tibia and fibula and interosseous membrane.	Tuberosity of navicular bone and gives slips to other neighbouring tarsal bones, except talus.	Most deeply palced muscle of flexor group.	Tibial nerve	Invert foot and weak plantar fle Support medial longitudinal arch and transverse ar of foot.

Muscles of Gluteal Region (Figs 4.11A and B)

Muscle	Origin	Insertion	Description	Nerve supply	Action
Gluteus maximus	• From area behind the posterior gluteal line of hip bone. • Outer sloping surface of dorsal segment of iliac crest.	3/4th fiber in ilio tibial tract and gluteal tuberosity of femur.	Largest and more superficial of gluteal muscle. From bulk of buttock; fibers are thick and course and runs downwards and laterally.	Inferior gluteal nerve	Extends and lat rotates the hip jo
Gluteus medius	From outer ilium, surface between anterior and posterior gluteal lines.	Gluteal tuberosity of femur.	Thick muscle; its posterior 1/3rd is covered by gluteus maximus. It is superficial in its anterior 2/3rd. Inter muscular injection is given in anterior part of outer and upper part of hip region.	Superior gluteal nerve	• Abducts thigh (acting from pelvis) and rot it medially. • Take an essen part in maintain the trunk upri when the foot the opposite sit raised from ground.
Gluteus minimus	Between anterior and inferior gluteal line.	Anterior surface of greater trochanter of femur.	Fan shaped smallest and deepest gluteal muscle.	Superior gluteal nerve	• Abducts thigh (acting from p vis) and rotate medially. • Take an essen part in maintain the trunk uprig when the foot the opposite site raised from t ground.

Con

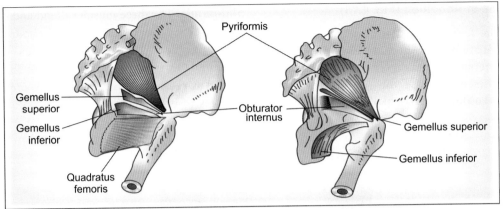

Fig. 4.11B: Insertion at the upper end of femur (muscle seen after removal of gluteus maximus + gluteus medium)

uscle	Origin	Insertion	Description	Nerve supply	Action
iformis	From anterior surface of sacrum by three steps:	Upper border of greater trochanter of femur.	Pyramidal muscle; located on posterior aspect of hip joint; comes out from pelvis via greater sciatic foramen.	First and second sacral nerve (nerve to pyriforms).	• Rotates thigh laterally • Assists abduction of thigh when hip is flexed • Stabilizes hip joint
turator ernus	• Inner surface of obturator membrane. • Greater sciatic notch and margins of obturator foramen.	Upper border of greater trochanter of femur.	Surrounds their obturator foramen within pelvis. Leaves pelvis via greater sciatic foramen along with two small gemelli muscle.	From sacral plexus.	• Rotate thigh laterally.· • Stabilizes hip joint.
turator ernus	• Medial 2/3rd of the external surface of obturator mem-brane. • From pubis and ischium.	By a tendon into trochanteric fossa.	Flat, triangular muscle deep in upper medial aspect of thigh.	Obturator nerve	• Rotate thigh laterally. • Stabilizes hip joint.
nsor fasica a	From anterior 5 cm of outer aspect of iliac crest.	In iliotibial tract.	Fibers run downwards and backwards.	Superior gluteal nerve.	Extends knee and laterally rotate the leg.
adratus noris uadrate uare aped)	From femoral surface of body of ischium.	Quadratus tubercle of femur.	Short, square muscle, lies between gemelli above and upper border of adductor magnus below in deeper plane.	Nerve of quadratus femoris.	Lateral rotator of thigh.

Muscles of Abdomen (Fig. 4.13)

There are four pairs of flat muscle in abdomen. They protect the anterior abdominal wall from external injury as there is no bony support. The muscles are from outside inwards **external oblique, internal oblique, transverses** **abdominis**. The three muscles blend and for broad sheat (aponeurosis). The aponeurosis turn, encloses the fourth muscles re abdominis in front like a sheath. This sheat known as **rectus sheath**. They are the additio muscles of expiration.

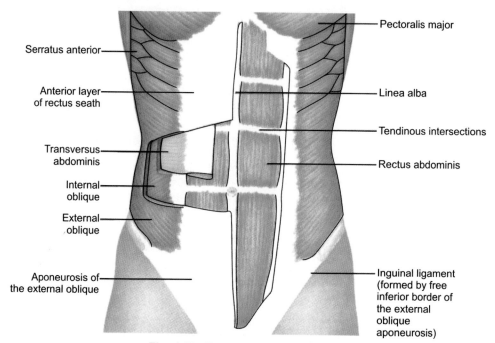

Fig. 4.13: Exposure of rectus sheath

Muscle	Origin	Insertion	Description	Nerve supply	Action
External oblique (outer layer)	By fleshy slips from outer surface of lower eight ribs.	Most fibers inserted in linea alba (white line) some into pubic crest, tubercle and iliac crest.	It is most superficial muscle. Fibers run downwards and medially and end in aponeurosis, which folds upon inferiorly and forms inguinal ligament	By T7 to T12 intercostal nerve.	It compresses abd minal wall a increases the int abdominal press (which helps micturition, defae tion, sneezing, et along with t muscles of back, helps in tru rotation and late flexion.
Internal oblique (Middle layer)	Arises from a thoracolumbar fascia, iliac crest, inguinal ligament	Inserted in linea alba, pubic crest and last three ribs.	Fibers run upwards and forward at right angle to those of external oblique.	T7 – T12 intercostal and L1 nerves.	Same as extern oblique.

Cont

uscle	Origin	Insertion	Description	Nerve supply	Action
iseversus ominis hermost er)	Arises from thoraco-lumbar fascia, inguinal ligament, cartilage of last six ribs, iliac crest.	In linea alba and in pubic crest.	Fibers run horizon-tally and its deep surfaces lined by transversalis fascia.	T7 – T2 intercostal nerve and L1 spinal nerve.	Compresses abdo-minal contents.
:tus lominis	Arises as tendon from public crest and symphysis pubis	Inserted in xiphoid process (anterior sur-face) and 5–7 ribs (as fleshy fiber).	It is vertically placed straight muscle of abdomen situated on either side of midline intersected by tend-inous intersection	T7 – T12 intercostal nerves.	Flex and rotate the lumbar region of vertebral column.
vator pulae vator – vator or ses)	Transverse process of first four cervical vertebrae.	Located in the back and side of neck, deep to trapezius.	Medial border of scapula.	Elevates the medial border of scapula.	C3 and C4 spinal nerve and dorsal scapular nerve.

lied: Due to repeated childbirth in a woman, it is seen that the rectus muscle of abdomen is weak there is herniation between two recti. This is known as ventral hernia or abdominal hernia.

scles of Head (Fig. 4.14)

scles of scalp

Muscle	Origin	Insertion	Description	Nerve supply	Action
:cipito-ntalis has o parts: Frontalis Occipitalis	Epicranial aponeurosis	Skin, superficial fascia of eyebrows.	Bipartite muscle connected by epicarnial aponeurosis (galea aponeurotica).	Facial nerve.	Pull scalp forward.
		From lateral 2/3rd of superior nuchal line of occipital and from mastoid part of temporal bones.		Facial nerve.	Move scalp backwards.

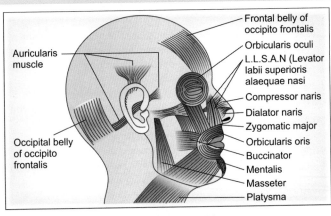

Fig. 4.14: Muscle of face

Muscles of Facial Expression

Muscle	Origin	Insertion	Description	Nerve supply	Action
Orbicularis occuli – two parts 1. Palpebral part 2. Orbital part	Medial palpebral ligament. Frontal and maxillary bones.	Lateral palpebral raphe. Loops return to origin.	Thin, flat, circular muscle around eye. Paralysis lead to drooping of eyelid and spilling of tears.	Facial nerve.	1. Closes eyelid 2. Protects eye f intense light and injury.
Corrugator superciliarils.	Superciliary arch.	All muscles of face inserted in facial skin except masseter.	Small muscle; actively associated with orbiculari occuli.	Facial nerve.	Draws eyebrows together. Vertical wrinkling in forehead.
Orbicularis oris	Maxilla, mandible and skin.	Encircle oral orifice.	Thin, flat muscle encircling the oral aperture.	Facial nerve.	Compresses lips together.

Other small muscles are, procerus (situated at root of nose), dilator naris (dilates nostrils), compressor naris (reduces nostril), need not know in details.

Dialator Muscles of Lip

They are levator labii superioris et alaequae nasi,

levator labii superioris, zygomaticus ma zygomaticus minor, levator anguli oris, riso depressor anguli oris, depressor labii infer and mentalis. They arise from bones and fa around oral aperture and inserted into subst of lip. They separate lips and supplied by fa nerve.

Muscles of Mastication

Muscle	Origin	Insertion	Description	Nerve supply	Action
Masseter	Zygomatic arch	Angle and ramus of mandible.	Powerful muscle that covers lateral aspect of mandibular ramus. This muscle is covered on its lateral aspect by tough masseteric fascia.	Branch of mandibular nerve.	Elevates mandibl and clenches teel
Temporalis	Temporal fossa	Coronoid process (its top and anterior border).	Fan shaped muscle. Its contraction is easily felt during clenching of teeth.	Branch of mandibular teeth.	
Medial pterygoid	• Medial surface of lateral pterygoid plate. • Tuberosity of maxilla.	Medial surface of mandible near its angle.	Thick, quadrilateral muscle with deep origin. The insertion of the muscle makes the mandible rugged upto mylohyoid line.	Mandibular nerve.	• Synergist to temporalis and masseter in elev tion of mandibl • With lateral pte goid it produ side to side mo ment.

Con

Muscle	Origin	Insertion	Description	Nerve supply	Action
Lateral pterygoid 1.Upper head	Infra temporal fossa of greater wing of sphenoid.	Pterygoid fovea at the neck of mandible and articular disc.	It is a short, thick muscle. Maxillary artery either crosses super-ficial or deep to the muscle.	Mandibular nerve.	Pulls mandible forward (protrudes lower jaw) and helps side to side chewing movement.
2.Lower head	Lateral surface of lateral pterygoid plate.				
3.Buccinator	Linear origin from the region of molar teeth of maxilla and mandible.	The central fiber decussate and upper and lower horizontal fiber blends with orbi-cularis oris.	It is a thin, quadrilateral muscle of cheek that occupies the interval between maxilla and mandible. A large mass of fat separate it from mandible. The muscle is pierced by parotid duct.	Buccal branch of facial nerve.	• Compresses cheek against the teeth and gums.

Muscles of Neck (Fig. 4.15)

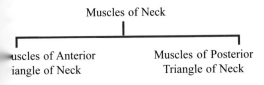

Muscles of Neck
- Muscles of Anterior Triangle of Neck
- Muscles of Posterior Triangle of Neck

Muscles of Anterior Triangle of Neck

Most important muscle is Sternocleidomastoid which forms the posterior boundary of anterior triangle.

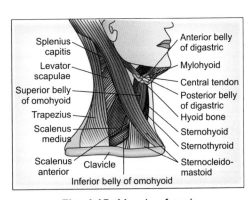

Fig. 4.15: Muscle of neck

Muscle	Origin	Insertion	Description	Nerve supply	Action
Sternocleido mastoid	• Anterior surface manubrium sterni. • Medial 1/3rd of cervicle.	Mastoid process of temporal bone.	Two headed muscle, located deep to platy-sma on antero lateral surface of neck. Key mascular landmark in neck. Spasm of this muscle cause wryneck.	Accessory nerve (11th cranial nerve)	Both sided muscle acting together extend head and flex neck. Acting alone one muscle, tilt head towards same side.

Suprahyoid Group (Lies Superior to Hyoid Bone)

Muscle	Origin	Insertion	Description	Nerve supply	Action
Digastric – two bellies Anterior belly	Impression on body of mandible (lower part).	Inserted intermediate tendon which is held from hyoid by a fascial ring.	Di – two; gaster – belly. The muscle arises as two bellies. Two bellies from a V shaped area under the chin.	• From nerve to mylohyoid. • From facial nerve.	• Elevate hyoid bone and steady it during swallowing and speech. • Depress mandible.
Posterior belly	From deep groove on the medial aspect of mastoid process.				
Stylohyoid	Styloid process of temporal bone.	Body of hyoid.	Slender muscle below angle of mandible parallel to posterior body of digastric.	Facial nerve	Elevates hyoid bon
Mylohyoid	Myloid line on the body of mandible.	Body of hyoid bone and fibrous raphae.	Flat, triangular muscle just deep to disgastric; this muscle pair form the floor of anterior mouth.	Nerve to mylohyoid coming from inferior alveolar nerve.	Elevates floor mouth and hyo bone in first stage deglutition depress mandible.
Geniohyoid	Lower genial tubercles	Body of hyoid.	Narrow muscle, in contact with its fellow on medial side, runs from chin to hyoid.	First cervical nerve.	Elevates hyoid bo and draws depre mandible.

Infrahyoid Group

Muscle	Origin	Insertion	Description	Nerve supply	Action
Sternohyoid	• Upper part of posterior surface of manubrium sternal. • Medial end of clavicle.	Lower margin of body of hyoid bone.	Narrow, strap and medial most, muscles of neck. Superficial muscle except inferiorly where it is covered by sternocleidomastoid.	Through ansa cervicalis (slender nerve root of cervical plexus).	• Depress hyo bone. • Plays a part speech and mas cation.
Sternothyroid	From posterior surface of manubrium inferior to origin of sternohyoid known as details.	Oblique line on lamina of thyroid cartilage.	Shorter and wider than sternohyoid lies deep and partly medial to it.	Through ansa cervicalis slender nerve root of cervical plexus).	Draw hyoid bone and the thyroid cartilage (i.e. larynx) inferiorly.
Thyrohyoid	Oblique line on anterior surface of lamina of thyroid cartilage.	Lower border of body of hyoid bone.	Appear as a superior continuation of sternothyroid muscle; quadrilateral in shape.	First cervical nerve via hypoglossal.	Depress hyoid bo and elevates laryn

Con

uscle	Origin	Insertion	Description	Nerve supply	Action
ohyoid uperior y	Lower border of body of hyoid.	Intermediate tendon is held to clavicle and first rib by a sling of deep fascia.	Thin, strap like muscle. The inferior belly divides the posterior triangle of neck into two – upper occipital and lower supraclavicular triangle.	Ansa cervicalis.	Depress hyoid bone.
nferior y	Upper border of scapula near scapular notch.	— Do —			

scles of Posterior Triangle of Neck (Fig. 4.15)

uscle	Origin	Insertion	Description	Nerve supply	Action
rnocleido-stoid	Trapezius • Medial 1/3rd of superior nuchal line of occipital bone. • Ligamentus nuchae. • Spines of C7 and all the thoracic spine.	• A continuous insertion along acromin and spine of scapula (upper border of crest).	Most superficial muscle of back of neck, and thorax. Rhomboid in shape; upper fibers run downwards and middle fibers run horizontally. Lower fibers runs upwards and laterally.	Accessory nerve.	• The upper fibers elevates the scapula. • Middle fibers pull the scapula medially. • Lower fibers pull the medial border of scapula downwards.
alenus erior hough s is not in sterior angle – in section it shown in s region)	Transverse process of third to sixth cervical vertebrae.	Scalene tubercle of first rib.	Located lateral neck deep to sternocleido-mastoid.It is small vertical muscle.	Ventral rami of C4, C5, C6.	• Elevates first rib (and inspiration).· Bends the cervical • Portion vertebral column.
alenus edius	Transverse process of upper six cervical transverse process (posterior tubercle).	First rib between tubercle of rib and groove for subclavian artery.	The largest and longest of scalene. It is sepa-rated from scalenus anterior by the subcla-vian artery, levator scapulae and scalenus posterior.	Ventral rami of C3 to C8th spinal nerves.	• Bends cervical part of vertebral column of same side. • Elevates first rib during active inspiration.
calenus; osterior	Posterior tubercle of 4th, 5th and 6th cervical vertebrae	In second rib	Smallest and most deeply situated among the scalene.	Ventral branches from 6th, 7th and 8th cervical · nerve.	• Elevates second rib. • Bends cervicle part of vertebral column to the same side.

Extrinsic Muscles of Tongue (Fig. 4.16)

Muscle	Origin	Insertion	Description	Nerve supply	Action
Genio-glossus	Uppergenial tubercle of body of mandible.	Blends with other muscle of tongue.	Fan shaped muscle, forms part of tongue and lies on either side of mid line.	Hypoglossal (12th cranial)	• Protrude tong • Acting bilate it depress the central part o tongue.
Hyoglossus	Body and greater cornu of hyoid bone.	Inferolateral aspect of tongue; blends with other muscles	Flat quadrilateral muscle.	Hypoglossal (12th cranial nerve)	• Depress tong and draws its sides downwa
Styloglossus	Styloid process of temporal bone.	Inferolateral aspect of tongue; blends with other muscle.	Slender muscle, running superiorly to hypoglossal nerve, shortest and smallest of all muscles arising from styloid process.	Hypoglossal (12th cranial nerve)	Draws tongue upwards and backwards.
Chondro-glossus	Medial side and base of lesser cornu of hyoid.	Blends with other muscles between hyoglossus and genioglossus.	Sometimes described as part of hyoglossus; sometimes separated from it by fibers of genioglossus.	Hypoglossal (12th cranial nerve)	Assists hyoglos in depressing the tongue.
Palato-glossus	Palatine aponeurosis.	Side of tongue.	Form palatoglossal fold of mucous membrane; and anterior boundary of tonsillar fossa.	Pharyngeal plexus	Pulls root of the tongue upwards backwards; narr or opharyngeal isthmus.

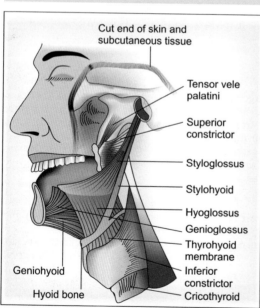

Cut end of skin and subcutaneous tissue

Tensor vele palatini

Superior constrictor

Styloglossus

Stylohyoid

Hyoglossus

Genioglossus

Thyrohyoid membrane

Inferior constrictor

Cricothyroid

Geniohyoid

Hyoid bone

Fig. 4.16: Muscles of tongue and pharynx (lateral view)

Nervous System

5

RODUCTION

nervous system is controlling and
municating system of our body. Its main
tions are to monitor, integrate, and response
formation on the environment.

is *divided into two major parts:*
'entral nervous system [including brain and
al cord] and *Peripheral nervous system* [12
s of cranial nerves, 31 pairs of spinal nerves
their associated ganglia].

unctionally, the nervous system is again
ded into *Somatic nervous system* [which
trols *voluntary* function] and *Autonomic*
'ous system [control *involuntary* function].

pinal Nerves: Spinal nerves are united ventral
dorsal roots, attached in a series, to the side of
the spinal cords. There are 31 pairs; 8 cervical, 12
thoracic, 5 lumbar, 5 sacral, 1 coccygeal. These
emerges through intervertebral foramina. Except
T2 – T12, all ventral rami join one another forming
nerve plexuses. This plexuses occur in the cervical,
brachial, lumbar and sacral regions. *The ventral
rami of spinal nerves supply the limbs and the
anterolateral aspect off the trunk.*

Cervical Plexus and its Branches
(Figs 5.1A to C)

The cervical plexus is formed by ventral rami of
C1 – C4. It lies deep to the internal jugular vein,
sternocleidomastoid, and anterior to scalenus
medius, levator scapulae. Its branches are:

Nerves	Comments	Structure served
erficialis branches [cutaneous]	Ascending (Figs 5.1A to C)	
sser occipital nerve	It is second cervical ventral ramus mainly. It hooks round the accessory nerves and ascends along the posterior border of sternocleidomastoid.	Skin on posterolateral aspect of neck.
eater articular nerve	It is the largest ascending branch encircles the posterior border of sternocleidomastoid.	Skin of the ear over mastoid process, and skin over parotid gland.
ansverse cutaneous terior] nerve	Curves around the midpoint of the posterior border of sternocleidomastoid and runs horizontally deep to the external jugular vein.	Skin on anterior and lateral aspect of neck.

Contd...

Nerves	Comments	Structure served
Descending Supraclavicular	It arises as a common trunk, and later divides into medial, intermediate, and lateral division at the posterior border of sternocleido-mastoid.	Skin of shoulder and ant aspect of the chest.
Deep branches [motor] Phrenic nerve Rectus capitis nerve Anterior nerve	It lies over scalenus anterior muscle.	Supplies diaphragm.
Rectus capitis nerve Lateralis nerve Longus capitis nerve Longus coli nerve Inferior root of ansa nerve	Very slender branch	Supplies respective muscles

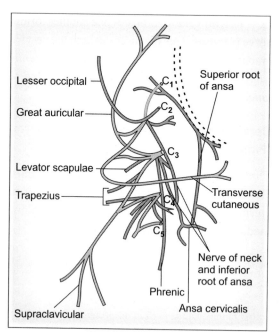

Fig. 5.1A: Cervical plexus and its branches

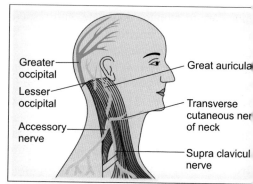

Fig. 5.1B: Cutaneous nerve supply of face, scalp and neck

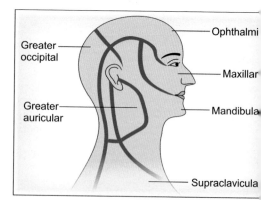

Fig. 5.1C: Distribution of cutaneous nerves

ied Anatomy

n of the phrenic nerve – division of phrenic in neck during operation, procedures complete ysis of the diaphragm of that side identified g X-ray screening of chest. If accessory phrenic sent, complete paralysis will not occur.

Brachial Plexus and Its Branches (Fig. 5.2)

The large important brachial plexus is situated partly in the neck and partly in the axilla. The plexus is formed by the ventral rami of the C5, C6, C7, C8 and the major part of T1.

Nerves	Comments	Structure served
ches from root		
al scapular	Arises from the root of brachial plexus, pierce the scalenus medius.	Rhomboids muscles.
thoracic	Arises from the root of brachial plexus.	Serratus anterior muscle.
e to subclavius	Arises from the trunk of brachial plexus. Very slender nerve.	Subclavius muscle.
ascapular nerve	Arises from the trunk of brachial plexus. Large branch.	Shoulder joint; supraspinatous and infraspinatous muscle.
nches from the lateral cord		
culocutaneous	Arises opposite lower border of pectoralis minor.	Biceps brachii, brachialis, coracobrachialis muscle and elbow joint.
ral pectoral	Small branches; pierces the clavipectoral fascia.	Pectoralis major and minor. Muscle of thumb to skin of lateral 2/3rd of palm.
ral root of median	Discussed along with the medial root. The two roots combine to form the median nerve.	
cular branches to elbow and wrist		
or carpi ulnaris and medial part exor digitorum profundus		
nches from the medial cord		
lial pectoral	Small branches, arise from medial cord, where it lies posterior to axillary artery.	Pectoralis minor.
dial cutaneous nerve of arm	Communication with intercostobrachial nerve coming from T2.	Supplies skin of upper and medial side of the arm.
dial cutaneous branch of forearm	The nerve situated medial to brachial artery.	Supplies skin of upper and medial side of the front of forearm and skin over front of arm.
dian nerve	Arises as two roots from lateral and medial cord of brachial plexus lies in front of or slightly lateral to the axillary artery.	It gives no branch in arm. Muscular branches to pronator teres, pronator quadratus, flexor

Contd...

Nerves	Comments	Structure served
		carpi radialis, the palmaris lo and flexor digitorum su ficialis, lateral half of fl digitorum profundus (i.e. deep muscle of flexor com ment except flexor carpi ul and medial part of fl digitorum profundus.
Ulnar nerve	It is the terminal branch of medial cord; run along the medial aspect of arm and passes behind the medial epicondyle to enter forearm.	Flexor carpi ulnaris, medial of flexor digitorum profur most intrinsic muscle (about of hand, skin of medial 1/3 hand (both palm and dorsun

Branches from posterior cord

Nerves	Comments	Structure served
Upper subcapular	It is a slender nerve, passes posteriorly and difficult to trace in axilla dissection; when clavicle is present.	Subscapular muscle.
Thoracodorsal	Arises between upper and lower subcapular, runs inferolaterally.	Latissimus dorsi.
Lower subcapular	Passes inferolaterally deep to subscapular artery and vein.	Inferior portion of subscapul and teres major.
Axillary	Terminal branches, passes to posterior aspect of arm through quadrangular space, winds round the surgical neck of humerus.	Deltoid, teres minor, shoul joint, skin over the inferior of deltoid.
Radial	Terminal and largest branch; passes posterior to axillary artery enters radial groove with anteria profunda brachii.	Triceps, anconeus, brach radialis and extensor muscles forearm. Skin of posterior asp of arm and forearm.

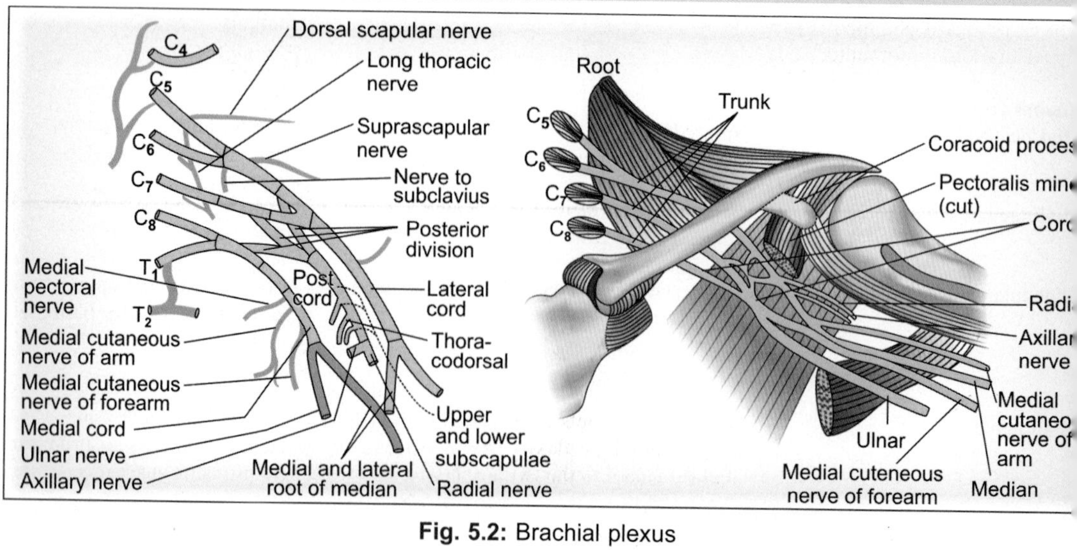

Fig. 5.2: Brachial plexus

on of Important Nerves of Brachial us (Fig. 5.3)

rachial plexus is deeply placed in the root of the neck but can be injured in penetrating injuries (in war) can be avulsed (in birth trauma and motor cycle accident).

Names	Site of injury	Effect (Manifestation)
ascapular e	At the suprascapular notch, [entrapment neuropathy] or trauma in this region.	Weakness of supraspinatous and infraspinatous muscle and gradually muscle wasting.
g thoracic e (Fig. 5.3)	Blow in the posterior triangle of the neck or during surgical procedure.	Paralysis of the serratus anterior, muscle. So there is difficulties in arising arm above head. There is winging of scapula.
er lesion of hial plexus or Erb henne palsy nly C5 and partly s involved] . 5.4)	In mortorbike accident when there is abnormal separation of head and shoulder, during delivery (the same cause), the region of Erbs point (meeting of six nerve) is involved.	Supraspinatous, infraspinatous, subclavius, biceps brachii and greater part of brachialis, coracobrachialis and deltoid are paralysed. So the arms hang by the side of the trunk and rotated medially, elbow extended and forearm pronated, as if some body is taking the tips. Movements of the wrist and fingers are not lost.
er plexus paralysis mpkee] involves and T1	It occurs in the lower part of the neck, and axilla (upper part) by cancerous infiltration from apex of lung, of breast, cervical rib, etc.	Progressive weakening of small muscles of hand and wasting of muscle gradually. Hypothenar emences become wasted. This is known as claw hand [due to hyperextension of metacarpophalangeal joint and flexion of interphalangeal joint].
lary NV lesion	Fracture at the surgical neck of humerus	Paralysis of deltoid with dropping of shoulder as first initiator of abduction is lost (deltoid).

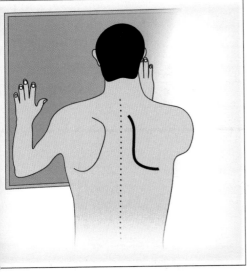

5.3: Winging of right scapula due to paralysis of thoracic nerve which supplies serratus anterior

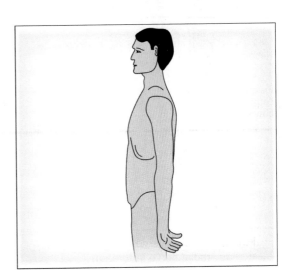

Fig. 5.4: Erb-Duchenne paralysis (waiters tip)

Important Nerves of Brachial Plexus (More Details) Median Nerve (Figs 5.5 to 5.7)

Origin	Course	Branches	Applied
From lateral and medial cord of brachial plexus in axilla.	It embraces the third part of axillary artery in the axilla. In the arm it is lateral to brachial artery, near the insertion of coraco-brachialis it crosses in front of the artery and in cubital fossa it is medial to the artery. It enters the forearm by passing between two heads of pronator teres, separated from ulna art by deep head of pronator teres. In the forearm lies deep to flexor digitorum superficialis and profundus. The nerve enters the hand by passing deep to flexor retinaculum (in the carpal tunnel) and it divides into two, to supply the lateral 3½ digits.	Muscular to the superficial flexor muscles of forearm except the flexor carpi ulnaris. Anterior interosseous branch, supplies flexor pollicis longus. Palmar cutaneous branch – arises above the flexor retinaculum, supplies the skin of thenar eminence. It gives articular to elbow joint, the proximal radio-ulnar joint; vascular to radial and ulnar artery.	Injury, above elbow, (as in supracondylar fracture) – produce paralysis of all the flexor muscles of forearm except, flexor carpi ulnaris. In the hand, thenar muscles and first and second lumbricals paralysed. So forearm lies in supine position, hand is adduced flexion at interphalangeal joint index and middle finger is lost. When the patient tries to make fist, the index and middle finger tend to remain straight. The muscles of thenar eminence paralysed and the eminence flattened. The thumb is adducted and laterally rotated (ape-like hand). There is sensory loss lateral 3½ finger.

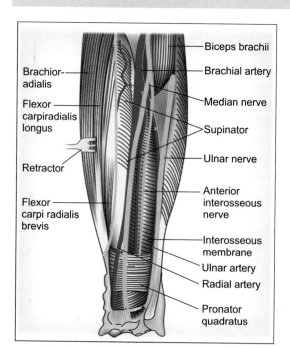

Fig. 5.5: Median nerve, ulnar nerve and radial nerve in forearm

Biceps brachii

Brachial artery

Median nerve

Supinator

Ulnar nerve

Anterior interosseous nerve

Interosseous membrane

Ulnar artery

Radial artery

Pronator quadratus

Brachior-adialis

Flexor carpiradialis longus

Retractor

Flexor carpi radialis brevis

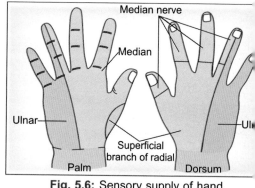

Fig. 5.6: Sensory supply of hand

Median nerve

Median

Ulnar

Superficial branch of radial

Palm

Dorsum

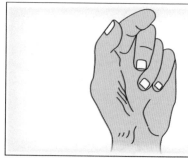

Fig. 5.7: Median nerve palsy

r Nerve (Figs 5.5 and 5.9)

Origin	Course	Branches	Applied
the continu- n of medial l of brachial us.	In the axilla it runs downwards between axillary artery and vein; then medial to brachial artery in the arm. At the middle of the arm the nerve pierces the medial intermuscular septum, descends in the back of arm up to medial epicondyle. Here nerve can be felt against the bone. The nerve enters the forearm between two heads of flexor carpiulnaris, runs between flexor digitorum profundus (on medial aspect) and flexor digitorum superficialis (on medial aspect). The nerve enters the palm by passing superficial to flexor retinaculum lateral to pisiform bone	• Articular to elbow, wrist. • Muscular to flexor carpi ulnaris and flexor digitorum profundus. • Superficial – sensory supply to medial 1½ digit and mascular to palmaris brevis. • Deep terminal branch –muscular to adduc- tor pollicis, all palmar and dorsal interossei and third and fourth lumbricals	Ulnar nerve paralysis commonly occurred behind the medial epicondyle of humerus. • There is impairment of power of adduction at the wrist due to paralysis of flexor carpi ulnaris and medial ½ of flexor digitorum profundus flattening of medial side of forearm. • Paralysis of interosseous muscle produces claw hand (hyper extension of metacarpo- phalangeal joint and flexion of interphalangeal joint). • Inability to adduct the thumb. • Wasting of hypothenar muscle. • Sensation is impaired in the ulnar 1½ fingers on both palmar and dorsal surfaces.

l muscles of hand are supplied by ulnar nerve except muscle of thenar eminence and first and second lumbricals (supplied median nerve).

ial Nerve (Figs 5.5 and 5.8)

Origin	Course	Branches	Applied
se from post l; largest ich of hial plexus.	In axilla it descends behind the third part of axillary artery. In between long and lateral head of triceps, it enters the spiral groove with arteria profunda brachii. It pierces the lateral intermuscular septum to enter the anterior compartment. In front of lateral epicondyle it divides into superficial and deep branches. The superficial branch lies in front of supinator muscle deep to brachioradialis and descends lateral to radial artery. In the middle third of arm the artery is medially situated; it quits the artery about 7 cm above the styloid process of radius. Deep terminal branch is known as posterior interosseous nerve.	Muscular: 1. Triceps 2. Anconeus 3. Brachioradialis 4. Brachialis (lateral part) 5. Extensor carpi radialis longus posterior inteross- eous nerve supplies. 6. Supinator 7. Extensor carpi radialis brevis. 8. Extensor digitorum 9. Exterior carpi ulnaris 10. Exterior pollicis longus 11. Abductor pollicis longus Articular to radio carpal joint.	Radial nerve palsy commonly occurs due to compression of nerve in axilla (malfitted crutchs at armpit); arm thrown carelessly by drunkers over a chair [Saturday night palsy]. • Elbow and wrist extension is impaired. • So there is wrist drop, fingerdrop due to weakness of extensor tendon. • Sensory impairment in lower part of arm, back of forearm, lateral part of dorsum of hand. Post interosseous palsy. This is due to compression of nerve within the extensor muscles. • No sensory impairment since the superficial branch arises above this level. • There is weakness in finger and thumb (extensions and abduction).

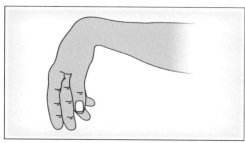

Fig. 5.8: Wrist drop due to radial nerve palsy

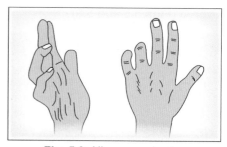

Fig. 5.9: Ulnar nerve palsy

Musculocutaneous

Origin	Course	Branches	Applied
Arises from lateral cord of brachial plexus at the level of lower border of pectoralis minor.	It runs down between the axillary artery and coracobrachialis, leaves the axilla by piercing the coracobrachialis. It descends laterally between biceps and brachial is to the lateral side of the arm; just below elbow it pierces the deep fascia, lateral to tendon of biceps, continued as lateral cutaneous nerve of forearm.	• Muscular to biceps brachii. • Lateral half of brachialis. Cutaneous branch to forearm	Rarely injured, as it is prote by biceps brachii. If it is inju it is injured high up in the arr Biceps and coracobrachialis be paralysed resulting in ma weakness in elbow flexion. Sensory impairment on extensor aspect of forearm.

Lumbar Plexus and its Branches

The plexus is formed by union of ventral rami of L1, L2, L3 and L4. It lies in the posterior part of psoas major muscles anterior to lumbar transv processes. Branches come out from lateral bo of psoas major (Figs 5.10A and B).

Nerves	Comments	Structure served
Ilio hypogastric	It comes out from upper part of psoas major, crosses obliquely behind the lower pole of kidney, then it lies in front of quadratus lumborum; pierces internal and external oblique muscle near iliac crest.	Muscles of anterolateral al minal wall (internal oblique transverses) abdominal skir lower abdomen, lower back and
Ilio inguinal	It comes out below and parallel to ilio hypogastric, cross obliquely the quadratus lumborum, pierces the roof of inguinal canal and comes out through superficial inguinal ring.	Skin of the external genitalia upper medial aspect of thigh internal oblique muscle.
Lateral femoral cutaneous	Runs inferolaterally in front of iliacus muscle, enters thigh behind the inguinal ligament, just medial to anterior superior iliac spine. It may be compressed by inguinal ligament or through fascia lata. There is tingling sensation in the area served by this nerve.	Skin of the lateral side of thigh.
Femoral (Fig. 5.11)	Largest branch of lumbar plexus. Emerging low, from lateral border of psoas major, enters thigh behind the inguinal ligament, lies in ilio psoas groove. Splits into anterior and posterior divisions.Branches of anterior division-(a) Two cutaneous (b) One muscular Branches of posterior division- (a) Four muscular – to vasti and rectus femoris. (b) One cutaneous – saphenous nerve.	Skin of the anterior and me side of the thigh. Skin of medial side of the leg and foo also supplies hip joint, knee jc Motor to quadriceps femo sartorius, pectineus and iliac

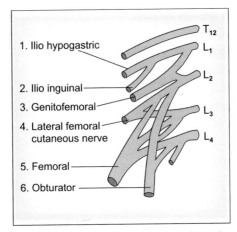

Fig. 5.10A: Lumbar plexus and its branches

1. Ilio hypogastric
2. Ilio inguinal
3. Genitofemoral
4. Lateral femoral cutaneous nerve
5. Femoral
6. Obturator

Branches comes out from medial border of psoas major (Figs 5.10B and 5.11)

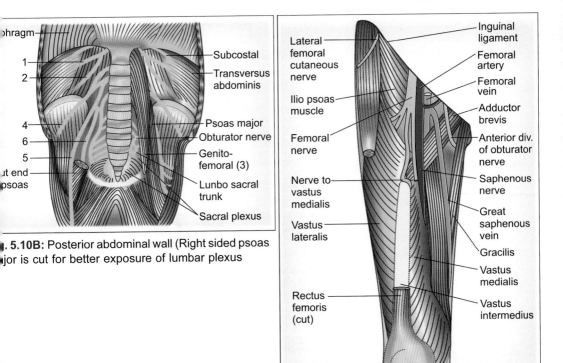

Fig. 5.10B: Posterior abdominal wall (Right sided psoas major is cut for better exposure of lumbar plexus

Fig. 5.11: Femoral nerve and its branches in thigh (right)

Branches Come Out from the Medial Border of Psoas Major

Nerves	Comments	Structure served
Obturator (Fig. 5.11)	It emerges near pelvic brim passes behind the common iliac vessels. It enters in obturator canal and divides into anterior and posterior division.	Motor to adductor long, adductor brevis, pubic fibe, adductor magnus, gracilis obturator externus. It supp, articular branches to hip and l, joint, cutaneous branch to skin of medial thigh.
Accessory obturator	Not always present. When present it is very thin and small.	It supplies pectineus muscle, hip joint.
Lumbosacral trunk (Fig. 5.11)	Thick nerve trunk descends in front of ala of sacrum and joins with ventral rami of sacral nerve form.	

Sacral Plexus and its Branches

It is formed by lumbosacral trunk (part of L4 and whole of L5), the first to third sacral ventral rami, and part of the fourth sacral ventral rami. It lies in posterior pelvic wall and in front of pyriformis mu

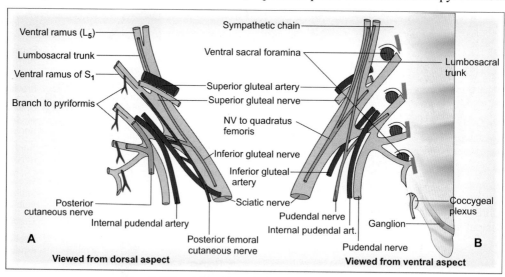

Figs 5.12A and B: Sacral plexus and its branches

Nerves	Comments	Structure served
Superior gluteal (Figs 5.12A and B)	Comes out through greater sciatic forearm above pyriformis and immediately divide into superior and inferior branch.	It is motor to gluteus medius, minimus, tensor fascia lata.
Inferior gluteal	Comes out through greater sciatic forearm below pyriformis and supply the gluteus maximus from its deep surface	Gluteus maximus.

Nerves	Comments	Structure served
...erior femoral ...neous	It descends under cover of gluteus maximus, lying postero-medial to sciatic nerve.	Skin of buttock, posterior thigh, popliteal region.
...endal	It leaves the pelvis via greater sciatic foramen below pyriformis and lies over the tip of ischial spine along with the internal pudendal vessels – re-enter pelvis through lesser sciatic foramen runs in pudendal canal.	Supplies the most of the skin and muscles of perineum and external anal sphincter.
...tic nerve Tibial component (Figs 5.13A and B)	Broadest nerve of the body; comes out through greater sciatic foramen below pyriformis. It lies in between ischial tuberosity and greater trochanter. It descends in the back of thigh and divides into tibial and common peroneal component. In the popliteal fossa, this nerve supplies to popliteal vessels and in the distal part of the fossa, it is continued as tibial nerve of leg.	Hamstrings muscles, gastrocnemeus, soleus, plantaris, popliteus, deep muscles of posterior tibio-fibular region and muscles of sole and foot. To knee joint To skin of posterior surface of leg and foot.
...Common peroneal component	It is half the size of the tibial; situated at the medial border of the biceps femoris in the popliteal fossa, and at the neck of fibula it divides into superficial and deep peroneal branch.	Gives cutaneous branch to skin of anterior surface of leg and dorsum of foot. Motor to short head of biceps femoris, peroneal muscles, muscles of anterior compartment of leg (tibialis anterior, extensor hallucis longus, extensor digitorum longus and peroneus tertius).

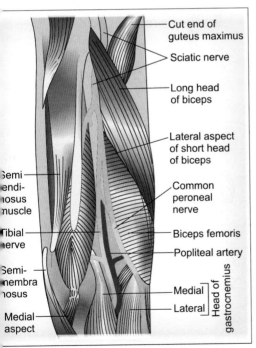

Fig. 5.13A: Sciatic nerve and hamstring muscle in back of thigh (right)

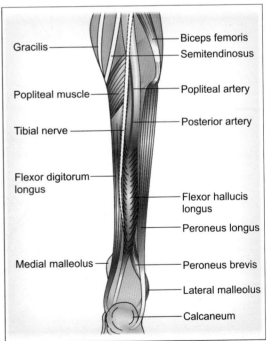

Fig. 5.13B: Tibial nerve and muscles of right leg (soleus and plantaris removed)

Applied Anatomy – Sciatic Nerve

1. Shooting pain along the distribution of sciatic nerve is known as sciatica. Injection Novocain is given midway between ischial tuberosity and greater trochanter of femur around the sciatic nerve, to get relief from sciatica pain.
2. Damage of the individual component of sciatic nerve takes place by bullet wounds in the region of back of thigh. If tibial component is injured, paralysis of the superficial and deep muscles of calf and sole takes place. There is loss of plantar, flexion of the ankle joint and toes. So the foot is held in calcano-valgus position and walking is difficult.
3. The common peroneal component most

frequently injured during fracture of the of fibula or a badly fitting leg plaster. Com division produces paralysis of muscle anterior and lateral compartment of leg an short extensor of toes. The dorsiflexion eversion is lost, so there is foot drop inversion.

AUTONOMIC NERVOUS SYSTEM

It is the part of nervous system that con automatic activity of our body (i.e. involu activity) like heart, smooth muscles and glar is divided into two parts sympathetic parasympathetic and both parts have afferent efferent nerve fibers (Figs 5.14A and B).

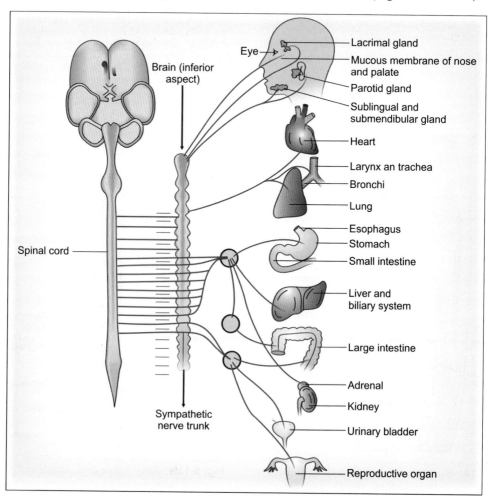

Fig. 5.14A: Autonomic nervous system (sympathetic division)

Characteristic	Sympathetic	Parasympathetic
...ion	It prepares body for emergency.	Maintenance functions, i.e. conserves and stores.
...gin (outflow)	Arises from thoracolumbar outflow (lateral horn of grey matter of spinal chord).	Craniosacral outflow (i.e. brainstem nuclei of third, seventh, tenth cranial nerves and S2, S3, S4 segments of spinal cord).
...ganglionic fiber	Myelinated	Myelinated.

Contd...

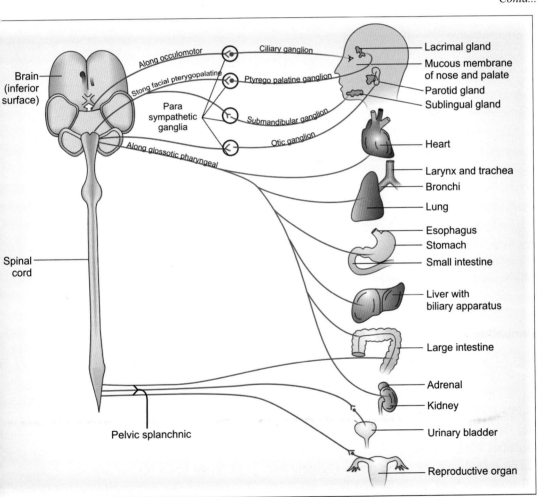

Fig. 5.14B: Autonomic nervous system (para sympathetic division)

Characteristic	Sympathetic	Parasympathetic
Location of ganglia	Paravertebral (sympathetic trunk), prevertebral coeliac, superior mesenteric, inferior mesenteric.	Small ganglia close to viscera (e.g. otic,cili or ganglion cells in plexuses (cardiac and monary plexus).
Relative length of preganglionic and postganglionic fibers	Short preganglionic, long postganglionic.	Long preganglionic Short postganglionic.
Degree of branching of preganglionic fibers	Extensive	Minimal
Neurotransmitters	All preganglionic fiber release acetylcholine. Most postganglionic fibers liberate norepinephrine (nor-adrenaline). So it is adrenergic except sweat glands (cholinergic).	All fibers release acetylcholine (choline fibers).
Physiological	• Reaction is mass response. • Increase heart rate, increase blood pressure, constriction of cutaneous arteries (increase blood supply of heart, muscle, brain), decrease peristaltic activity of gut. All structures are supplied by postganglionic fiber except suprarenal medulla (supplied by preganglionic as it is a sympathochromaffin organ).	• Reaction is localized. • Decrease heart rate • Increase glandular secretion. • Increase peristaltic activity of gut. All structured are supplied by postganglic fibers.
Higher control	Hypothalamus	Hypothalamus

Sympathetic Trunk (Fig. 5.14A)

They lie on either side of vertebral column; extends from base of the skull to the coccyx. It looks like a knotted thread. There are three cervical (superior, middle and inferior), eleven thoracic, four lumbar, four sacral ganglia. The sympathetic ganglions are structures where synapse (white rami) between pre and postganglionic fiber takes place. The right and left trunk coverage medially and form ganglion impar (unpaired) in front of coccyx. Most preganglionic fibers reach the sympathetic trunk, they have three types of termination:

1. They may terminate in the ganglion they h entered. These postganglionic nerve fi (known as rami), now pass through the thor spinal nerve and supply the smooth muscl blood vessels and sweat glands.

2. The fibers may ascend high up and terminat cervical ganglia or lower fiber may desc down in lower lumbar and sacral ganglia.

3. Some of the preganglionic fibers may p through the ganglia on thoracic part sympathetic trunk without synapsing. Th fibers form *three splanchnic nerve.*

Greater splanchnic nerve – Arise from fifth to ninth thoracic ganglia pierces the diaphragm and synapses (neuro – neuronal junction) with coeliac plexus.

Lesser splanchnic nerve – Arise from tenth and eleventh thoracic ganglia, pierces diaphragm and synspses with lower part of plexus.

Least splanchnic nerve – Spinal nerve correspond to the same segment of spinal cord, but the sympathetic path ways do not correspond with the segment of spinal cord.

T1 segment – Passes up and goes to head region

T2 segment – goes to neck.

T3 – T6 segment – into thorax

T7 – T11 segment – for abdomen

T12 – L2 segment – for leg.

reganglionic fibers are cholinergic in both pathetic and parasympathetic; postganglionic pathetic fiber are adrenergic except for sweat d and arrector pili muscle. Postganglionic one of parasympathetic is cholinergic. Parapathetic are essential for life.

lied

onomic Nervous System is involved in every ortant process that goes in our body. Most nomic disorders reflect, excess, or deficient trols of smooth muscle activity.

- Hypertension (high blood pressure) – May result from excessive sympathetic activity. It is known as stress-induced hypertension.

- Vaso-occlusive disease – They are Raynaud's disease affecting the upper limb, Buerger's disease affecting the lower limb. It is characterized by gradual cyanosis (bluish coloration), pain in the affected region in severe cases gangrene (tissue death) may result. To treat severe cases, sympathectomy is done. The involved vessels dilate, re-establishing adequate blood delivery to the affected region.

- Congenital megacolon (Hirschsprung's disease) – In this condition, parasympathetic innervation of the distal part of colon fails to develop. As a result, distal colon is immobile and dilated. The condition is corrected surgically.

- Achalasia (Not relaxed) – A condition where oesophagus is unable to propel food in the lower part due to parasympathetic neuron deficiency. The distal esophagus becomes dilated and vomiting is common.

- Horner's syndrome – Results from an interruption of the sympathetic nerve supply to head and neck. The effected person exhibits contriction of pupil (myosis), slight drooping of eye lid (ptosis), vasodilatation of skin arterioles and loss of sweating (anhydrosis).

CRANIAL NERVES (12 pairs)

Name and components	Origin and course	Function	Clinical testing	Applied
Olfactory (special sensory) No. I (Figs 5.15 and 5.16)	Olfactory nerve fibers arise from olfactory receptor cells located on olfactory epithelium of nasal cavity and pass through cribriform plate of ethmoid and synapse in olfactory bulb. The bulb end posteriorly as olfactory tract, which runs beneath the frontal lobe and terminate in the olfactory cortex.	Smell from nasal mucosa of roof of each nasal cavity and superior sides of nasal septum and superior concha.	Person is asked to sniff the aromatic substance like clove oil, vanilla, etc and to identify each.	Fracture of ethmoid or lesion of olfactory fibers may result in partial or total loss of smell (anosmia).
Optic (special sensory) No. II (Fig. 5.16)	Fibers arise from eye forms optic nerve, which passes through optic foramen of orbit; the nerve converge to form optic chiasma where the nasal fiber crosses over. The nerve continue and as optic tract – enters thalamus and synapses there. Thalamic fibers run as optic radiation to occipital cortex where visual interpretation occurs.	Vision from retina	Acquity of vision and visual fields are determined with eye chart and by testing the point at which the person first sees an object moving into the visual field.	Damage leads to blindness in eye served by the nerves.
Occulomotor (somatic motor and visceral motor) No. III (Fig. 5.15)	Fibers arise from ventral aspect of midbrain and junction of pons and pass through superior orbital fissure to eye.	Somatic motor to four intrinsic muscle of eye (superior, inferior, medial recti, inferior oblique) and levator (palpebral superioris) elevates eyelid and accommodates eye. Parasympathetic motor – to constrict muscle of iris, and to ciliary muscle (for changing the shape of lens).	Pupils are examined for size, shape and equality. Papillary reflex is tested with pencil torch. Convergence for near vision is tested (ability to follow object near the eye).	In this nerve paralysis, eye cannot move up, down or inward and at rest, eye rotates laterally (external strabismus), drooping of upper eyelid. Person has double vision and trouble on focusing near object.

Eyeball
Optic nerve
Optic canal
Anterior clinoid process
Optic chiasma
Optic tract
Mid brain
Lateral geniculate body

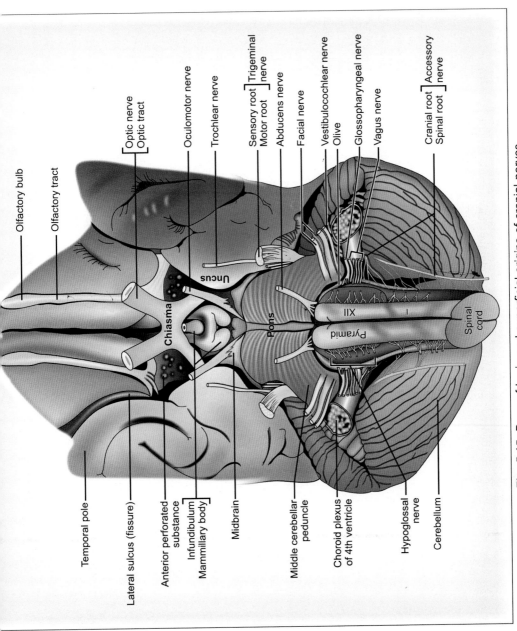

Fig. 5.15: Base of brain and superficial origins of cranial nerves

Name and components	Origin and course	Function	Clinical testing	Applied
Trochlear (motor) No. IV (Figs 5.15 and 5.17)	Fibers emerge from dorsal midbrain and course ventrally around the midbrain, to enter orbit through superior orbital fissure along with oculomotor nerve.	Motor to superior oblique that assist in turning eye inferolaterally.	Like cranial nerve III.	Trauma or paralysis results in double vision and reduced ability to rotate eye inferolaterally.
Trigeminal (largest cranial nerve) No. V (mixed) nerve three divisions: Ophthalmic division (sensory)	Fibers arises from the junction of pons and middle cerebellar peduncle and enter the face via superior orbital fissure (Figs 5.15 and 5.18A)	Convey sensory impulse from skin of forehead, scalp, eyelid, cornea, mucosa of nasal cavity and para nasal sinuses.	Corneal reflexes tested by touching cornea by wisp of cotton – it elicit blinking.	Injury to terminal branches (particularly maxillary) in roof of maxillary sinus, pathologic process affecting trigeminal nerve – produce loss of pain and touch sensation. Paresthesia of face; loss of corneal reflex
Maxillary division (sensory) (Fig. 5.18B)	Fibers run from pons to face via foramen rotundum.	Sensory impulse from nasal cavity, palate, upper teeth and skin of cheek, upper lip and lower eyelid.	Sensation of pain, touch, temperature are tested by safety pin and by touching hot and cold objects.	
Mandibular division (motor + sensory). (Fig. 5.18B)	Fibers pass through foramen ovale.	Convey sensory impulse from out 2/3rd of tongue except taste buds, lower teeth, skin of temporal region of scalp, supplies motor fibers to muscles of mastica-tion.	Motor activity can assessed by asking the person to clench his teeth, open mouth against resistance and move jaw side to side.	Paralysis of masticatory muscles, derivation of mandible to the side of lesion, when the mouth is opened.
Abducent No. VI Mainly motor (Figs 5.15 and 5.17)	Fibers leave inferior aspect of pons and pass through superior orbital fissure and supply lateral rectus muscle.	Lateral rectus muscle turns eyeball laterally.	Patient is asked to rotate the eye laterally. Person can move, if the nerve is all right.	Injury to base of brain or fracture involving cavernous sinus or orbit. Cause no movement of eyes on lateral side and diplopia on lateral grazing.

Contd...

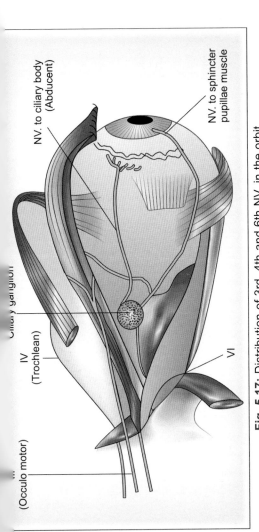

Fig. 5.17: Distribution of 3rd, 4th and 6th NV. in the orbit

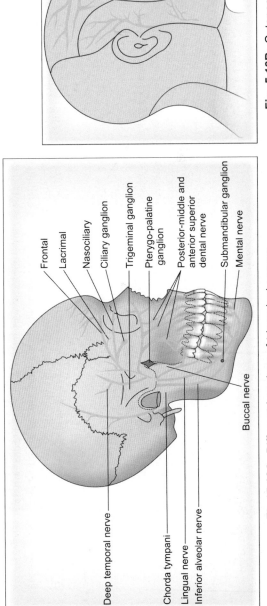

Fig. 5.18B: Cutaneous distribution of trigeminal nerve

Fig. 5.18A: Different banches of trigeminal nerves

Name and components	Origin and course	Function	Clinical testing	Applied
Facial (mixed) nerve No. VII (Figs 5.19A to C)	Fibers arise from pons just lateral to abducent nerves, enter temporal bone through internal auditory meatus and run within internal ear before emerging through stylomastoid foramen, nerve then passes to lateral aspect of face and supplies muscles of facial expression.	It is the chief motor nerves of face have five major branches – temporal, zygo-matic, buccal, mandibular and cervical. It also transmit parasympathetic motor impulse to lacrimal, nasal and palatine glands. Convey sensory impulse from taste bud of anterior 2/3rd of tongue.	Anterior 2/3rd of tongue is tested for ability to taste sweet, salty, sour and bitter substances. Symmetry of face is checked. Subject is asked to close eyes, smile, whistle and so on.	Laceration in parotid region produces paralysis of facial nerve results in paralysis of facial muscles, eye remains open, angle of mouth droops, Bell's palsy – characterized by paralysis of facial muscle, partial loss of taste sensation, may develop rapidly in Herpes Zoster infection.
Vestibulocochlear No. VIII (Sensory)	Fiber arises from hearing, organ of corti, forms cochlear division and equilibrium (semicircular canals) from vestibular division apparatus located within internal ear of temporal bone and pass through internal acoustic meatus and enter brainstem at pontomedullary junction.	Purely sensory. Cochlear division is responsible for hearing and vestibular division for sense of equilibrium.	Hearing (air and bone conduction) is checked usually by tuning fork.	Lesions (due to infection) of cochlear nerve produce nerve deafness. Where as damage to vestibular division produce tinnitus, vertigo, nausea, vomiting.
Glossopharyngeal No. IX (Secretomotor, parasympathetic sensory)	Fibers emerge from medulla and leave skull through jugular foramen.	Motor to stylopharyngeus muscle (assists swallowing); secretomotor to parotid gland. It covers general sensation and taste sensation from posterior 1/3rd of tongue.	Position of uvula is checked. And swallowing reflexes are checked. Subject is asked to speak and cough. Posterior 1/3rd of tongue may be tested for taste.	Injury or inflammation of glossopharyngeus pain in swallowing and taste is lost (particularly bitter).

Contd...

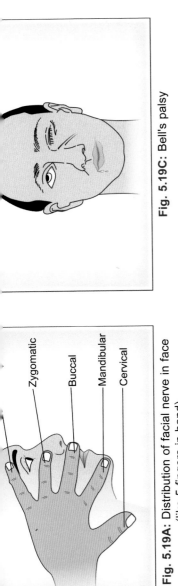

Zygomatic

Buccal

Mandibular

Cervical

Fig. 5.19A: Distribution of facial nerve in face (like 5 fingers in hand)

Fig. 5.19C: Bell's palsy

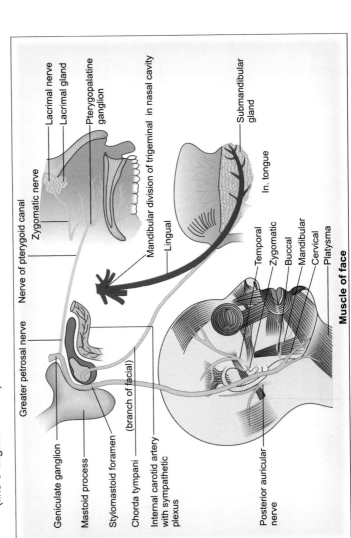

Lacrimal nerve

Lacrimal gland

Pterygopalatine ganglion

Zygomatic nerve

Nerve of pterygoid canal

Mandibular division of trigeminal in nasal cavity

Submandibular gland

In. tongue

Lingual

Temporal

Zygomatic

Buccal

Mandibular

Cervical

Platysma

Greater petrosal nerve

Geniculate ganglion

Mastoid process

Stylomastoid foramen

Chorda tympani (branch of facial)

Internal carotid artery with sympathetic plexus

Posterior auricular nerve

Muscle of face

Fig. 5.19B: Distribution of facial nerve (7th cranial)

Name and components	Origin and course	Function	Clinical testing	Applied
Vagus (mixed) No. X (Figs 5.20A and B)	The only cranial nerve that extends beyond head and neck region. Fibers emerge from medulla, pass through jugular foramen and descends through neck region into thorax and abdomen.	Mixed nerves; nearly all motor fibers are sympathetic efferent, except muscles of pharynx and larynx. Parasympathetic motor supply to heart, lungs and abdominal viscera (from pharynx to splenic flexure of colon, liver and kidneys).	Like cranial nerve IX.	Brainstem lesion or deep laceration of neck produce sagging of soft palate, deviation of uvula to unaffected side, hoarseness due to para-lysis of vocal fold. Diffi-culty in swallowing and speaking.
Accessory (cranial root and spinal root) No. XI Motor (Figs 5.15 and 5.21)	Cranial root emerges from lateral aspect of medulla. Spinal root arises from superior region of spinal cord enter skull via foramen magnum and temporally joins spinal root; the resulting nerve comes out through jugular foramen, the cranial and spinal root diverge. Cranial root fibers joins the vagus to supply larynx and spinal root supplies the sternomastoid and trapezius.	Muscle of soft palate except tensor vele palatine; pharynx (except stylopharyngeus). Larynx (except cricothyroid) and sternocleidomastoid and trapezius.	Sternocleidomastoid and trapezius muscle are checked for strength by asking person to rotate head and shrug shoulder against resistance.	Laceration of neck produces paralysis of sternomastoid and superior fibers of trapezius. There is drooping of shoulder.
Hypoglossal No. XII Motor (Fig. 5.22)	Fibers arise by a series of rootlets from medulla and exit from skull via hypoglossal canal and supplies tongue muscles.	Supplies muscles of tongue (except palao glossus) and controls its shape and movement.	Person is asked to protrude tongue. Any deviation can be noted.	In lesion of hypoglossal nerve, protrude tongue deviates toward affected side. It causes difficulty of speech (moderate dysar-thria).

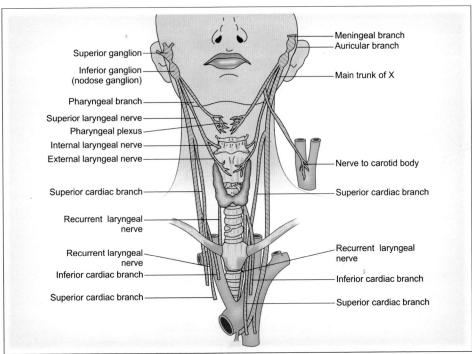

Fig. 5.20A: Vagus nerve (branches arising in the head and neck)

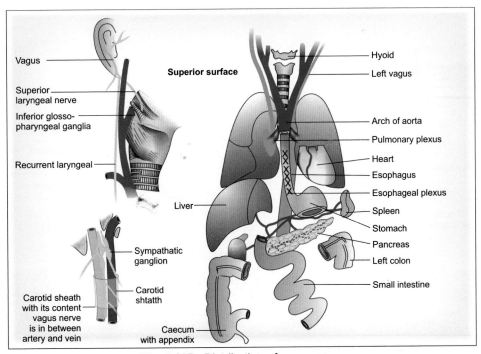

Fig. 5.20B: Distribution of vagus nerve

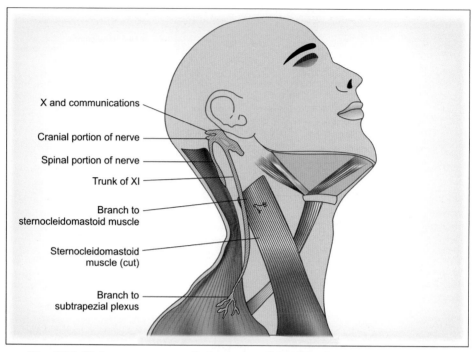

Fig. 5.21: XI Accessory nerve: that spinal portion ascending into the cranium to join the cranial portion before exiting the jugular foramen

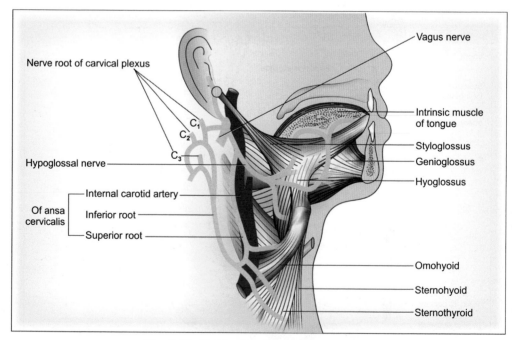

Fig. 5.22: Distribution of hypoglossal nerve

Chapter

6

Heart and Arterial System

Angina pectoris – chest pain
Artery – carries more oxygenated blood away from the heart.
Embolous – plug.
Infarction – virtually blood less area.
Ischemia – lacking adequate blood supply.
Stenosis – narrowing.
Vein – carries poorly oxygenated blood towards the heart.

TRODUCTION

tal amount of blood in our body is 5.5 litres, but
as to do tremendous function (supply nutrient
d O_2) continuously from birth up to death, so
od must circulate. The function of heart is to
culate blood by pumping action. Its size is about
's close fist; situated in middle mediastinum,
losed in a double sac of pericardium – outer
rous and inner serous (parietal and visceral

layer). It has four chambers – right atrium, right ventricle, left atrium and left ventricle. The two atria are separated from ventricle by an incomplete c-shaped sulcus – atrioventricular groove. Right atrium receives poorly oxygenated blood through superior vena cava, inferior vena cava and coronary sinus. Blood passes from atria to ventricle by right atrioventricular orifice (tricuspid orifice) and thence ejected to pulmonary trunk for oxygenation (pulmonary circulation). The left atrium receives oxygen rich blood via four pulmonary veins. From left atrium, blood passes to left ventricle and thence ejected to ascending aorta for systemic circulation. The heart wall is composed of (from inside outwards) endocardium – (inner thin layer); middle thick myocardium (muscle coat) and outer thin epicardium (visceral layer of serous pericardium).

Heart (Figs 6.1A and B)

It has three surface, three borders, an apex and a base.

Name	Important points
Apex	Pointed, formed only by left ventricle, directed downwards, forwards and to the left 9 cm away from midline (just below and medial to the left nipple). Apex beat (downmost and outermost point of definite cardiac pulsation) is palpable here.
Base (anatomical)	Formed solely by two atria (right and left); directed upwards, backwards and towards right

Contd...

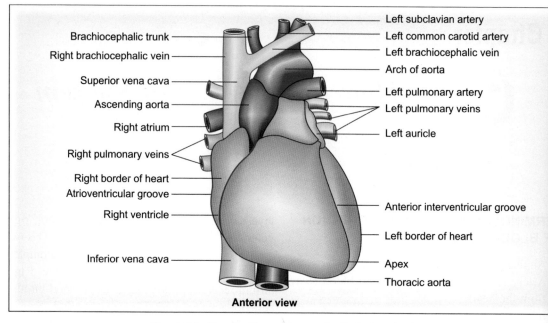

Fig. 6.1A: Heart with great vessels (Anterior view)

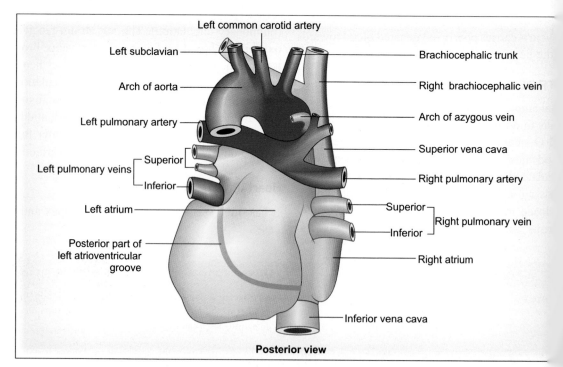

Fig. 6.1B: Heart with roots of great vessels (Posterior view)

Name	Important points
ase (clinical) terno-costal urface Figs 6.1A and .2)	Corresponds to parasternal part of right second intercostal space, examined by auscultation Formed by left (1/3rd) and right ventricle (2/3 part), right atrium with auricle. The surface is covered by lungs and plura, except the area of cardiac dullness. If there is excess fluid in pericardium; it is drained through this area. Anterior interventricular groove is situated here 1. lodges anterior interventricular branch of left coronary artery. 2. great cardiac vein (drains in coronary sinus).
Diaphragmatic urface	Formed by right (1/3 part) and left (2/3 part) ventricle – there is a flat surface rest on diaphragm. This surface present posterior interventricular groove which lodges posterior interventricular branch of right coronary artery and middle cardiac vein.
Left surface	Formed by left auricle and left ventricle
Right border separate sterno-costal from base)	It extends from right side of superior vena cava to inferior vena cava, it correspond to sulcus terminalis outside.
Left border separate sterno-costal from left surface)	It is formed mainly by left ventricle and partly by left auricle. Each borders formed angle with diaphragm called right and left cardiophrenic angle (in X- ray flim).
nferior border separate sterno-costal from diaphragmatic surface)	It formed mainly by right ventricle and partly by left ventricle near its apex.Medial to the apex lies a notch (incisura apicis codis). At this border lies right marginal vessels.
interior of right atrium (Fig. 6.2)	It has two parts – anterior rough part (where comb-like musculae pectinati present), – posterior smooth part. It is separated from rough part by a muscular ridge – crista-terminalis. It receives superior vena cava, inferior vena cava (guarded by semiulnar valve) and coronary sinus (guarded by semi-circular valve). Right side of intra-atrial septum present • Fossa ovalis – oval depression. • Limbus fossa ovalis – crescentic margin, surrounding upper, anterior and posterior part of fossa ovalis.
Interior of right ventricle (Fig. 6.3A)	It has inflowing rough part – in it, present ridges (supraventricular crest – an important ridge which separates inflowing rough from outflowing smooth part) bridges, out of which septomarginal trabecula or moderator band is important. It extends from right side of interventricular septum up to base of anterior papillary muscle. Papillary muscles – finger like projections, three in number, anterior, posterior and septal – attached to tricuspid valve by chordae tendineae. Anterior papillary muscle arises from sternocostal surface, attached to anterior and posterior valve cusp. Posterior papillary muscle arises from diaphragmatic surface, attached to posterior and septal cusp.Septal papillary muscle – very small, often absent. If present, it is attached to septal and anterior cusp.

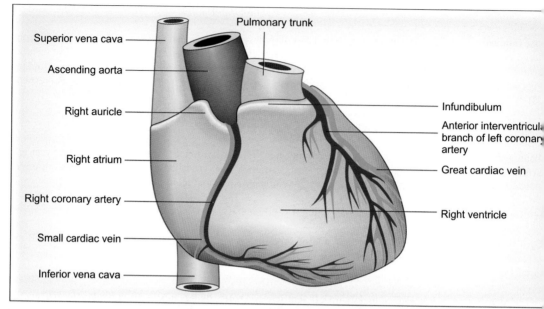

Fig. 6.2: Sternocostal surface of heart showing coronary arteries

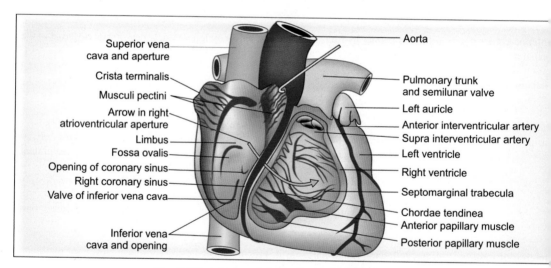

Fig. 6.3A: Interior of right atrium and right ventricle

rtery Supply of Heart (Coronary Circulation) ig. 6.3B)

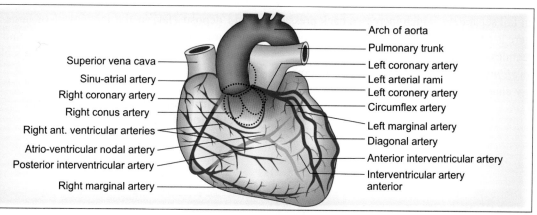

Fig. 6.3B: Coronary arterial system

Name	Begining	Course	Branches	Area supplied
Right coronary artery (smaller than left coronary artery)	Arises from ascending aorta from the anterior aortic sinus.	It passes downwards in between the root of pulmonary trunk and the right auricle, winds the inferior border, passes in the posterior part of atrioventricular groove and terminate by anastomosis with left coronary artery.	• Marginal • Posterior interventricular· Nodal (60% case)	Supplies all of the right ventricle, the variable part of diaphragmatic surface of left ventricle, post 1/3rd of interventricular septum, the right atrium part of left atrium and nodal tissue.
Left coronary artery	Arise from ascending aorta from left posterior aortic sinus.		• Anterior inter-ventricular. • Branch to diaphragmatic surface of left ventricle.	Supplies most of left ventricle, small area of right ventricle, anterior 2/3rd of interventricular septum, most of left atrium.

plied Anatomy (Heart and Pericardium)

Pericardial Effusion: When excess fluid is accumulated (more than 300 c.c.), it is known as pericardial effusion. There is compression symptoms (cardiac temponade). The cardiac output is reduced and heart beats in, abnormal rhythm; and eventually, cardiac arrest. To relive pain, a tapping is done through left costo-xyphoid angle.

• *Angina Pectoris:* It is an intermittent, transient, central chest pain. It is due to coronary artery insufficiency.

• *Valvular Disease:* It is commonly seen in rheumatic fever, produces valvular incompetence (incapability), seen most commonly in mitral and aortic valves.

Heart Failure: When diastolic pressure of ventri increases (normal pressure 0) – there is gradual heart failure. Any one of the four chambers of heart can fail separately, which increases back pressure. There is edema (accumulation of fluid) of feet and breathlessness on exertion.

Developmental Anomalis: Discussed in embryology chapter, i.e. Chapter 10.

Arterial Aneurysm: Abnormal dialation of segment of main artery is known as aneurysm.

Atherosclerosis: It is characterized by irregula lipid deposit (fat) in the inner wall of large an medium size artery. Common in middle, and o aged group; produces partial ischemia, (less bloc supply) of the region supplied.

Aorta and Major Arteries of Systemic Circulation (Fig. 6.4)

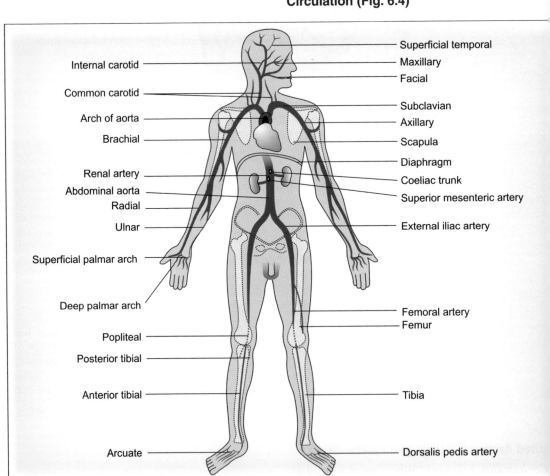

Internal carotid
Common carotid
Arch of aorta
Brachial
Renal artery
Abdominal aorta
Radial
Ulnar
Superficial palmar arch
Deep palmar arch
Popliteal
Posterior tibial
Anterior tibial
Arcuate

Superficial temporal
Maxillary
Facial
Subclavian
Axillary
Scapula
Diaphragm
Coeliac trunk
Superior mesenteric artery
External iliac artery
Femoral artery
Femur
Tibia
Dorsalis pedis artery

Fig. 6.4: Major arteries of systemic circulation

Name	Begining	Termination	Branches	Area supplied
..ending aorta	Left ventricle of heart	Sternal angle	Right and left coronary arteries	Heart
..h of aorta	Sternal angle (right side)	Sternal angle (left side)	• Brachiocephalic • Left common carotid • Left subclavian	Whole of superior extremity and head and neck region.
..chiocephalic	Arch of aorta	Upper border of right. Sternoclavicular joint.	• Right subclavian. • Right common carotid and occasionally arteria thyroidemia.	Right side of head and neck, right superior extremity.
..t common ..otid	Arch of aorta	Upper boarder of thyroid cartilage.	• Left external and left internal carotid arteries.	Left side of head and neck.
..scending ..racic aorta	Sternal angle on the left side	Continuous as abdominal aorta at the level of T12 vertebra.	• Parietal – posterior intercostal; superior phrenic • Visceral – mediastinal esophageal; bronc-hial, pericardial.	Supplies intercostal muscles, spinal cord, vertebrae, pleura, skin, posterior and superior diaphragm.
..dominal aorta	Arises at the T12 level, as a continuation of thoracic aorta.	Terminates at the level of L4 by dividing into right and left common iliac arteries.	Ventral → Coeliac → Superior mesenteric → Inferior mesenteric Lateral → Interior phrenic → Gonadal → Suprarenal → Renal Dorsal–4 lumbars	Supplies whole of the abdominal organs and parietes.
..ft and right ..mmon iliac	At L4 level	At the level of sacroiliac joint	• External iliac • Internal iliac	Mainly supplied pelvic structure and inferior extremity.

..ries of Superior Extremity (Fig. 6.5)

Name	Begining	Termination	Branches	Area supplied
..bclavian ..ght and left)	Right from brachiocephalic and left from arch of aorta.	At the outer border of first rib, continues as axillary artery.	• Vertebral • Internal thoracic • Thyrocervical • Costacervical • Dorsal scapular (Total – 5 branches)	Neck and upper limb

Contd...

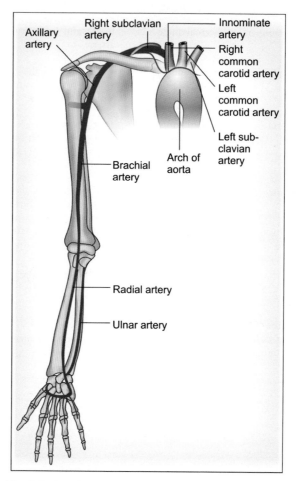

Fig. 6.5: Arterial supply superior extremity (upper limb)

Name	*Begining*	*Termination*	*Branches*	*Area supplied*
Axillary artery	Outer border of first rib	At the lower border of teres major.	• Superior thoracic – from first part. • Acromio thoracic – from 2nd part • Lateral thoracic. • Subscapular • Anterior humeral circumflex. • Posterior humeral circumflex – from third part. (Total – 6 branches)	Shoulder, axilla, chest wall.

Co

Name	Begining	Termination	Branches	Area supplied
chial ry . 6.5)	At the lower border of teres major	As ulnar and radial artery at the level of neck of radius.	• Arteria profunda brachii. • Nutrient artery to humerus. • Superior ulnar collateral artery. • Interior ulnar collateral artery. (Total 4 branches)	Supplies anterior flexor muscles and posterior extensor muscle (triceps) of arm, by small branches; to elbow joint, by anasto-mosis.
lial artery	At the level of neck of radius from brachial artery.	At the fifth meta-carpal base, after passing through first dorsal inter-metecarpal and also through two heads of adduc-tor pollicis, form deep palmar arch	• Radial recurrent arteries. • Muscular branches· • Palmar carpal branch· • Superficial palmar branch· • Dorsal carpal branch· • First dorsal metacarpal artery. • Arteria princeps pollicis.· • Arteria radialis indicis (Total 8 branches)	Supplies lateral muscles of forearm, the wrist and the thumb and index finger.
ar artery	At the neck of radius from brachial artery	At the level of pisiform bone	• Anterior ulnar recurrent artery • Posterior ulnar current artery • Common interosseous artery • Muscular • Palmar carpal branch • Dorsal carpal branch • Deep palmar branch • Superficial palmar arch.	Muscles of medial side of forearm three to fifth fingers medial aspect of index finger, elbow joint, wrist joint.

·ries of Thorax (Figs 6.6 and 6.7)

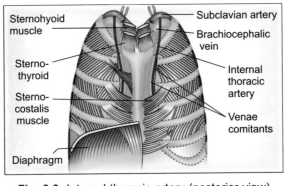

Fig. 6.6: Internal thoracic artery (posterior view)

Name	Begining	Termination	Branches	Area supplied
Descending thoracic aorta (Fig. 6.5)	Arises from arch of aorta at external angle (lower border of fourth thoracic vertebra).	At the T12 vertebra passing through aortic opening of diaphragm. (2 cm above the transpyloric plane in the midline).	• Pericardial. • Bronchial. • Esophageal. • Mediastinal. • Superior phrenic. • Posterior intercostals (except first two) (6 branches) • First two are the branches of costo cervical trunk.	Thoracic wall diaphragm and thoracic viscera except mammary gland.
Internal thoracic artery	From lower border of first part of sub clavian artery about 2 cm above the sternal end of clavicle.	At the level of sixth intercostal space 1 cm from the lateral sternal border, it ends by dividing into two branches.	• Pericardio phrenic • Mediastinal. • Pericardial. • Sternal. • Anterior intercostals • Perforating • Musculo phrenic • Superior epigastric. (8 branches)	Thoracic wall, thoracic viscera, diaphragm and mammary gland.

Arteries of Abdomen
Abdominal Aorta and Its Branches (Fig. 6.7)

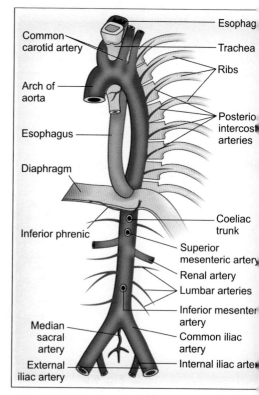

Fig. 6.7: Major arteries of thorax and abdome

Ventral Branch

Name	Begining	Termination	Branches	Area supplied
Coeliac trunk	Wide, unpaired ventral branch of abdominal aorta. It lies 1.25 cm above the transpyloric plane slightly to the left of mid line.	Passes almost horizontally towards and slightly right, above pancreas and splenic vein, dividing into three branches.	1. Left gastric 2. Common hepatic 3. Splenic	Stomach, liver and spleen.
Superior mesenteric	Unpaired ventral branch of abdominal aorta, at the level of first lumbar vertebra, just below the coeliac trunk.	The artery crosses in front of inferior vena cava, right ureter and psoas major, narrows down and anastomoses with its own ileo-colic branch.	1. Inferior pancreaticoduodenal. 2. Jejunal and ileal. 3. Middle colic. 4. Right colic 5. Left colic.	Whole of the small intestine from superior part of duodenum up to right 2/3rd and left 1/3rd of transverse colon (large gut).
Inferior mesenteric	Unpaired Ventral branch arises at the level of third lumbar vertebra.	Continues at superior rectal artery within lesser pelvis.	Sigmoid. Superior rectal.(3 branches)	Left 1/3rd of transverse colon and most of the rectum.

Lateral Branches (Paired)

Name	Begining	Termination	Branches	Area supplied
Inferior phrenic rtery	At the level of T12 from aorta just inferior to diaphragm.	End by supplying the inferior surface of diaphragm.	• Small branches to liver. • To spleen. • Superior suprarenal.	Under surface of diaphragm and suprarenal gland only.
Middle suprarenal rtery	Paired small branches of abdominal aorta; arises at the level of superior mesenteric artery.	By supplying suprarenal gland.	No branch.	Suprarenal gland.
Renal artery	Two large arteries arise slightly below the superior, mesenteric artery (between L-1 and L-2).	Near the renal hilum, it divides into four to five branches.	• Inferior suprarenal • Ureteric • Muscular	Kidney, Suprarenal gland, Upper part of ureter and muscles of posterior abdominal wall.
Gonadal rtery	Paired, long slender artery; arises little below the renal arteries.	End by supplying gonads.	• Ureteric	In case of males supplies testis, perirenal fat, ureter and iliac lymph nodes. In case of females, ovary, skin of labia majora, inguinal region.

Contd...

Name	Begining	Termination	Branches	Area supplied
• Lumbar artery	These are in series with posterior intercostal arises from lumbar region.	Ends by supplying muscles of lumbar region.	• Muscular branches	These segmental arteries supply the posterior abdominal wall.
• Common iliac	At the level of 4th lumbar vertebra as terminal branch of abdominal aorta.	At the level of 5th lumbo sacral disc (sacroiliac joint) it terminate into two arteries: 1. Internal iliac artery 2. External iliac artery	• Peritoneal • Branch to psoas major • Ureteric • Loose aveolar tissue	
• Internal iliac artery (right and left)	At the level of sacroiliac joint from common iliac.	At the greater sciatic foramen by dividing into anterior trunk and posterior trunk.	Branches from anterior trunk Superior vesical. Inferior vesical. Middle rectal. Uterine. Obturator. Internal pudendal. Muscular. Inferior rectal. Perineal. Urethral. Deep artery of penis. Dorsal artery of penis. Branches from posterior trunk: Iliolumbar. Lateral sacral. Superior gluteal (total 15 branches)	

N.B. – The testicular artery is not the sole supply to the testis. It also receives some blood from branches of inferior epigastric artery. Thus, injury to the artery high in the abdomen usually leaves the testis unharmed; whereas injury in the region of spermatic cord involves both the vessel and leads to gangrene of testes.

Arteries of Inferior Extremity (Figs 6.8A and B)

Name	Begining	Course	Branches	Area supplied
Femoral artery	Continuation of external iliac at the level of inguinal ligament.	At the fifth osseoaponeurotic opening continued as popliteal artery.	1. Superior epigastric 2. Superficial circumflex iliac 3. Superficial external pudendal 4. Muscular 5. Arterioprofunda femoris (main branch)	Muscle of thigh head and neck region of femur.

Con

Name	*Begining*	*Termination*	*Branches*	*Area supplied*
Popliteal artery	At the fifth osseoaponeurotic opening from femoral artery.	At the lower border of popliteus by dividing into anterior and posterior tibial.	• Cutaneous branches. • Superior muscular branches. • Superior genicular (medial and lateral).	By arterial anastomsis, supplied knee joint. By terminal branches supplied to the

Contd...

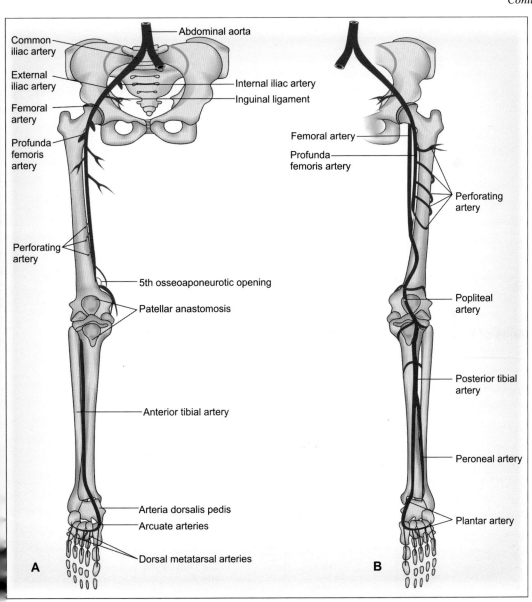

Figs 6.8A and B: Arteries of lower limb (inferior extremity)

Name	Begining	Termination	Branches	Area supplied
			• Middle genicular (small in size). • Inferior genicular (medial and lateral).	muscles and joints of leg region.
Anterior tibial artery	At the lower border of popliteus from popliteal artery.	At the level of ankle continued as dorsalis pedis artery.	• Posterior tibial recurrent. • Anterior tibial recurrent. • Muscular. • Arteria dorsalis pedis	External muscle of anterior compartment of leg.
Posterior tibial artery	Larger terminal branches of popliteal artery, at the lower border of popliteus.	At the ankle, midway between medial tubercle of calcaneum and medial malleolus, it end by dividing into medial and lateral plantar arteries.	• Peroneal largest branch • Circumflex fibular. • Nutrient artery to tibia. • Muscular. • Medial malleolar. • Calcaneal. • Medial plantar. • Lateral plantar	Flexor and peroneal muscles of leg, sole.
Dorsalis pedis artery	At the ankle beyond inferior extensor retinaculum, and medial to the tendon of extensor hallucis longus.	At the first intermetatarsal space.	• Tarsal. • Arcuate. • First dorsal metatarsal.	Ankle joint, dorsum of foot.

Arteries of Head and Neck (Fig. 6.9)

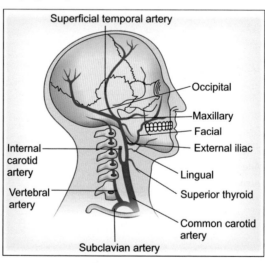

Fig. 6.9: Arteries of head and neck

Name	Begining	Termination	Branches	Area supplied
ght and external otid eries	Common carotid; arteries at the upper border of thyroid cartilage.	In the substance of parotid gland behind the mandibular neck; terminates by dividing into superficial temporal and maxillary arteries.	• Superior thyroid. • Ascending pharyngeal. • Lingual. • Facial. • Occipital. • Posterior auricular. • Superficial temporal. • Maxillary.	Thyroid, pharynx, tongue, face, occipital region behind the ear, temple, meninges of brain, external ear (i.e. most tissue of head except orbit and brain).
ernal rotid artery ght and t)	Larger than external carotid arises at the upper border of thyroid cartilage. It is divided into four parts, cervical, petrous, cavernous and cerebral.	At the medial end of base of lateral sulcus of brain.	Cervical part – No branch • Tympanic • Pterygoid • Cavernous • Hypophyseal • Meningeal • Ophthalmic • Anterior cerebral • Middle cerebral • Posterior communication • Anterior choroids (Total 10 branches)	Supplies orbit and 80% of cerebral hemisphere.
rtebral teries (right d left)	From subclavian arteries at the root of the neck.	At the base of brain (near ponto-medullary junction) the two arteries unite and form basilar arteries.	• Spinal branch • Muscular • Meningeal • Posterior spinal • Anterior spinal • Posterior interior cerebella • Medullary arteries (Total 7 branches)	Spinal cord occipital lobes and part of (interior) temporal lobe of cerebral hemisphere

erial Circle Of Wills: It is polygonal rather than ular. It is bounded arterially by anterior cerebral eries (from internal carotid) are joined by erior communicating artery. Posterior the basilar ry divides into two posterior cerebral arteries, h joined to the same sided internal carotid by a terior communicating artery.

Applied Anatomy

Angiogram: Visualisation of arterial tree by radio-paque dye is known as angiogram. At the upper limb brachail artery (just above the cubital fossa) and radial artery (region where radial pulse is felt) are the common site, common carotid artery in neck (near its bifurcation) and femoral artery in lower limb (just below the inguinal ligament) in the site of choice for angiography. Various regions in the body where arterial pulsations can be felt are shown in Figure 6.10.

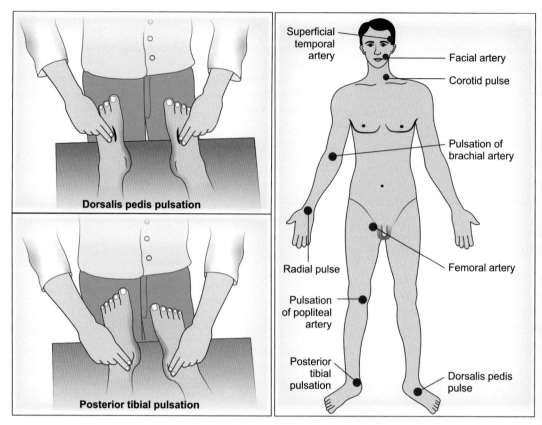

Fig. 6.10: Regions where arterial pulsation is felt (Peripheral arterial pulse)

Chapter

7

Veins

INTRODUCTION

Veins are the channels that carry blood towards the heart. Poorly oxygenated blood is carried by all veins in the body except pulmonary veins which carries oxygenated blood. It posses thin muscle wall and are wider and numerous than the arteries. It is formed from capillary tissue fluid (micro molecular in nature). In human body four types of venous system present 1) Caval system, 2) Portal venous system, 3) Azygos venous system, 4) Para vertebral veins.

The Venae Cavae (Figs 7.1 and 7.2)

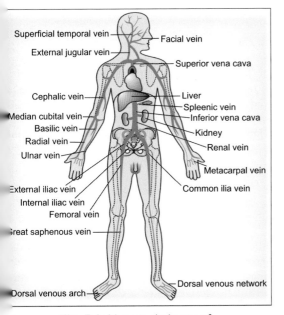

Fig. 7.1: Venous drainage of whole body (anterior aspect)

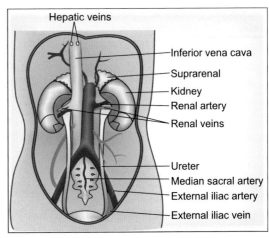

Fig. 7.2: Inferior vena cava along with aorta

Name	Formation	Termination	Tributaries	Area of drainage
Superior vena cava	By union of two brachio-cephalic vein at the lower border of first right costal cartilage.	At the posterosuperior aspect of right artrium.	• Two brachiocephalic. • Arch of azygos vein.	Drains blood from a areas superior t diaphragm exce from the pulmo-na circuit.
Inferior vena cava	Formed by union of right and left common iliac vein at the level of L5 to the right of the midline.	It terminates at the postero- inferior part of right atrium just after passing through vena-caval opening of dia-phragm at the level of T8.	• Two common iliac (for-mative) tributary. • Lumbar veins. • Ascending lumbar vein. • Gonadal (testicular in male, and ovarian vein in female) • Renal • Suprarenal • Inferior phrenic • Hepatic	From all th structures of boc below dia-phragm.
External jugular	By union of posterior division of retroman dibular and posterior auricular vein near mandibular angle.	Passing super ficial to sternocleido mastoid, pierce the deep fascia and drain into subclavian vein.	• Posterior division of retromandibular • Posterior auricular. • Posterior external jugular • Transeverse cervical. • Supra scapular. • Sometimes anterior jugular. (6 tributaries)	Drain the supply region of head (scalp and face) to some exten deepar part.
Vertebral veins	Arises as a plexus in the suboccipital tri-angle and lies over the posterior arch of atlas.	Drains into brachio-cephalic veins of corres-ponding side at the root of neck.	• Connected to sigmoid sinus by a tributary. • Occipital vein. • Veins from pre-vertebral muscles. • Internal and exter-nal vertebral plexus (4 tributaries)	Drains from th region of **** vertebrae, th spinal cord and small neck muscles. [Unlike vertebra arteries the verte bral vein do no much of th branch).
Internal jugular vein	It begins at jugular foramen cranial base as a continuation of sigmoid sinus.	Joined with subclavian vein at the posterior end of sternoclavicular joint of corresponding side forming brachiocephalic vein.	• Inferior petrosal sinus. • Facial vein. • Lingual vein. • Pharyngeal vein. • Superior and middle thyroid vein. • Some times occipital (6 tributaries)	Drains fror region of sku (superficial par face, and majo structures o neck.

...s of Thorax (Fig. 7.3A)

Name	Formation	Termination	Tributaries	Area of drainage
...achio- ...phalic ...in (inno- ...nate) ...void of ...ves	By union of internal jugular and subclavian	At the sternal end of right costal cartilage two brachiocephalic vein unites to form superior vena cava.	• Two brachio-cephalic • Left vertebral • Internal thoracic (internal mammary) • Inferior thyroid • Superior intercostal • Thymic and pericardial veins (6 tributaries)	Blood from whole of head and neck and superior extremity and thorax.
...zygos vein	Arises in abdomen as lumbar aszygos vein, from inferior vena cava.	It ends in superior vena cava; at the junction of its intra and extra pericardial part, at the level of sternal angle.	• Right posterior inter-costal veins except the first. • Right superior intercostal vein. • The hemiazygos. • Accessory hemiazygos vein • Esophageal	Right sided parietes of thorax, mediastinal structures and bronchus.
...uperior ...emiazygos ...ein.	Formed by union of fourth to eighth inter-costal vein.	It joins the azygos at the level of T7 vertebra.	• Mediastinal • Pericardial • Bronchial (right) • Ascending lumber • Subcostal. • Four to eight intercostal vein. • Sometimes left bronchial.	Left upper part of thorax and sometimes the left bronchus.
...nferior ...emiazygos ...ein.	Formed by the union of left ascending lumbar vein and left subcostal vein.	At azygos vein at about T8 level.	• Lower three posterior intercostal vein. • Common trunk formed by ascending lumbar and subcostal, esophageal, and mediastinal veins.	Lower parietes of thorax, structures of mediastinum.

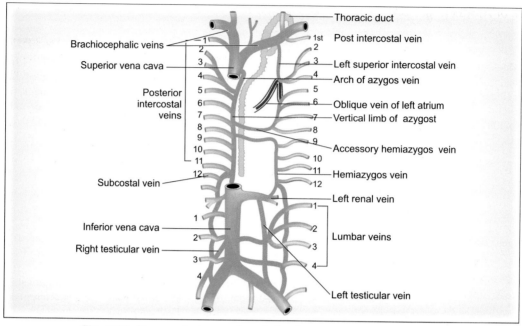

Thoracic duct
Brachiocephalic veins — 1, 2
Superior vena cava — 3, 4

1st
2
Post intercostal vein
3 — Left superior intercostal vein
4 — Arch of azygos vein

Posterior intercostal veins — 5, 6, 7, 8, 9, 10, 11, 12

5
6 — Oblique vein of left atrium
7 — Vertical limb of azygost
8
9 — Accessory hemiazygos vein
10
11 — Hemiazygos vein
12

Subcostal vein —
Left renal vein

Inferior vena cava — 1, 2
Right testicular vein — 3, 4

1
2
3 — Lumbar veins
4

Left testicular vein

Fig. 7.3A: Venous drainage of posterior thoracic and abdominal wall

Cardiac Veins (Venous Drainage of Heart) (Fig. 7.3B)

Name	Formation	Termination	Tributaries	Area of drainage
Coronary sinus	Formed behind the left atrium and left ventricle; 2-3 cm long.	Open in the right atrium between the opening of inferior vena cava and right atrioventricular orifice.	• Great cardiac vein (begin at cardiac apex, ascends in anterior inter ventricular sulcus). • Small cardiac vein. • Middle cardiac vein (begin at cardiac apex ascends in posterior inter ventricular groove). • Posterior vein of the left ventricle, oblique vein of left atrium.	Whole heart.
Thebesian vein or inferior cardiac vein	Situated in sub-pericardial tissue.	End in right atrium through foramina venerum minimerum.		Anterior part of right ventricle.

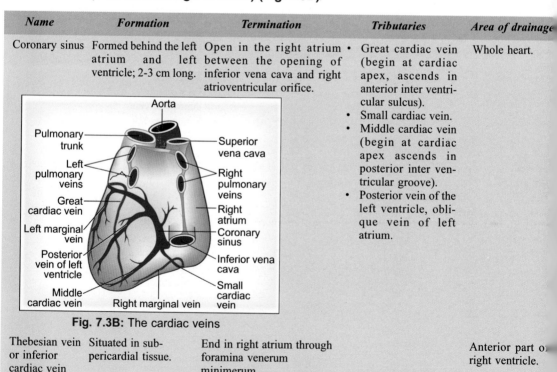

Aorta
Pulmonary trunk
Left pulmonary veins
Great cardiac vein
Left marginal vein
Posterior vein of left ventricle
Middle cardiac vein
Right marginal vein

Superior vena cava
Right pulmonary veins
Right atrium
Coronary sinus
Inferior vena cava
Small cardiac vein

Fig. 7.3B: The cardiac veins

s of Abdomen and Pelvis (Fig. 7.2)

s from whole of abdomen and pelvis are
ed by inferior vena cava which has discussed
iously. Here we discuss the portal vein.

tal Vein (Figs 7.4A, B and 7.5A)

hepatic portal system collect blood from
stive tract, and are valve less. They form a
k – the portal vein, which enter into the liver
breaks up again into capillaries. Thus, the
d have to passed through capillaries in the gut
, again passes through capillaries (sinusoids)
e liver.

ortant Porto-systemic Anastomosis
. 7.5A)

der normal condition portal blood passes
ugh the liver and drains in the inferior
a cava (systemic vein) by hepatic veins.

This is the direct route. But when this route is
blocked (by chirrosis of liver), other smaller
communication exists between the portal and
systemic system and bypass the blood from liver
and drains into systemic vein. These communication exists at:

1. *Lower end of esophagus* – Communication of
   esophageal branch of left gastric (portal system)
   with esophageal veins of azygos system
   (systemic). An abnormally large amount of
   blood passes through these channels forms
   esophageal varices. Channels may rupture and
   produce severe hemorrhage.

2. *In the distal part of anal canal* – The superior
   rectal vein (portal system) anastomoses between
   the middle and inferior rectal vein (systemic).
   In portal hypertension these veins dilated and
   protruded through mucosa and form internal
   piles (hemorrhoids) which may rupture during
   passage of stool.

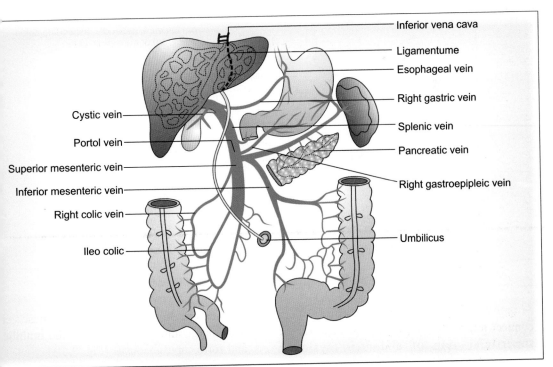

Fig. 7.4A: Tributaries of portal vein

Formative tributaries

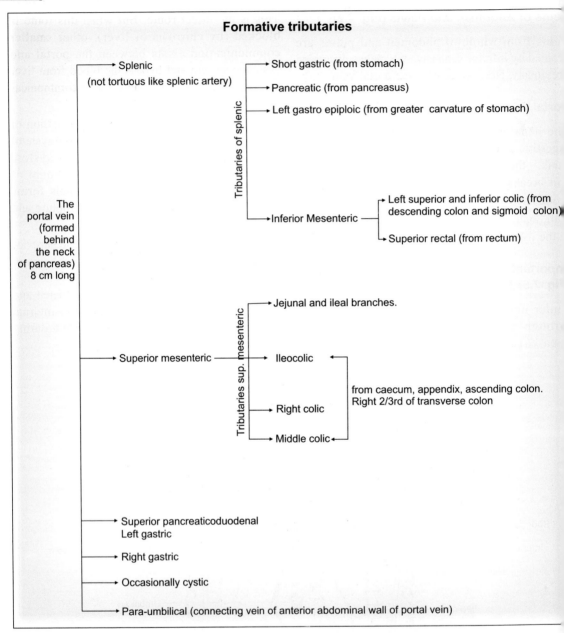

Fig. 7.4B: The veins forming portal system and their tributaries

3. *In umbilical region* – The paraumbilical vein connect left branch of portal vein between the superficial vein of abdomen (systemic Circulation). In portal hypertension these veins are enlarge and radiates around the umbilicus and form caput medusae (Fig. 7.5B).

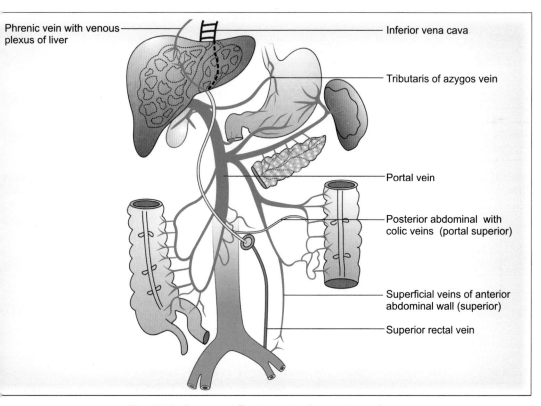

Phrenic vein with venous plexus of liver

Inferior vena cava

Tributaris of azygos vein

Portal vein

Posterior abdominal with colic veins (portal superior)

Superficial veins of anterior abdominal wall (superior)

Superior rectal vein

Fig. 7.5A: Important Proto-systemic anastomosis

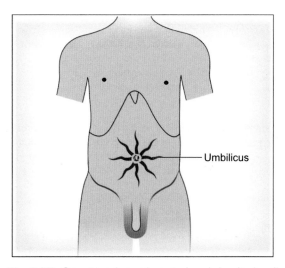

Umbilicus

Fig. 7.5B: Caput medusae in anterior abdominal wall

Name	Formation	Termination	Tributaries	Area of drain
External iliac	Continuation of femoral vein from the level of inguinal ligament.	At the corresponding sacroiliac joint by joining with internal iliac.	• Inferior epigastric vein. • Deep circumflex iliac vein. • Pubic vein. (3 tributaries)	Lower part anterior abdominal w of pelvis.

> Disease of external iliac artery may cause adherence with the external iliac vein. Dissection in this region there produces severe venous hemorrhage which is difficult to control.

Name	Formation	Termination	Tributaries	Area of drain
Internal iliac	Veins from different viscera of pelvis; converge near the region of greater sciatic foramen to form the internal iliac vein.	At the corresponding sacroiliac joint it joins with internal iliac vein to form the common iliac vein.	• Superior gluteal v. • Inferior gluteal v. • Middle rectal v. • Internal pudendal v. • Obturator vein. • Lateral sacral v. • Vesical v. • Uterine and vaginal v (in case of female). • Prostatic venous plexus. • Dorsal vein of penis. (10 branches)	Gluteal region and structure lesser pelvis a external genitalia.
Lumbar vein	Four pairs from lumbar muscles and skin.	At inferior vena cava except the first one, drains into ascending lumbar and lumbar azygos.	• Lumbar. • Abdominal.	Lumbar musc and skin, from wall of abdomen.
Gonadal or testicular veins	Emerge posteriorly from testis, as pampiniform plexus and in case of ovary from ovarian plexus.	The right vein ends in inferior vena cava, below renal vein, at an acute angle. Left one drain in left renal vein at 90° angle.	Veins from all the structres of spermatic cord.	From gonads.
Renal vein (right 2.5 cm and left 7.5 cm long)	Within renal sinus by union of lobar veins.	Into inferior vena cava at right angle just below the origin of superior mesenteric artery.	Left receives left gonodal and left suprarenal vein.	Drains the kidney.
Suprarenal (right and left)	Form from, numerous small veins from supra-renal medulla and cortex.	Right drain into inferior vena cava. Left into left renal vein.		From suprarenal glands.
Hepatic veins (right and left)	Within the substance of liver commences as intra lobular veins.	Opens in inferior vena cava in the groove on the posterior surface of liver.	Cystic vein.	Liver, gallbladder

ous Drainage of Inferior Extremity

e are three types of veins in lower limb. rficial (lies in superficial fascia), deep (lies to deep fascia) and a connecting channel n as perforating veins.

orating Veins

perforating veins are those veins which ects the superficial and deep vein. There are perforating veins in femoral region, adductor canal, a little above knee, little below knee and ankle perforation. The flow of blood is from superficial vein to deep vein. It is provided with valves.

Deep Veins (It lies along the arteries)

Veins are drained from below upwards. Anterior tibial venae comitants, posterotibial venae comitants, popliteal vein, femoral vein.

Superficial veins (Fig. 7.6)

Jame	Formation	Termination	Tributaries	Area of drainage
g saphe-s vein gest vein he body)	Arises from medial marginal vein which is the continuation of medial part of dorsal venous network. It goes upward accom-panied by saphenous nerve, bends behind the medial condyle of femur; ascends in the medial side of thigh.	It ends in femoral vein about 3 cm below the inguinal ligament.	• From sole of foot by medial marginal vein. • Communicating vein from small saphenous vein. • Accessory saph-onous vein. • Superficial epigas-tric • Superficial circum-flex iliac. • Superficial external pudendal vein. • Thorace epigastric vein – It is a connec-ting link between superior and inferior vena cava.	From superficial structures of whole of lower limb except back of leg.
all saph-us vein rd sap- means ly seen)	Arises from lateral border of foot as a continuation of lateral end of dorsal venous network.	It ascends upwards in the back of by perforates deep fascia on the back of knee and terminates in popliteal vein between the two heads of gastroc nemius.	• Veins from back of leg. • Communicating vein with the great saphonous vein. • From lateral part of the foot.	From superficial structures of back of leg.

plied

Vene section—When patient is in collapse state (in shock), it is not easy to get superficial vein. Vene section is lone near the region or great saphenous veins (in front of ankle) for therapeutic (treatment) purpose.

Varicosity—Dilatation and tortuasity of veins is known as varicosity. Common sites of varicose veins are lower imb veins (person with long standing habit, in pregnancy, etc.) superficial abdominal veins (in portat hypertension —as in caput medisae), testicular vein (pampiniform plexus—dilatation known as varicocele).

Intravenous injection—Common site—(a) Median cubital vein in front of elbow, (b) Cephalic vein (near its formation in hand), used as diagnostic purpose (Blood T.C, D.C, E.S.R., Sugar, Urea, etc.)

Therapeutic purpose—Fluid transfusion.

Spread of cancer by vein—Act as a vehicle for spread of cancer, e.g. cancer prostate spread from prostate to ertebrae by veins of Batson.

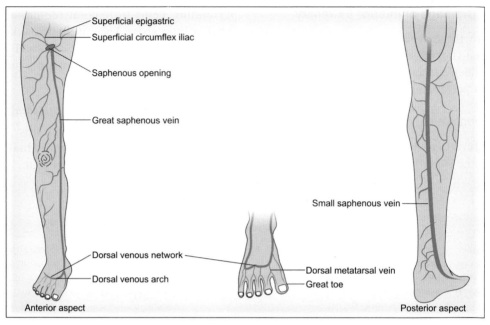

Fig. 7.6: Superficial venous drainage of inferior extermity (lower limb)

Veins of Superior Extremity (Fig. 7.7)

The deep veins of upper limb follows the paths of their companion arteries and have the same na Most are paired that lies by the side of the a except longest one.

Name	Formation	Termination	Tributaries	Area of drain
1. Cephlic vein—It is used for cardiac catheterisation	It is formed over the anatomical snuff box as a continuation of lateral part of dorsal venous network.	It pierces the clavi-pectoral fascia, crosses the axillary artery and end in axillary vein below the clavicle.	Many tributaries from lateral and posterior surface of limb.	Lateral and pe erior surface limb.
2. Baisilic vein.	Continuation of medial part of dorsal venous network.	Reaching the lower border of teres major, it is joined by venae comitantes of brachial artery and continued as axillary veins.	• Medial cubital vein. • Various tributaries on medial and posterior surface of limb.	Medial and pe erior surface limb.
3. Medial veins of forearm	Arises from palmar venous plexus.	Terminate either in basilic or cephalic vein or into median cubital vein.	• Numerous unnamed tributaries.	Palm and from forearm.
4. Median cubital vein	Communication bet-ween cephalic and basilic vein just below the crease of elbow. It is used in intravenous injection, blood trans-fusion.			

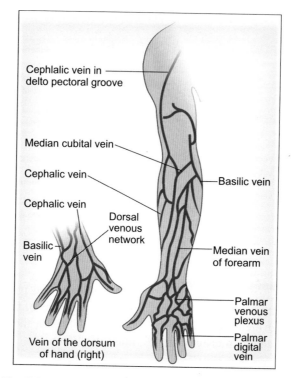

Fig. 7.7: Venous drainage of superior extremity (right)

ins of Head and Neck (Figs 7.8A and B)

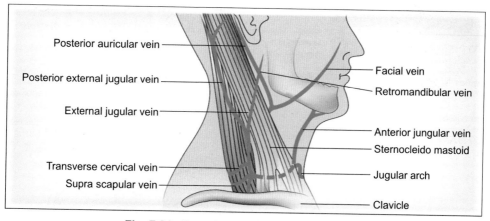

Fig. 7.8A: Superficial veins of head and neck

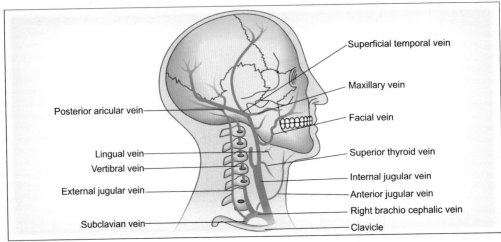

Fig. 7.8B: Major veins of head and neck

Cranial Dural Venous Sinuses (Figs 7.9A to C)

The dural venous sinuses are blood filled spaces between the endosteal and meningeal layer of duramaters except straight sinus, inferior sagittal sinus, anterior and posterior intercavernus sin Most of the veins of the brain drains into it. Th have no valves in their wall, and also devoid muscular tissue.

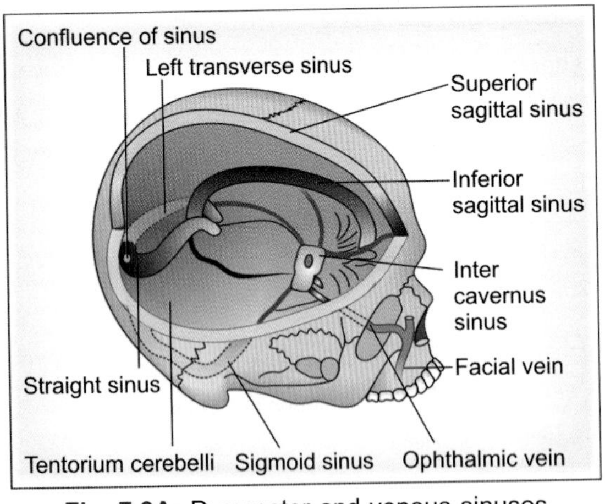

Fig. 7.9A: Duramater and venous sinuses (lateral view)

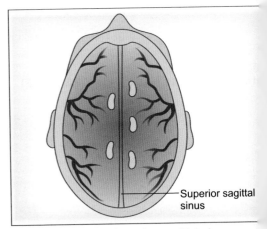

Fig. 7.9B: Superior sagittal sinus after removal of cranial vault

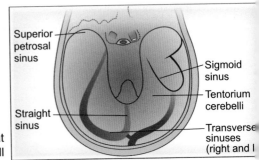

Fig. 7.9C: Venous sinus at the base of skull

Name	Situation	Beginning	End	Tributaries
⸱perior ⸱gital ⸱us ⸱paired)	It is situated at the attached, or convex margin of falx cerebri	Begin near the crysta gali of ethmoid bone.	At the internal occipital protuberence, it is continuous as right transverse sinus.	• Superior cerebral v. • Parietal emissary v. • Diploic and meningeal vein (3 tributaries)
⸱erior ⸱ittal sinus ⸱paired)	In the posterior half or 2/3rd of free margin of falx cerebri.	At the anterior part of lower folded part of meningeal layer of dura mater	In straight sinus.	• Veins from falx cerebri. • Sometimes from medial surface of brain (2 tributaries).
⸱aight ⸱us ⸱paired)	Lies at the site of attachment falx cerebri, with tentorium cerebelli	Union of inferior sagittal sinus and the great cerebral v.	Normally it will continued as left transverse sinuses.	• Great cerebral vein
⸱nsverse ⸱us ⸱ired)	It lies along the attached margin of tentorium cerebelli	Begins at the internal occipital protuberance	Continued as sigmoid sinus at the postero-lateral part of temporal bone.	• Superior petrosal sinus. • Inferior cerebral v. • Inferior cerebellar v. • Diploic v. (4 tributaries)
⸱gmoid ⸱us ⸱ired)	It lies along the inner surface of mastoid angle of temporal bone.	As a continuation of the transverse sinus	It comes out at posterior compartment of jugular foramen as superior bulb of internal jugular vein.	• Mastoid • Chondylar emissary vein.
⸱cipital ⸱us ⸱paired)	Smallest of the sinuses situated at the attached margin of tentorial cerebelli	Begins near the foramen magnum	Straight sinuses.	• Connects with vertebral venous plexus.
⸱vernus ⸱us	Situated at the sides of body of sphenoid bone.	Begins from superior orbital fissure	At the apex of petrous part of temporal bone.	• Spheno parietal sinus. • Superior ophthalmic vein. • A tributary of inferior ophthalmic vein. • Crntral vein of retina. • Middle meningeal sinus. • Inferior cerebral veins. • Superficial middle cerebral vein.

Lymphatic System

INTRODUCTION

Apart from artery and vein, there exist another channel in our body, i.e. lymphatic system. Lymphatic system is accessory to venous system. It also drains tissue fluid from the tissue spaces like veins, but the difference is that it carries protein and fat macromolecules from tissue spaces. The veins carries micromolecular substance from tissue space. Lymphatic tissue is essential for immunological defence of the body from bacteria and viruses.

Lymph is the name given to the tissue fluid, once it has entered a lymphatic vessel. Before lymph is drained into the blood stream, it passes at least one lymph node (small masses of lymphatic tissue),

sometimes several. The lymph vessels ▮ numerous valves. The lymph vessels that ᴄ lymph towards the LN is known as afferent ve and that carries lymph away from LN is know efferent vessel. The lymph reaches the blood st▮ at the root of the neck by large lymph vessels c▮ right lymphatic duct and thoracic duct. The tho▮ duct begins in the abdomen as a sac; cysterna c and enters the thorax through a opening (a▮ opening) of diaphragm. It ascends through th▮ lies in front of thoracic vertebrae. It then asc▮ into neck and drain into the angle, formed by▮ internal jugular and left subclavian vein.

The right lymphatic duct drains lymph from body's right upper quadrant (right side of head▮ neck, right upper limb and right half of tho▮ The thoracic duct drains lymph from remaind▮ the body (Fig. 8.1).

The central nervous system, the eyeball; internal ear, the epidermis of skin, cartilage bone are devoid of lymphatic vessels.

Applied

1. *Lymphangitis.* It is the inflammation of ly▮ vessel. When lymph vessels are seve▮ inflamed, the vasa vesorum (vessel supplyi▮ vessel) become congested with blood. ▮ result the pathway of the associated lymph▮ become visible through skin as red line▮ painful to touch.

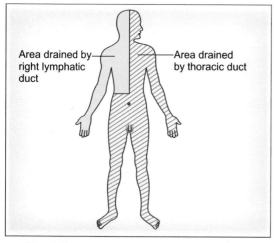

Area drained by right lymphatic duct — Area drained by thoracic duct

Fig. 8.1: Lymphatic drainage of whole body

mphadenitis. It is the inflammation of lymph de. This two phenomenons may occur when e lymphatic system is involved in the spread cancer cell.

mphoedema. The accumulation of lymph in sue space. When lymph does not drain from area of the body. It is seen in coastal region Orissa, there is repeated attack by a bacteria. he lower limb is most commonly affected and e condition is known as elephantiasis, edema upper limb occurs due to removal of axillary mph node after cancer of breast.

he LN are bean shaped structures having a n (depression) on one side. They are not so inent in health, but during inflammation it is nguishable. A numerous afferent lymphatics the node from periphery. The single (usually) ent vessel leaves the LN through helium. A h vessel in its course passes through different of lymph nodes before it reaches the final ination.

ional Lymph Nodes

important regional lymph nodes are:
ymph nodes of head and neck
ymph nodes of axilla (armpit)
ymph nodes of inguinal region.

4. Lymph nodes of mediastinum.
5. Lymph nodes of mesentery.

Lymph Nodes of Head and Neck (Figs 8.2A and B)

It divides into two division, superficial (lies in the superficial fascia) and deep (lies beneath the deep fascia). The members of superficial sets are arranged in circular chain along the base of mandible. They are named as follows:

1. Occipital LN—One to 2 in number (in back of head – often enlarged due to dandruff in the head).
2. Mastoid LN—Two to 3 in number (behind the auricle – postauricular).
3. Parotid LN—Three to 4 in number (in front of auricle – preauricular).
4. Buccal (facial) LN—Two to 3 in number lies along the facial vein.
5. Submandibular LN—Eight to 10 in number, situated in the submandibular region – Enlarged in tongue disease.
6. Submental LN—One to 2 in number, situated below the chin (enlarged commonly in tongue disease).
7. Deep cervical LN—Twenty to 30 in number – It is a long chain of LN situated along side the

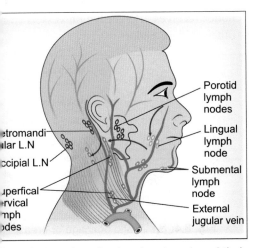

labels: Porotid lymph nodes, Lingual lymph node, Submental lymph node, External jugular vein, etromandi-lar L.N, ccipial L.N, uperfical rvical mph des

Fig. 8.2A: Lymph nodes head and neck and their areas of drainage (superficial)

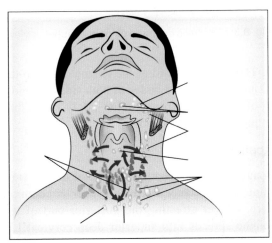

Fig. 8.2B: Lymph nodes of neck: Arrows indicate the lymphatic drainage of thyroid gland, larynx and trachea

carotid sheath deep to sternocleido mastoid. They form superior (jugulodigastric) and inferior (jugulo-omohyoid) groups.

Lymphatic Drainage of Tongue (Fig. 8.3)

1. Lymphatics from the tip of tongue drains to submental lymph nodes (of both sides).
2. The right and left halves of remaining part of anterior 2/3rd of tongue drain to the sub mandibular lymph node of the corresponding side. A few central lymphatics drain to the same nodes of both sides.

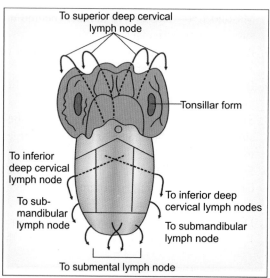

Fig. 8.3: Lymphatic drainage of tongue (superior view)

3. The posterior 1/3rd of the tongue drains to the jugulo-omohyoid nodes of both sides. As most of the lymph from tongue lately drain into jugulo-omohyoid nodes.

Applied

Tongue—The lymphatic drainage of tongue is of clinical importance because cancer is common here. Cancer affecting the posterior part of the tongue spreads into superior deep cervical LN

(jugulo-digastric group) on both sides. Whe cancer from anterior part of tongue spread inferior deep cervical lymph nodes (jug omohyoid group). Cancer in the tip of tongue spread into submental and submandibular g of lymph nodes and in all cases nodes are enla and feel stony hard.

Axillary Lymph Nodes (Fig. 8.4)

These nodes lie in axilla. They are divided in groups.

1. Anterior (pectoral) group—Three to number – lying along the lower border o pectoralis minor.
2. Posterior (subscapular) group—Six to number – lying in front of the subscapu muscle.
3. Lateral (humeral) group—Six to 7 in num lying along the medial side of axillary vein. T nodes receives most of the lymphatics of u limb.
4. Central group—Three to 4 in number – L in size lying in the center of axilla wthir axillary fat.
5. Infra clavicular (delto pectoral) group—T nodes are not strictly axillary nodes because are located outside.
6. Apical group—Lying at the apex of axilla. T nodes receives efferent lymph vessels fror other axillary nodes.

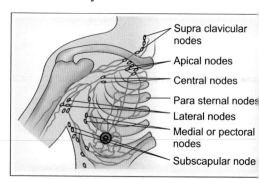

Fig. 8.4: Lymphatic drainage of breast

...phatic Drainage of Breast
(...nmary Gland)

...phatic drainage of breast is clinically important ...use cancer is common in this gland and ...lly, spread of cancer takes place through ...phatics. For the anatomical location and ...iption of tumors, the surface ultimately drain ...jugulo-omohyoid nodes.

...mph passes from nipple, areola and lobules ...e gland pass to the subareolar lymph plexus ...rom it most lymph (more than 75%) drains to ...ary LN Remaining (25%) lymph, mainly ...oral, some also passes directly to detopectoral ...p, supraclavicular particularly from medial ...rant of breast, drains to parasternal nodes of ...e side or opposite side. Lymph from lower ...rant passes to the abdominal nodes (inferior ...nic). Axillary tail drains directly into posterior ...scapular) group of lymph node.

...lied

...axillary LN enlarge and become painful when ...tion of upper limb occur. The lateral group is ...first one to be involved. Excision (cut) and ...ologic analysis is often necessary for treatment ...reast cancer. During the removal of node two ...es are in danger; long thoracic nerve (supply

serratus anterior) and thoracodorsal nerve (supply latissimus dorsi) and to be carefully presented.

Inguinal Lymph Nodes
(Figs 8.6A and B)

They lie below the inguinal ligaments and divided into two groups—superficial and deep.

- Superficial group—Lies in superficial fascia and around like letter T. It is divided into a horizontal (lies below and parallel to inguinal ligament) and vertical group (lies along the upper part of great saphenous vein).

The superficial inguinal LN drain the following area:

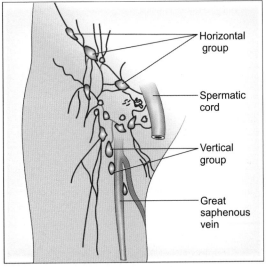

Fig. 8.6A: Distribution of inguinal lymph nodes

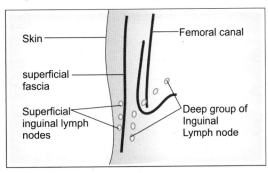

Fig. 8.6B: Relation of superficial and deed inguinal lymph nodes

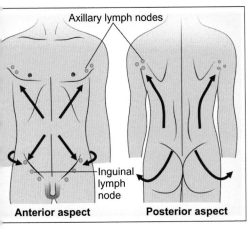

Fig. 8.5: Lymph drainage of skin of trunk

a. Superficial lymphatics from skin and subcutaneous tissue of lower limb (Fig. 8.5).
b. Gluteal region.
c. Anterior abdominal wall below the level of umbilicus.
d. Perineum and external genitalia except glans penis.
e. Vagina and lower part of anal canal.

• Deep inguinal lymph nodes—They are few lymph nodes lying along the upper part of femoral vein. All the vessels from superficial nodes drain into deep group; in addition they receive deep lymphatics from the lower limb. The glans penis also drain into deep inguinal lymph nodes. The efferents from deep inguin LN draind into the external iliac lymph nod (lies along the external iliac artery).

Applied

1. Any infection in the foot, even sometimes tig shoes produce (blister) enlargement of inguin L nodes (superficial group).
2. In cancer of glans penis, deep inguinal lym nodes are enlarged.
3. In carcinoma of body of uterus superfic inguinal lymph nodes (medial group) will enlarged.

Viscera

...IORAX (FIG. 9.1)

...ngs: They are essential organ in respiration; ...nical in shape, covered by thin serous membrane ...sceral pleura), floats in water. It has following ...senting features:

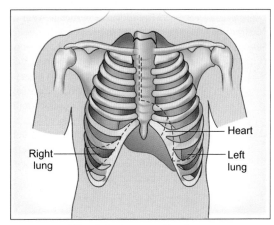

Fig. 9.1: Lungs with pleura

Name	Right lung	Left lung
...pex	Conical; lies above the impression of first rib; covered by cervical pleura (part of parietal pleura) and Sibson's fascia; extends into anterior aspect of root of neck.	Same
...ase	Concave, semilunar, related to liver separated by the diaphragm.	Concavity is less, semilunar, related to left lobe of liver, stomach and spleen separated by diaphragm.
...nterior ...rder	Thin, descends from apex, downwards and medially upto sternal angle, then vertically downwards upto xiphisternal junction slightly right of midline.	Thin, descends from apex, downwards and medially upto sternal angle (slightly left to midline). Then descends vertically downwards upto fourth space. It then deviates towards left 3 to 4 cm away from

Contd...

Name	Right lung	Left lung
		midline producing cardiac notch and lingula and end at left sixth costal cartilage.
Posterior border	Thick, rounded, extends from apex to base and fits in para vertebral gutter.	Same
Costal surface	Identified by impression of ribs, covered by costal pleura (part of parietal pleura).	Same
Medial surface (Mediastinal surface + Vertebral part) Mediastinal surface (Figs 9.2 and 9.3) (Fig. 9.3)	Identified by several impression. Impressions are: • Hilum - Triangular nonpleural impression in which structures of lung root enter and leave the lung. These are from above downwards bronchus, artery, (pulmonary) bronchus, vein (pulmonary vein). • Cardiac impression – lies below and infront of hilum. It is concave, related to sternocostal surface of heart. • Groove for azygos vein – slender groove above the hilum for terminal part of azygos vein. • Groove for superior vena cava – it is the upwards continuation of cardiac impression, wide shallow groove. • Groove for esophagus lies behind the hilum. • Impression of inferior vena cava – thumb like impression lies at the posteroinferior part of the cardiac groove.	• Hilum – triangular nonpleural impression through which the structures passes, related from above downwards are (pulmonary) artery, bronchus, vein (pulmonary). • Cardiac impression – lies below and in front of hilum more concave than right side, related to sternocostal and left surface of heart. • Groove for arch of aorta – deep impression arching above the hilum. • Groove for descending thoracic aorta behind the hilum – it is deep groove.

Contd

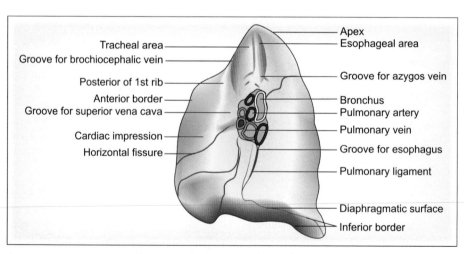

Fig. 9.2: Medial surface of right lung

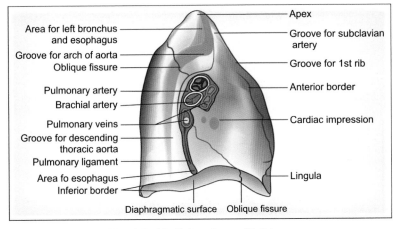

Area for left bronchus and esophagus
Groove for arch of aorta
Oblique fissure
Pulmonary artery
Brachial artery
Pulmonary veins
Groove for descending thoracic aorta
Pulmonary ligament
Area fo esophagus
Inferior border

Apex
Groove for subclavian artery
Groove for 1st rib
Anterior border
Cardiac impression
Lingula

Diaphragmatic surface Oblique fissure

Fig. 9.3: Medial surface of left lung

ame	*Right lung*	*Left lung*
res oblique	Lined by visceral pleura, extends from above and behind the hilum. Cuts the posterior border and descends obliquely downwards and forwards; again it cuts the inferior border, goes to medial surface and end below and infront of hilum.	Same as right lung but obliquity is more marked.
verse e	Lined by visceral pleura, extends from anterior border (at the fourth sternocostal junction) to oblique fissure in mid axillary line.	Not present.
s	3 in number	2 in number
chopul-ry segment n of lung d by ry hus 9.4A and	10 in number • In upper lobe 1. Apical, 2. Anterior, 3. Posterior • Middle lobe 1. Medial, 2. Lateral. • Lower lobe 1. Superior, 2. Anterior basal, 3. Posterior basal, 4. Medial basal, 5. Lateral basal.	10 in number • Upper lobe 1. Apical, 2. Posterior, 3. Anterior, 4. Superior lingular, 5. Inferior lingular. • Lower lobe 1. Superior, 2. Anterior, 3. Posterior, 4. Medial, 5. Lateral basal. Here medial basal segment is suppressed.
y supply	By one right brochial artery branch of third posterior intercostal artery.	By two brachial arteries branch of descending thoracic aorta.
e supply	Both lung by pulmonary plexus formed by, sympathetic (derived from T1–T4 ganglia), parasympathetic from vagi. The sympathetic efferent fibers produce bronchodilatation and vasoconstriction. The parasympathetic efferent fibers produces, bronchoconstriction, vasodilatation and increase glandular secretion.	

Contd...

Name	Right lung	Left lung
Anatomical position / side determination	• Conical apex should be placed above. • Convex base should be placed below. • Thin anterior border should be placed anteriorly. • Thick posterior border should be placed posteriorly. • Medial surface with hilum should be placed medially.	

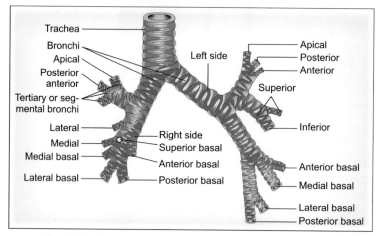

Fig. 9.4A: Bronchi and its divisions (segmental bronchi)

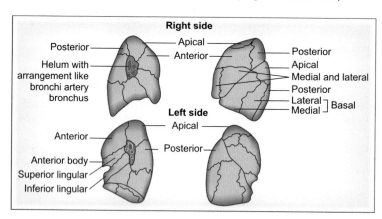

Fig. 9.4B: Bronchopulmonary segments

Applied

1. Pneumonia—Infective inflammation of lung; in which fluid accumulated in the alveoli area. It is cured by proper antibiotics.

2. Asthma—An obstructive condition, which is characterized by coughing, difficult breathing (dyspnea), wheezing and chest tightne partially relieved by antibiotics and bronc dialators.

3. Tuberculosis (TB)—It is an infectious dise caused by bacteria (mycobacterium tube losis). Most common lung disease in country.

ural drainage—Excessive accumulation of
into a lobe or bronchopulmonary segments
interfere with breathing. To facilitate normal
nage a medical person often advise to
ge the posture of patient, so that gravity
sts in process of drainage.

g cancer—It is dangerous and spread rapidly
known as bronchogenic carcinoma.

Important Notes

- In every case of lung disease respiration is impaired.
- Lung is divided functionally into conducting zone (upto terminal bronchiole, which filter, moisten and warm air) and respiratory zone, (respiratory bronchioles to alveoli—where gaseous exchange occur).
- Heart—written in chapter of arteries pg. 119.

minal Viscera (Figs 9.5 and 9.6A to C)

Position of abdominal viscera in relation to regions of abdomen

Viscera	*Quadrants of abdomen*
ch	Right and left hypochondrium and epigastrium.
	Epigastrium, left hypochondrium and umbilical region.
enum	First part extends into epigastrium rest of the parts in umbilical region plastered with the posterior abdominal wall.
eas (Figs 9.6A and B)	It is retroperitoneal and is situated in the epigastrium and left hypochondrium
n	Left hypochondrium and against the nineth, tenth and eleventh rib.
m with appendix	Right iliac fossa.
verse colon	Right lumbar, umbilical and may extend upto hypogastrium, left lumbar, left hypochondrium.
m and anal canal	Pelvic cavity

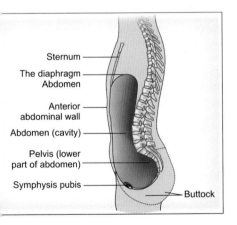

g. 9.5: Abdominal cavity (sagittal section)

Sternum
The diaphragm
Abdomen
Anterior abdominal wall
Abdomen (cavity)
Pelvis (lower part of abdomen)
Symphysis pubis
Buttock

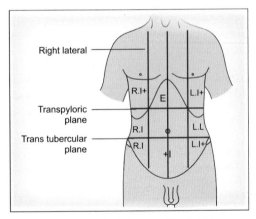

Fig. 9.6A: Regions of abdomen RH-right hypochondrium E–Epigastrium, LH–Left hypocondrium, RL–Right lumbar, U–Umbilical, LL–Left lumbar, RE–Right iliac, H–Hypogastrium, LI–Left iliac

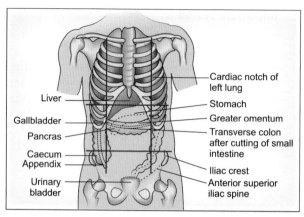

Fig. 9.6B: Postions of viscera in different quadrants of abdomen

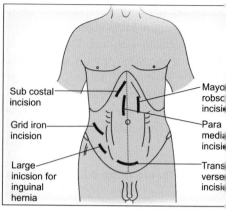

Fig. 9.6C: Abdominal incisions

Name	Features
GI Tract stomach shape	J shaped in normal built.
Capacity (in adult) and newborn	1500 cc usually empties food after 3 hours capacity is 50 cc, that's why infant requi more frequent meals.
Situation	Epigastrium, umbilical, and left hypochondrium
Two orifices 1. Cardiac orifice 2. Pyloric orifice	Deeply placed, lies 1 inch left of the median plane at the level of seventh cos cartilage. Superficially situated; 1inch to the right of the median plane and transpyloric line.

Two borders
1. Lesser curvature
  (right border)
 	
2. Greater curvature
  (left border)
  (Figs 9.7 and 9.8A)
	Start from the right margin of esophagus, goes towards the right upto pylorus.
	• At the most dependent part there is an angular notch known as incisura angular
	• Lesser omentum is attached here.
	• Anastomosis of right and left gastric artery lies in this border.
	  Start from cardiac notch; ascends upwards, backwards and to the left upto
	  fifth intercostal space, then runs downwards, forwards and to the right upto pylor
	• From above downwards gastrophrenic, gastrosplenic and greater omentum attached.

Two surfaces
1. Anterosuperior
2. Posteroinferior
  surface
  (Fig. 9.8A)
	Related to diaphragm, liver and anterior abdominal wall.
	Lies on following structures that constitute the stomach bed:
	1. Left kidney
	2. Left suprarenal gland
	3. Left crus of diaphragm.
	4. Pancreas (body)
	5. Left colic flexure
	6. Transverse mesocolon.
	7. Splenic artery.

Cont

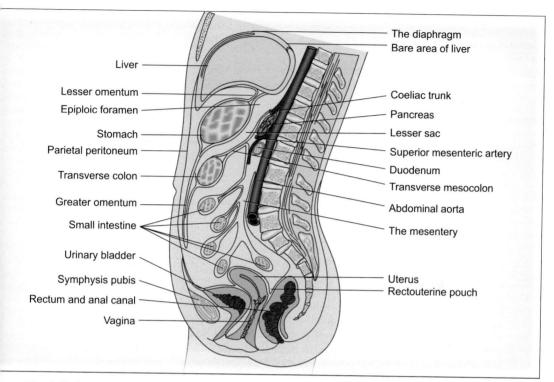

Fig. 9.7: Sagittal section of abdomen showing peritoneal cavity and the folds of peritoneum

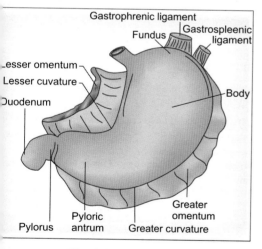

Fig. 9.8A: Stomach

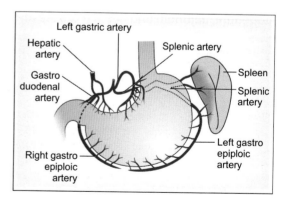

Fig. 9.8B: Arteries of stomach and spleen.

Name	Features
Cavity of stomach has three parts:	
Fundus	• It is the part above the horizontal line, from cardiac notch to greater curvature. Normally it contains gas. In X-ray film it looks black.
Body (Fig. 9.8A)	• From fundus upto a line that extends from incisura angularis vertically downwards. Inside which, there are temporary fold (rugae) in mucous membrane which disappear when stomach is full.
Pyloric part.	• Extends from right side of body to pyloric (proximal part) constriction. Pyloric part is further subdivided into pyloric autrum and pyloric canal (distal part).
Artery supply (Fig. 9.8B)	• Principal supply by left gastric – branch of coelic trunk. • Right gastric – branch of hepatic • Short gastric – branch of splenic, supply the fundus of stomach
Venous drainage	Correspond to arteries.
Nerve supply	Autonomic nervous system – Sympathetic from celiac plexus (T6 segment). Parasympathetic – From vagi via anterior and posterior gastric nerves.
Applied	• Gastric ulcer – Breach (break in continuity) in mucus membrane occur along the lesser curvature very common disease in case of low income groups. • Malignancy (cancer) – Affects stomach, readily spread to surrounding viscera, i.e. esophagus, pancreas due to profuse lymphatics. • Gastric pain – It is felt in the epigastrium, due to same segmental supply. The sensation of visceral pain is caused by the distention or spasmodic contraction of smooth muscle
Anatomical position	• Place stomach on left hand with lesser curvature facing towards right. • Thin cardiac end should be above, and directed to left side. • Thick pyloric end (occasionally bile stained) should be placed below and to the right of the midline.

Duodenum, Jejunum and Ileum (Figs 9.9 and 9.10)

Features	Duodenum	Jejunum	Ileum
Situation	In posterior abdominal wall.	Between the outline of large gut.	Between the outline of large gut and in pelvis.
Shape	C shaped and consists of four parts – First (2 inches in length), Second (3 inches in length), Third (4 inches in length) and Fourth (1 inch in length).	Proximal 2/5th (8 inches) is jejunum.	Distal 3/5th (12 inches) of small intestine is ileum.
Mesentery	No mesentery, so less mobile.	Present (highly mobile).	Present (highly mobile).
Wall	Thick	Thicker	Thin
Lumen, circular folds	Absent in first 1 inch of duodenum. In the second part of	Permanent, very thick and closely placed and due to this	Permanent, thin and li at a distance from o

Contd

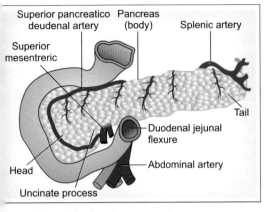

Fig. 9.9: Duodemum and pancreas

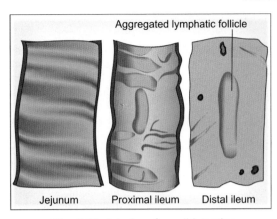

Fig. 9.10: Interior of small intestine

Features	Duodenum	Jejunum	Ileum
	duodenum in postero medial aspect there is a papilla (major duodenal papilla) on which, common bile duct and pancreatic duct open, unitedly or separately.	reason it feels like two tubes on palpation.	another. Feeling of single tube on palpation.
eritoneal ·indow and ascularity	Not present	Thinner near gut due to absence of fat. • Arterial arcades are less (1 or 2 in number). • Vasa recti (long)	Thicker near gut due to presence of fat. • Arterial arcades are more (5 or 6 in number). • Vasa recti (short).
·rterial supply	Auperior and inferior pancreatico duodenal.	Jejunal branch of superior mesenteric.	Ileal branches of superior mesenteric.
·pplied	The first part of duodenum is the common site for duodenal ulcer. In barium to med X-ray first 1 inch of first part of duodenum shows a triangular white shadow called duodenal cap. In duodenal ulcer there is defective duodenal cap.	Because of its extent and position traumatic injury is common here. Small penetrating injuries may self- healed but in large bullet wound, material leaks freely into the peritoneal cavity. Small bowel content have nearly neutral pH and produce slight irritation in the peritoneum.	• Meckel's diverticulum – It is a diverticulum present in 2% of cases 2 feet away from ileocaecal junction, 2 inches in length and lies in antimesenteric border. • The payer's patches get ulcerated in typhoid fever. There may be perforation of intestine.
·portant features note	There is no sharp demarcation between jejunum and ileum. The change from jejunum to ileum is a gradual structural change.		

Name and features	Description

Pancreas (Fig. 9.9)	It is a mixed gland, soft and lobulated, placed transversely along the posterior abdominal wall. It occupies epigastrium and left hypochondriac region. It has four parts – flattened globular head, small constricted neck, prismoid body (with three surfaces and three borders) and a small tail. Important structures related to pancreas
	1. Head – Lies in the concavity of duodenum. Anteriorly lies transverse colon; posteriorly related with inferior vena cava.
	2. Neck – Behind it lies portal vein.
	3. Body – Presents three surfaces and three borders
	  a. Anterior surface - related to stomach and peritoneal.
	  b. Posterior surface – Nonperitoneal, related with abdominal aorta, left crus of diaphragm, left psoas major muscle, left kidney.
	  c. Inferior surface – Peritoneal, related to duodeno jejunal flexure, coils of small intestine. Three borders
	  a. Superior border – related to tortuous splenic artery.
	  b. Anterior border – transverse mesocolon is attached.
	  c. Inferior border – related to origin of superior mesenteric artery. Tail – lies within the lienorenal ligament.

Exocrine part of pancreatic ducts	Main pancreatic duct lies near its posterior surface, extends from left to right, receive small tributaries (looks like fish bone pattern). Within the head of pancreas common bile duct related to its right side. The two ducts, in the second part of duodenum, join and open over the major duodenal papilla 8 to 10 cm away from pylorus.
Endocrine parts	Consists of islets of Langerhans, secretes insulin (by β cells), glucagon (by α cells) gastrin and somatostatin (by δ cells).
Arterial supply	• Mainly by pancreatic branch of spelenic artery. • Superior and inferior pancreatic duodenal arteries.
Applied	1. Inflammation of pancreas is known as pancreatitis, which produces pain referred to back of abdomen. 2. Lack of insulin produces diabetes mellitus. 3. Deficiency of pancreatic juice produces digestive disturbances. 4. Carcinoma of the head of pancreas is quite common.
Anatomical position	It is always lies along with duodenum and spleen. • Hold the specimen in such a way that C shaped duodenum is on right hand and spleen on left hand. • If only pancreas is present then place globular head to right, triangular body in the middle, and tail towards the left hand. • Posterior surface, identified by splenic vein placed posteriorly.
Spleen (Fig. 9.11A)	It is soft, blood riched, pinapple colored, mobile and largest lymphoid organ in body located just beneath the diaphragm.
Situation and size	It is situated behind the stomach in the left hypochondrium. The size of the organ is 1 inch in thickness, 3 inches in breadth and 5 inches in length. It extends from left 9th rib to 11 rib of which 10th rib is the axis.

Conto

Name and features	Description
Presenting parts	It has 2 ends, 2 borders, 2 surfaces, 2 important ligaments and is completely covered by peritoneum except hilum. Two ends; medial (smaller and rounded) directed medially and upwards, lateral end is broader. Borders are 1. Superior – marked by notches anteriorly. 2. Inferior border – separates diaphragmatic surface from visceral surface. Diaphragmatic surface smooth and related to diaphragm. Visceral surface is marked near its middle by hilum which gives passage of splenic artery and vein. This surface is related to stomach (above hilum), left kidney, below hilum and at the lateral end with left colic flexure. Spleen is surrounded by splenic capsule which sends trabeculae inside the substance of spleen. In it rounded areas consists of lymphocytes and reticular tissue is white pulp, red pulp is the all other splenic tissues.
Applied	• Enlargement of spleen is known as splenomegaly. It is due to chronic maleria, chronic kalazar and leukemias (blood cancer). • As the splenic capsule is relatively thin, a direct blow or fall on the ground during playing may cause it, to rupture. The spleen is removed quickly and it is known as splenectomy. Care should be taken during removal, to avoid tail of pancreas.
Anatomical position	• Spleen should be placed on left hand with smooth convex surface lies over the palm. • Superior border identified by notches should be placed above. • Visceral surface (identified by hilum) should be placed above. • Rounded medial end (smaller) should be directed above and medially. • Large lateral end should be directed downwards and laterally.

LARGE INTESTINE

Large intestine (extends from caecum to anal orifice – 5 feet long).

Important Features (Cardinal Feature)

1. Presence of Tinea (longitudinal muscle aggrigation).
2. Sacculation (haustration).
3. Appendices epiploicae (peritoneal pocket containing fat).

Name and features	Description
Caecum (A blind pouch) (Fig 9.12A)	It is the commencement of large intestine, 6 cm long, 7 cm broad; lies in right iliac fossa. Caecum has a large right pouch and small left pouch with appendix hanging down from its posteromedial aspect. Ileum open in it through ileocaecal orifice, guarded by ileocaecal valve. The valves are formed by duplication mucous membrane containing submucous coat and circular muscle of ileum.
Applied (Figs 9.12A and B)	Caecum is often infected by amoebiosis. Carcinomas of caecum are also common.
Artery supply	Anterior and posterior caecal arteries branches of iliocolic branch of superior mesenteric artery.

Contd...

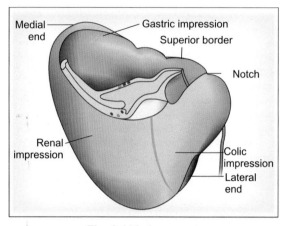

Fig. 9.11A: Large gut

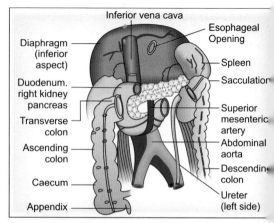

Fig. 9.11B: Spleen (visceral surface)

Name and features	Description
Appendix vermiform (worm like) (Fig 9.12B) (Fig. 10.18 in Embryology)	It is a blind diverticulum from the posterior medial aspect of caecum, 2 cm below th ileocaecal junction. Lengths 7 to 10 cm (average). It belongs to large gut, but without an haustration and appendices epiploicae. All the taenia coli starts from the base of appendi Commonest position of appendix is retrocaecal. Second common position is pelvic. Othe position is splenic (tip directed towards the spleen) – When lie in front of terminal ileu it is known as pre-ileal varity. This position is dangerous in appendicitis. Appendix has triangular fold of mesentry – mesoappendix, so it is highly mobile. It is supplied b appendicular artery – branch of posterior caecal. Appendicistis – Inflammation of appendix; which causes vague pain around the umbilicu at first (due to same segmental supply [T10]) next severe pain on Mc Burney's poir where maximum tenderness is felt.
Anatomical position	• Hold the viscera in such a way that cut end is above. • Appendix should be placed below and posteomedial to ileo-caecal orifice.
Ascending colon (Fig. 9.11B)	15 cm in length, wider than descending colon – It extend from ileocaecal orifice to rig colic flexure, supplied by right colic artery – branch of superior mesenteric.
Transverse colon (Figs 9.7 and 9.11B)	50 cm in length; extends from right colic flexure (1 inch below the transpyloric plane a 4 inches to the left of midline to left colic flexure. This flexure is 1 inch above t transpyloric plane and 4 inches away from midline. Artery supply–middle colic (bran of superior mesenteric).
Anatomical position	• Transverse colon is identified by two mesenterics, i.e. greater omentum and transver nesocolon. • Place the colon in such a way that right colic flexure (wider) should lies below the l colic flexure (narrower). • It has a mesentery– transverse mesocolon.
Descending colon	• 25 cm in length, narrower than ascending colon. • Extends from left colic flexure to sigmoid colon. • Artery supply – Sigmoid arteries – branches of inferior mesenteric.

Cont.

ame and features	*Description*
id colon	• 40 cm in length, extends upto third sacral vertebrae where it becomes rectum. It has a triangular sigmoid mesocolon. It is supplied by sigmoidal arteries. • Visualisation of interior of sigmoid colon by means of endoscope (an instrument) is known as sigmoidoscopy.
n).12B, 9.13 and	It begins at third sacral vertebra; passes downwards in the concavity of sacrum, and at the level of coccyx, it is dialated and form ampulla. At about 3cm in front of the coccyx it bends sharply backwards to become the anal canal. It has peritoneum of the upper third in anterior and lateral aspect, and on the middle-third in its anterior surface. Inferior 1/3rd is nonperitoneal. • It is related anteriorly rectovesical pouch, (peritoneal pouch) base of bladder, prostate, seminal vesicle and vas deferens in case of male, and pouch of Douglas (recto uterine pouch), post wall of vagina, in case of female. The rectum has three lateral bends. The highest and the lowest are concave to the left. Internally there are three horizontal shelves (valves of Houston) of mucosa. The upper part of rectum serves as faecal reservoir.

Contd...

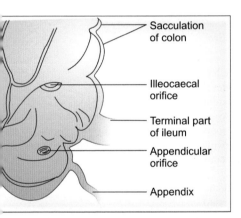

Fig. 9.12A: Interior of caecum

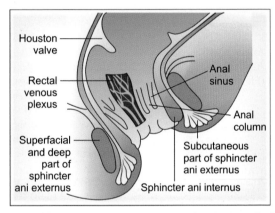

Fig. 9.12B Rectum and anal canal (sagittal section)

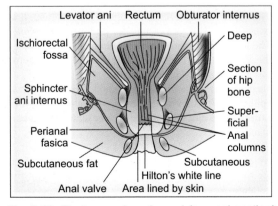

Fig. 9.13: Rectum and anal canal (coronal section)

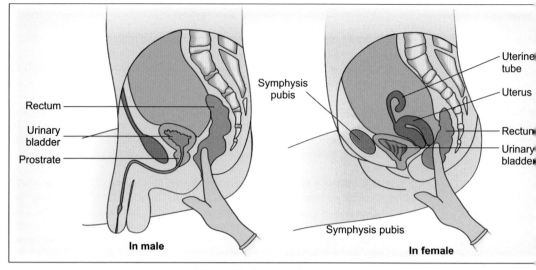

Fig. 9.14: Per rectal examination

Name and features	Description
Artery supply Applied (Fig. 9.14)	1. By superior rectal artery – branch of inferior mesenteric. 2. By middle rectal – branch of internal iliac. 3. By inferior rectal – branch of internal pudendal. Per-rectal examination (P/R) by means of finger is done to assess the anterior of rec as well as condition of the neighbouring structures specially the postrate in male, condition of genital tract in virgin women.To visualise the interior of rectum by mer an instrument is known as Proctoscopy.
Anatomical position	• Place peritoneal surface (shiny) anteriorly. • Nonperitoneal (dull) surface benind.
Anal canal. (Figs 9.12B and 9.13)	It is the last part of GI tract. It lies in the perineum, below the pelvic diaphragm 3.8 long.; the interior of anal canal is divisible into three parts: 1. The upper 15 mm is lined by columnar epithelium. It ends below at the pectinate (wavy line). This part of mucosa presents *anal columns* (longitudinal mucus fo The lower ends of anal column are united to each other by transverse fold of mu membrane; these folds are called *anal valves*. In between columns and valves t lies a depression called *anal sinus*. 2. Next 15 mm is the middle part known as *area pecten*, lined by stratified squan epithelium. Rectal venous plexus is situated in between mucosa and muscle coat. 3. Lower part 8 mm long, linned by true skin, present hair follicle, sebaceous and sv glands.
Nerve supply	Above pectinate line supplied by autonomic nerves which is insensitive to pain, to Below the pectinate line supplied by somatic nerve which is sensitive to pain, to temperature.

Con

...me and features	*Description*
...ed	1. Piles (Hemorrhoids) – Internal pile (true) – painless. They bleed profusely during straining due to passage of hard stool. The primary piles are seen in 3, 7, and 11 O' clock.region (in lithotomy posture, formed by enlargement of superior rectal vein).
...mical position	2. Fissure – It is due to tearing of one of the anal valves. • Lower end (identified by black stained skin) should be placed below. • Hold the specimen in such a way that upper part lies in the concavity of palm and lower end should be below the level of finger, producing perineal flexure.
...9.15)	The liver is the largest gland in the body, occupies mainly in the right hypochondrium, epigastrium and partly into left hypochondrium. It has manifold activities. It metabolises carbohydrate and protein after their absorption from intestine and secrete bile which digest fats. In natural state it is reddish brown, very soft like a jelly. Its weight is near about 1.5 kg and almost completely covered with peritoneum. In formalin hardened specimen it composed of 5 surfaces (follows the role of 5), 5 fissures, 5 borders, 5 bare areas (not covered by peritoneum). The surfaces are triangular (1) anterior (marked by saggitally placed falciform ligament – which divide the liver into right and left lobe). (2) Posterior (marked by a groove for inferior vena cava), (3) superior surface is convex (divided into two unequal lobes by attachment of falciform ligament), (4) inferior surface is uneven and slopping (most prominent surface) and (5) right lateral surface (forms the base and related to 7 to 11 ribs). The structure related to inferior surface from left to right side, stomach (gastric impression), pyloric impression (on the right side of ligamentum teres), duodenal impression (for 1st part of duodenum) in quadrate lobe. The fossa for the gallbladder, lies to the right of quadrate lobe, colic impression for right colic flexure

Contd...

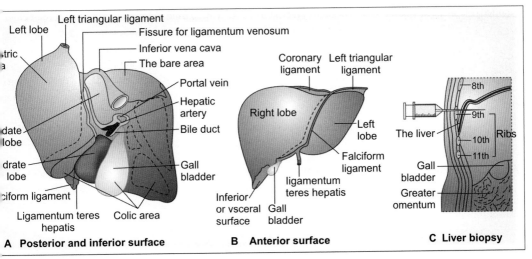

A Posterior and inferior surface   **B Anterior surface**   **C Liver biopsy**

Fig. 9.15: Liver and applied

Name and features	*Description*
	and the renal impression for right kidney. The 5 fissures are, fissures for ligamen venosum, ligamentum teres hepatis, groove for inferior vena cava, fossa gallbladder and porta hepatis (which is a gateway from where hepatic artery two division of portal vein goes in and two division of hepatic duct and lympha comes out).
	Out of 5 borders 3 are prominent, posterosuperior border, posteroinferior bo and inferior border (most prominent and sharp). It separates inferior surface f anterior surface and right lateral surface. Out of 5 bare areas 3 are important The bare area (triangular), present on posterosuperior aspect of right lobe of li demarcated by superior and inferior layer of coronary ligament; and groove inferior vena cava, (2) porta hepatis and fossa for gallbladder. Liver is broa subdivided into right and left lobe. Anatomical line of separation passes thro attachment of falciform ligament and behind by fissure for ligamentum venos and ligamentum teres. So, two other lobes quadrate and caudate lobes belong right lobe anatomically. But for practical purpose physiological division has tremendous importance and physiologic line of demarcation passes throu cholecysto vena caval line (i.e. groove for inferior vena cava and fossa gallbladder). So, physiological left lobe possess caudate and quadrate lobe. ligaments of liver are peritoneal, and nonperitoneal. Peritoneal ligaments (fa are falciform ligament, superior and inferior layer of coronary ligament, left right triangular ligament, lesser omentum. Non peritoneal (true) ligaments ligamentum teres hepatis and ligamentum venosum.
Arterial supply	Hepatic artery branch of caeliac trunk. Nutrition is carried to the liver by po vein. Venous drainage – Hepatic veins (2 to 3 in number) pierces the groove inferior vena and drain immediately into inferior vena cava.
Applied	1. Normally liver is palpable under costal margin in case of children below th years (because of huge size of the gland and small pelvic cavity). 2. Benign (not harmful) tumor of liver is known as hematoma. 3. Secondary metastasis (spread) of cancer cells are common. 4. Cirrhosis of liver – Detruction of liver tissue with haphazard degeneration (w out) and regenerations feature (growth). The liver is shrunken, and functions impaired. 5. Liver biopsy – Removal of small amount of liver tissue, from right lateral surfa of liver, between 8th and 9th rib is known as liver biopsy.
Anatomical position	Groove for inferior vena cava should be vertical. Inferior surface should be plac downwards, backwards and to the left.

Genitourinary System (Figs 9.16 and 9.17)

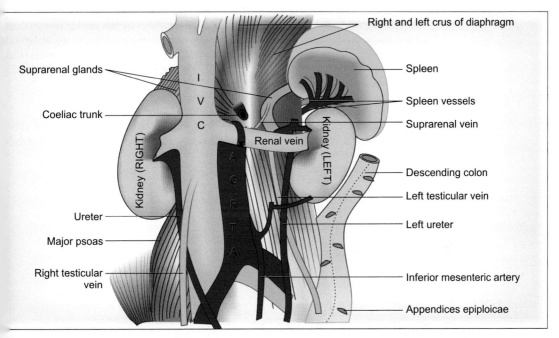

Fig. 9.16: Structures around the kidney (after removal of duodenum and pancreas)

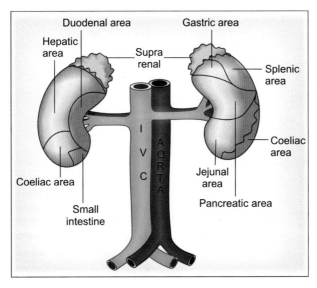

Fig. 9.17: Anterior surface of kidney with its relation

Name and features	Description
Kidney (Figs 9.18A and B)	The kidneys are bean shaped retro peritoneal suructure, which remove waste products (urea, uric acid, creatinine, etc) from the blood. It is highly vascular and has two surfaces, two poles, two borders (follow the rule of 2). Average length of kidney is 10 cm, breadth 6 cm and thickness 3 cm and weight roughly 150 gm. Left kidney is at higher level than right. It extends from T11 to L3 vertebra. The two kidneys are covered from inside outwards: 1. Renal capsule (easily stripped out) – goes into renal sinus. 2. Peri renal fat (perinephric fat) – it goes into the renal sinus. 3. Renal fascia – It consists of anterior and posterior layer. Upper part fuses above kidney and encloses suprarenal in separate compartment. The two layers remain separated in lower part. 4. Para renal fat – situated by the side of kidney. It acts as packing material.

The presenting features (Fig. 9.17)	Right	Left
Upper pole	• Related to triangular right supra-renal gland. • Right lobe of liver, second part of duodenum, right colic flexure, coils of small intestine.	Related to semilunar suprarenal (left) gland. Related to fundus of stomach, spleen, left colic flexure and coils of small intestine.

Posteriorly both kidneys are related with diaphragm. 12th rib, psoas major and quadratus lumborum muscles, su costal vessels and nerve, iliohypogastric vessels and nerve.

Coronal Section (Fig. 9.18A)	Coronal section of kidney presents two distinct area. Outer cortex and inner medull and a space known as renal sinus. In medulla few conical structures are seen which ar renal pyramids. In apices of pyramid 16-20 duct of Bellini opens. The papilla is receive by a cup like tube known as calices minor. In between two pyramid there are cortica

Contd

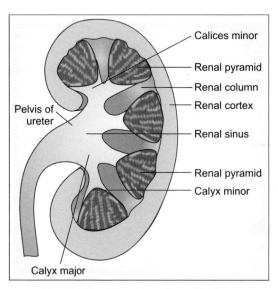

Fig. 9.18A: Coronal section of kidney

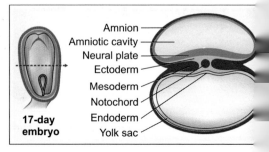

Fig. 9.18B: Development of kidney

Name and features	Description
	tissue, known as renal column; over the base of pyramid the cortical tissue is known as cortical arches. Several minor calices join and form major calyx. Two to three major calyces join to form pelvis of ureter.
Blood supply	1. By renal artery (right and left) – Lateral branch of abdominal aorta. 2. Accessory renal arteries (30% case) – usually supplies the lower pole.
Applied	In newborn/infant renal functions are weak. Similarly in old age due to destruction of nephrons renal function is weak. So in these extreme ages drug should be administered cautiously. • Renal stone – very common • Polycystic kidney
Anatomical position	• Anterior surface of kidney should be identified by relation of structures at hilum. Hold the kidney in such a way that long axis should be directed downwards and laterally. • Place right kidney at lower level than left.
Urinary bladder (Figs 9.19A to C)	The urinary bladder is a muscular sac, which stores urine. It lies behind the symphysis pubis, on the pelvic floor (formed by levator ani muscle). In male, rectum lies behind the urinary bladder but in females, uterus lies in between rectum and bladder. In contracted state, it presents three surfaces (superior, two inferolateral), an apex, base (posterior surface) and a neck. In case of male, neck is surrounded by prostate gland.
Presenting parts	1. Superior surface—peritoneal, related to coils of small intestine. 2. Two inferolateral surface—Nonperitoneal, related in front with a space known as space of retzius and loose areolar tissue. This space allows dilatation of urinary bladder. 3. Base of Posterior Surface—Situated behind, nonperitoneal. In male, this surface is related to seminal vesicle and ampulla of vas. The two ureters open in this surface. 4. Apex—Pointed and median umbilical ligament is attached. 5. Interior of bladder—The interior of bladder has openings for both ureters and the urethra. The smooth triangular region outlined by those three openings is the internal trigone (trigon – triangular). The trigon is important clinically because infections tend to persist in this region. The internal urethral opening is guarded by valve

Contd...

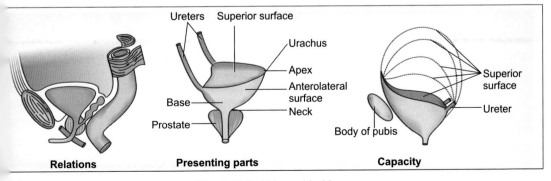

Fig. 9.19A: Urinary bladder

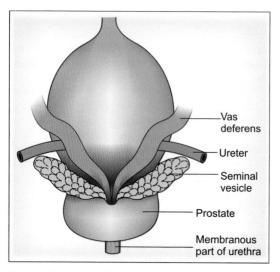

Fig. 9.19B: Male urinary bladder (posterior aspect)

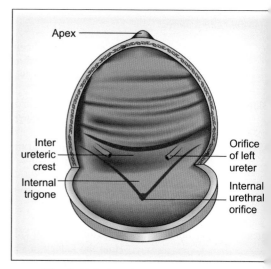

Fig. 9.19C: Interior of urinary bladder

Name and features	Description

(thickened detrusor muscle) – internal urethral sphincter is controlled involuntaril when bladder is disteneded with urine (more than 300 cc) it is palpable above symphysi When it is more distended, it loses its different surfaces and ovoid in shape. At th time, inferolateral surfaces become anterior surface and superior surface is posterio

6. CAPACITY – The mean capacity of adult urinary bladder is 220 ml. Bladder capaci and tone decreases with age leading to frequent micturation (emptying of bladder). newborn, bladder is small and further reason micturition is frequent.

Arterial supply
Applied
(Fig. 9.20)

Superior and inferior vesicle arteries.

• Urinary retention— Bladder is unable to expel its contained urine. It is normal after general anesthesia. Others causes of retention are enlarged prostate. Catheter must be inserted through urethra for drainage.

• Cystoscopy—Visualisation of interior of bladder mucosa by a thin viewing tube is known as cystoscopy.

• Bladder cancer is also not uncommon. It involves the bladder mucosa.·

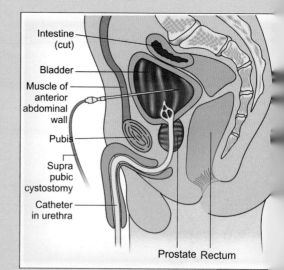

Fig. 9.20: Urethral and supra pubic catheterisation (sagittal section)

Name and features	Description
	Suprapubic cystostomy – When retention of urine is not relieved by catheter, suprapubic cystostomy (a wound done above the symphysis pubis and catheter is introduced in urinary bladder directly) is done
	• Atonic bladder – It is a condition in which bladder is flaccid and overfills, due to injury of spinal cord. It allows urine to dribble (to flow in drops) through sphincters due to temporary loss of micturition reflex.
...tomical position	• In contracted specimen place two inferolateral surface over the palm (like when you offering something to higher spirit).
	• Posterior surface (identified by two seminal vesicle and ampulla of vas) should place posteriorly.
	• Place bladder neck below.

...ale Reproductive System

Name and features	Description
...rus (womb) ...s 9.21, 9.22 and ...)	Nourishes the fertilized egg up to full form fetus. It is pear shaped and has a fundus (no lumen inside), body (where future baby is grown up) and cervix. It is located in pelvis in front of rectum, and postero superior to urinary bladder. In nulliparous woman (who do not give birth to child), it is anteflexed (angle between long axis of body and long axis of cervix) and anteverted (angle between long axis of uterus with that of vagina). The cavity of cervix is known as cervical canal which is almost closed by leaf like arrangement (arbor vitae uteri) of mucous membrane. The cervix communicates with the body by a narrow opening (internal os) and with the vagina by external os (another narrow opening). Cervical mucus also blocks the entry of sperms except at midcycle when the mucus thins out.
...ports of uterus ...s 9.22A to C)	1. Ligamentous – • Lateral aspect – Above, by the peritoneal broad ligaments. - Below, by Macken rod ligament (condensation of pelvic cellular tissue). • In front – Pubocavical ligament (from cervix to symphysis pubis). • Behind – Uterosacral ligament anchors uterus to sacrum. 2. Supports by pelvic floor muscles. The uterine wall is composed of outer serous lining the perimetrium, middle muscle coat (myometrium) and inner endometrium (mucous coat). The endometrium sloughs out periodically during reproductive period (extends from 10 to 50 years). 3. *Artery supply – By tortuous uterine artery –* branch of anterior division of internal iliac.
...plied	1. Uterine prolapse – Congenital weakness of pelvic floor muscle or tearing of muscles and ligaments due to repeated child birth produce prolapse of uterus (descends down of uterus through vagina). 2. Endometriosis – An inflammatory condition of endometrium characterised by abnormal uterine bleeding and pelvic pain. 3. Cancer of cervix is common in female (of 30-50 years age group) which is diagnosec by cervical smear test. 4. Hysterectomy – Surgical removal of uterus is known as hysterectomy.

Contd...

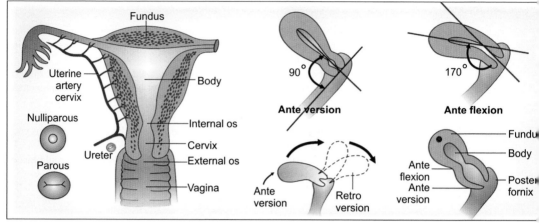

Uterus and vagina in coronal section

Uterus and vagina in sagittal section

Fig. 9.21: Presenting parts of uterus

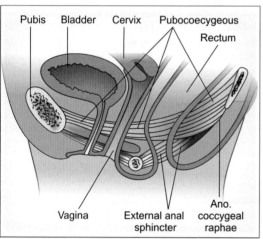

Fig. 9.22A: Supports of uterus (sagittal section)

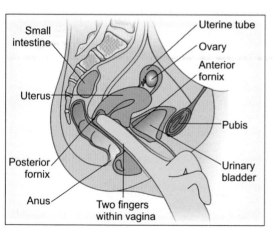

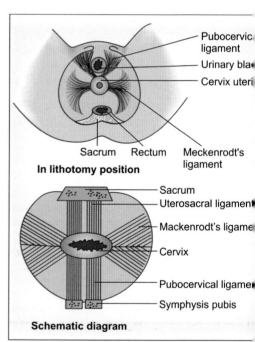

Fig. 9.22B: Ligamentous support

Fig. 9.22C: Per vaginal examination (sagittal section)

Name and features	Description
	5. Laparoscopy – Viewing of interior of abdomen and pelvis by means of instrumental (laproscope) through anterior abdominal wall is known as laparoscopy.
	6. PV Examination – Examination around the cervix (in married women) by passing two fingers in vagina is known as PV examination.
atomical position	• Place more convex anterior surface in front with a bend at the level of internal os.
	• Place uterine tube over the thumb of two hands.
	• Wider fundus is above.
	• Narrow cervix is below.

Reproductive System

Name and features	Description
tis gs 9.23A to C)	Testis (1 inch in diameter, and 1½ inch in length) is male sex gland, one on each side, and suspended by spermatic cord. It has three coverings – from outside inwards tunica Vaginalis, tunica albugenia and tunica vasculosa. The tunica vaginalis is smooth and shiny. The tunica albugenia is the fibrous capsule of testis. From the posterior part of it, an incomplete partition extends into testis known as mediastinum testis. From mediastinum, numerous partitions divide the testis into a number of lobules. Each lobule contains 1 to 3 tightly coiled seminiferous (sperm carrying) tubule. The seminiferous tubule of each lobule converge and form rete (network) testis, located in the mediastinum testis. From the rete testis, sperms ascend to epididymes through efferent ductules.
terial supply	By paired testicular artery – it is a lateral branch of abdominal aorta.
nous drainage	By pampiniform plexus of veins – through testicular veins. Left testicular vein drain into left renal vein at right angle and right one drain into inferior vena cava at acute angle.

Contd...

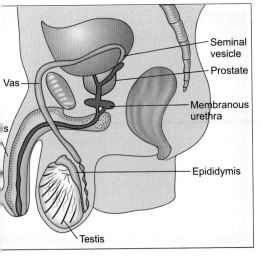

Fig. 9.23A: Male generative organ

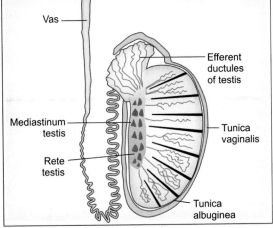

Fig. 9.23C: A semischematic diagram of testis to show its arrangement of tubules and ducts

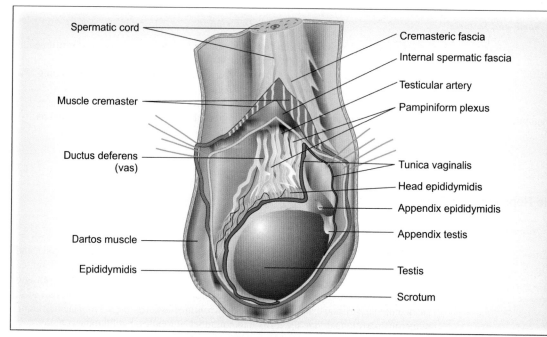

Spermatic cord

Cremasteric fascia

Internal spermatic fascia

Testicular artery

Pampiniform plexus

Muscle cremaster

Ductus deferens
(vas)

Tunica vaginalis

Head epididymidis

Appendix epididymidis

Appendix testis

Dartos muscle

Epididymidis

Testis

Scrotum

Fig. 9.23B: Testis and contents of spermatic cord

Name and features	Description
Applied	• *Varicocele*–Dilation and tortuosity of pampiniform plexus due to lack of drainage is known as varicocoele. Left sided varicocoele is more common. It results in elevation of scrotal temperature, which intereferes with sperm development. • *Orchitis*–Inflammation of testis is known as orchitis, commonly occur during mumps. Carcinoma testes is very common known as seminoma.
Anatomical position	• Place upper pole (identified by comma shaped epididymis) above. • Place lateral surface (identified by sinus of epididymis) laterally. • In this way you can determine the side also.

Viscera of Head and Neck

Name and features	Description
Tongue (Fig. 9.24)	The tongue occupies the floor of the mouth and fills the oral cavity when mouth is closed. It is a muscular (skeletal muscle) organ lined on both surfaces by mucous membrane.
Parts	It has two parts, anterior 2/3 (oral part) and posterior 1/3 (pharyngeal part).
Features	Tongue has dorsum, tip, inferior surface and a root.
Dorsum	Dorsum is divided by V shaped sulcus (sulcus terminalis) into two parts, anterior 2/3 and posterior 1/3, anterior 2/3 is roughened due to papillae of three types. In front of sulcus terminalis, lies twelve vallate papillae (biggest than other two, containing taste buds).

Contd...

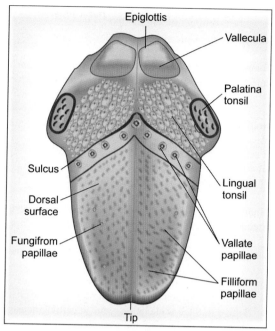

Fig. 9.24: Tongue (Dorsal surface)

Name and features	Description
	Filliform papillae are numerous pointed projection fills up the whole anterior part of tongue and fugiform papillae (club shaped). Fugiform papillae appears as reddish spot over the normal tongue (Fig. 9.24) In posterior 1/3 there are smooth elevation due to lymphoid tissue known as lingual tonsil.
ferior surface	The inferior surface is smooth and in the midline there is a fold of mucous membrane (frenulum linguae) which attaches tongue to the floor of mouth. On either side of frenulum, sublingual duct open over a papilla.
uscle of tongue	It has both extrinsic and intrinsic muscles. Intrinsic muscles mainly change the shape of tongue and there is no bony attachment. Extrinsic muscles change the shape as well as alter position; and anchors the organ to the bone. • Extrinsic muscles are discussed in chapter of muscles.
ood supply	By lingual artery branch of external carotid.
rve supply	Motor – All muscles of tongue (extrinsic and intrinsic) are supplied by hypoglossal (twelvth cranial) nerve except palatoglossus which is innervated by cranial accessory (eleventh cranial). Sensory (General) – Anterior 2/3rd by lingual except vallate papillae, posterior 1/3rd by glossopharyngeal including vallate papillae. Special sense (taste sensation) – Anterior 2/3rd by corda tympani through lingual nerve and posterior 1/3rd by glossopharyngeal.

Name and features	Description
Lymphatic drainage	Discussed in lymphatic system.
Applied	• Tongue tie – In tongue tie (ankyloglossia) frenulum is short due to developme defect. It affects speech depending upon the shortness of frenulum. • Cancer of tongue is also common.
Anatomical position	• Hold the specimen in such a way that rough superior surface (identified by papi placed above. • It is always associated with larynx and pharynx. • Glossy inferior surface lies over the palm. • Pharynx and larynx is directed below and behind.
Pharynx (Figs 9.25 and 9.26)	It is funnel shaped passage connecting nasal cavity to larynx and oral cavity to esopha It extends from base of skull up to sixth cervical vertebra.
Sub division	It has three sub divisions – Nasopharynx, Oropharynx and Laryngopharynx.
Nasopharynx (lining epithelium is ciliated pseudostratified columnar epithelium)	It lies posterior to nasal cavity and superior to soft palate. It is most dilated part and n of its walls are immovable. On its lateral wall opens the pharyngotympanic tube (eustac tube). Behind it, there is elevation – due to cartilaginous part of pharyngo tympanic (tubal elevation). In the roof and posterior wall of nasopharynx collection of lymp tissue known as nasopharyngeal tonsil.

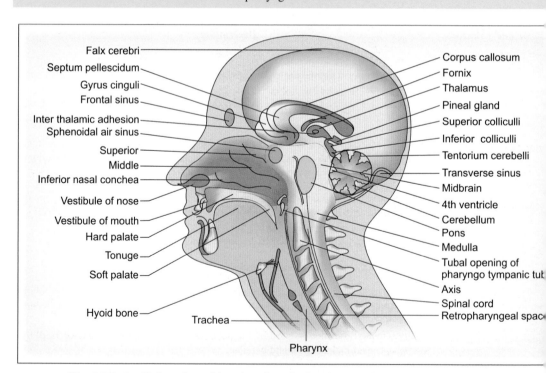

Fig. 9.25: Sagittal section of head and neck showing nasal cavity, pharynx and larynx

Name and features	Description
Oropharynx (Epithelium – stratified squamous epithelium)	Lies posterior to oral cavity; extends from soft palate to epiglottis. In its lateral wall lies palatine tonsil (the tonsil) in a fossa, known as tonsillar fossa. The fossa is between palatoglossal and palatopharyngeal fold.
Laryngopharynx (lined by stratified squamous epithelium)	Lies behind the larynx and extends from epiglottis to cricoid cartilage. The lateral wall of laryngopharynx present pyriform fossa (bounded by aryepiglottic fold on its medial aspect, laterally by mucous membrane lining the lamina of thyroid cartilage.
Pharyngeal muscles (Fig. 9.26)	There are 6 muscles, 3 constrictors (superior, middle and inferior constrictor) and stylopharyngeus, palatopharyngeus and salpingopharyngeus. The constrictors are circularly arranged and fits like three bucket where the superior one is the innermost and inferior one is the outermost. There is overlapping of fibers. All constrictors constrict pharynx and longitudinal muscle shortens the pharynx and propel the food to esophagus.
Artery supply	Ascending pharyngeal – branch of external carotid. Also supplied by branches of facial artery.
Nerve supply – motor	All pharyngeal muscles are supplied by cranial accessory through pharyngeal plexus except stylopharyngeus which is supplied by glossopharyngeal.

Contd...

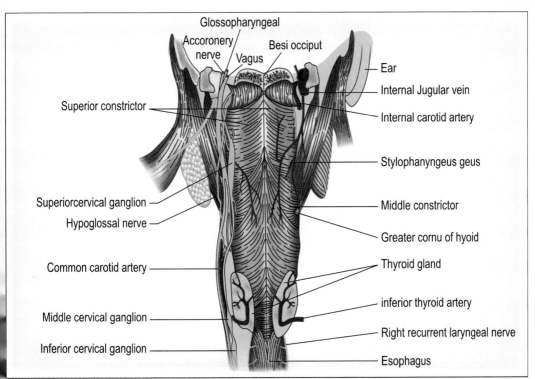

Fig. 9.26: Posterior view of pharynx with three constrictors

Name and features	Description
Applied	Inflammation of nasopharyngeal tonsil is known as adenoids which blocks the airway passage and leads mouth breathing. Common in children in the winter season.
Anatomical position	• Hold the specimen in such a way that rough superior surface of tongue (identified by papillae) placed above. • Glossy inferior surface lies over the palm. • Pharynx and larynx is directed below and behind.
Larynx (Voice box) (Figs 9.27 and 9.28)	Larynx extends from fourth to sixth cervical vertebra; 5 cm in length. It has a cartilaginous framework (epiglottis, thyroid, cricoid and a paired arytenoids cartilages). All cartilages are hyaline except epiglottis (elastic cartilage).
Cavity	The cavity of larynx (interior) is divided into three parts: (1) Vestibule (upper part), (2) sinus of larynx (middle part) and (3) infraglottic (lower part) region. • The laryngeal inlet is bounded by two folds (aryepiglottic fold) on either side, in front by epiglottis and posteriorly by transverse fold between two arytenoid cartilages. The vestibule is limited below by two vestibular fold. Between the vestibular fold (above) and vocal fold (below) lies sinus of larynx. The gap between the two vestibular folds is known as rima glottis or simply glottis. Anterior 3/5th of it is membranous (vocal cord) and posterior 2/5th is cartilaginous (in between vocal process of arytenoids cartilages). Vocal cord looks like pearly white when examined by indirect laryngoscopy.
Muscles (Fig. 9.29)	The muscles of larynx alter the size and shape of laryngeal inlet and causes movement of vocal ligament or changing the tension of vocal cord. There are 9 pairs of very thin muscles which control the phonations and breathing. Alteration of shape of glottis is done by abduction, adduction, tension and relaxation of vocal cord. **Abduction (separation)** – done by posterior cricoarytenoid (safety muscles of larynx). **Adductor (approximation)** – by lateral cricoarytenoid and transverse arytenoids. **Tension (elongation)** – done by cricothyroid and vocalis. **Relaxation (shortening)** – done by thyroarytenoid.
Nerve supply	**Sensory** – Above the vocal fold, mucous membrane is supplied by internal laryngeal branch of superior laryngeal and below the vocal by recurrent laryngeal nerve, branch of vagus. **Motor** – All intrinsic muscle of larynx is innervated by recurrent laryngeal nerve except cricothyroid which is supplied by external laryngeal.
Applied	• If there is damage of superior laryngeal (unilateral) during operation of thyroid cricothyroid muscle of the affected side is paralysed, there is temporary hoarsness of voice. • Bilateral damage of superior laryngeal nerve produces permanent hoarsness because rima glottis cannot close properly. Sensation of vallecula, pyriform fossa and vestibule of larynx is lost – therefore no cough reflex. • In cutting of recurrent laryngeal nerve (unilateral) there is weakness of voice. Bilateral cutting results in permanent hoarsness of voice and respiratory difficulty. • When both superior and recurrent laryngeal nerve is damaged, then there is complete paralysis of vocal cord called cadaveric position.
Anatomical position	• As above (like tongue)

Contd...

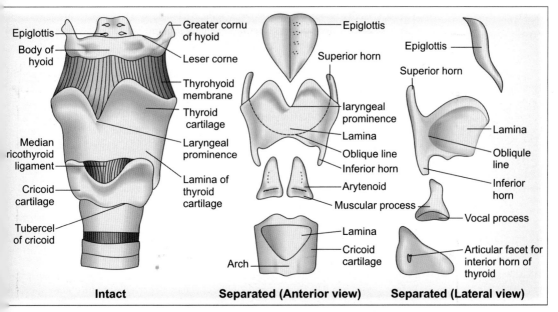

Fig. 9.27: Skeleton of larynx

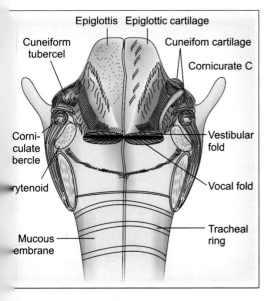

Fig. 9.28: Interior of larynx

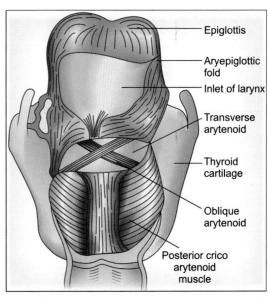

Fig. 9.29: Laryngeal musculative (posterior view)

Name and features	Description
Nasal cavity	The nasal cavity lies posterior to external nose. Air enters the nasal cavity through nostrils. The cavity is divided into two by a midline nasal septum. The nasal cavity is continuous behind with the nasopharynx by choanae (posterior nares).
Nasal septum Boundary (Figs 30A and B)	The septum is formed anteriorly by hyaline cartilage (the saptal cartilage) and posteriorly by perpendicular plate of ethmoid and vomer. The anteroinferior part of nasal septum is highly vascular where septal branch of facial artery, a branch from long sphenopalatine and greater palatine artery anastomoses. It is known as 'Little's area of epitaxis' which produce bleeding in children (commonly due to pricking of nose). The roof is bounded by ethmoid and sphenoid bone; floor is formed by palate (which separates it from oral cavity), the lateral wall is by medial wall of maxilla mainly.
Parts of nasal cavity	The portion of nasal cavity superior to the nostril is called vestibule, is lined by skin. Hair is present for filtering of dust and bacteria from inspired air. Small slit-like area at the roof is covered with olfactory mucosa (contains receptor for sense of smell). The rest of the area is covered with respiratory mucosa (lined by pseudostratified ciliated columnar epithelium). The paranasal air sinuses open into the respiratory region.
Nasal conchae (Fig. 9.31B)	Protruding medially from lateral wall of nasal cavity are three mucous-covered projection known as conchae. The superior and middle conchae are part of ethmoid bone and inferior nasal conchae is a separate piece of bone. The space under the conchae are named superior middle and inferior meatus respectively.Openings that are situated on the lateral wall of nasal cavity (A) Superior meatus – Opening of posterior ethmoidal sinus. (B) Middle meatus – 1. Contains ethmoidal bulla (elevation) – which contain middle group of ethmoidal air cells and it opens on it. 2. Hiatus semilunaris where maxilla sinus, frontonasal duct and anterior group of ethmoidal air cells open. (C) Inferior meatuses-Nasolacrimal duct opens here.
Applied	• Inflammation of nasal cavity is known as rhinitis.

Contd

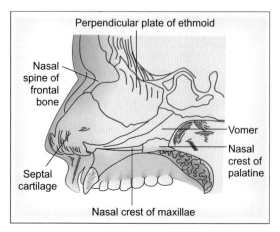

Fig. 9.30A: Nasal septum (sagittal section)

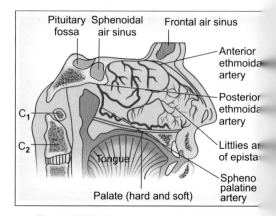

Fig. 9.30B: Blood supply of nasal septum

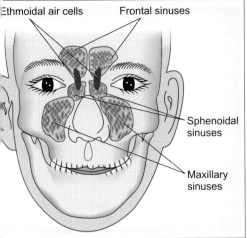

9.31A: Relative position of air sinuses in face

Fig. 9.31B: Paranasal air sinuses (coronal section)

Name and features	Description

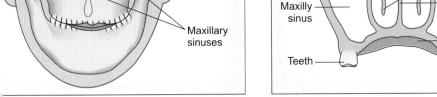

- The nasal septum is not truly median. Excessive deviation of nasal septum is known clinically as deflected nasal septum (DNS). Patients with DNS frequently suffer from common cold and often, respiratory difficulty.
- Benign growth in the nasal cavity is commonly known as polyps.
- Lesion of olfactory nerve due to breakage of cribriform place (usually in motor car accident) and CSF may dribble (drop by drop) through the breakage.

Paranasal air sinuses (Figs 9.31A to C)

The nasal cavity is surrounded by a group of air sinuses known as paranasal air sinuses (PNS). It makes the bone lighter and add moisture to the inspired air. Each sinus is lined by ciliated columnar epithelium. The sinuses are located in frontal, ethmoid, sphenoid and maxillary bones. The sinuses possess a sensory nerve supply and the mouth (ostium) of the sinus is more sensitive and other parts are relatively insensitive.

Maxillary sinus – Largest paired sinus whose floor is ½ inch deeper to floor of nasal cavity. Its opening to the nasal cavity is minimized by lacrimal (in front), palatine (from behind) uncinate process of ethmoid from above and a process of inferior nasal concea from below.

Ethmoidal air sinus (cells) – Lies within labyrinth of ethmoid bone. They are grouped into anterior, middle and posterior groups.

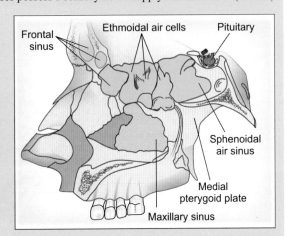

Fig. 9.31C: Paranasal air sinuses (in sagittal section)

Contd...

Name and features	*Description*
	Frontal air sinuses – Paired, unequal size, more prominent in male. It produces m⸱ prominent glabella and superciliary arch, in male and it is absent at birth. Sphenoidal sinus–Unpaired. Situated in middle, lies within the body of sphenoid. It is related pituitary above and cavernus sinus on both sides. It opens in sphenoethmoidal recess
Applied	• Inflammation of sinus due to common cold virus is known as sinusitis. It produ⸱ pain. • Accumulation of infected material in maxillary sinus produces much pain due to p⸱ natural drainage (as the floor of the sinus is deep). Surgical drainage is done by break⸱ the lateral wall of inferior meatus and middle meatus. • Paranasal air sinuses are well visualized in X-ray skull (in occipito-mental view).
Parotid gland (Para – near; otid – ear) (Fig. 9.32) So, gland near the ear	One of the salivary glands. Others are submandibular, sublingual. The large triangu⸱ parotid gland lies in parotid mould; (fossa) between masseter muscle and skin. The fo⸱ is bounded anteriorly by mandible, behind by mastoid process, medially by styloid proc⸱ and above by zygomatic arch. The gland is covered on lateral aspect by th⸱ parotidomasseteric fascia.
Presenting parts	The gland presents a tapering apex (placed downwards), a concave broad base (plac⸱ below the external acoustic meatuses) and three surfaces (A)superficial (related to sk⸱ and subcutaneous tissue), (B) anteromedial surface (deeply grooved by ramus of mandib⸱ and (C) posteromedial surfaces (large and related to mastoid process, styloid proce⸱ transverse process of atlas, facial nerve and external carotid artery).Facial nerve divic the gland into superficial and deep parts.
Parotid duct	By parotid duct the gland pours its secretion in the vestibule of mouth opposite the cro⸱ of upper second molar teeth. Length is 5 cm and can be palpable when teeth is clench⸱

Cont⸱

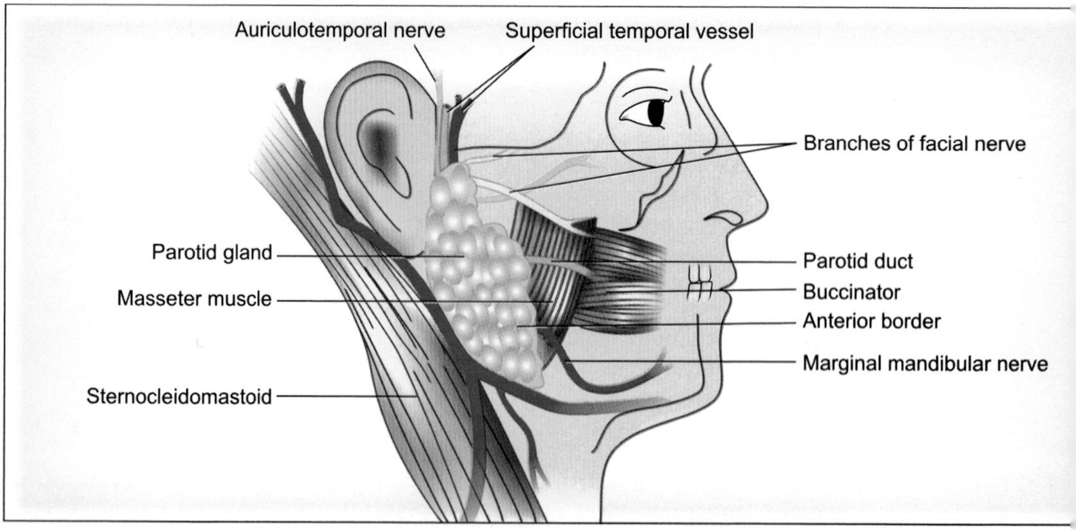

Fig. 9.32: Parotid gland and its relations

Name and features	Description
..tery supply	By external carotid artery and its branches.
..rve supply	By autonomic nervous system. Parasympathetic secretomotor passes through auriculotemporal nerve.
..plied	• Viral infection of parotid gland is known as mumps; common in children. • Inflammatory swelling of gland is very painful due to tough fascial covering. • Mixed parotid tumor – slow growing, benign, painless tumor and of huge size.
..atomical position	• Placed concave broad base, above (often external auditory meatus attached with it). • Tapering apex below. • Anterior border (identified by the presence of parotid duct) and it should be hold by other hand anteriorly. • Lateral surface is smooth and place outside. • Medial surface (identified by fossa and ridges) should be placed inside.
..yroid gland	Butterfly shaped largest endocrine gland situated in front of neck over trachea.
..rts (Fig. 9.33)	It has two lobes connected by median tissue mass called isthmus. The lateral lobe presents upper pole (extends up to oblique line of thyroid cartilage), lower pole (extends up to sixth tracheal ring), three surfaces – superficial (muscular surface), posterior (vascular surface) and medial (tubal surface) and three borders. Muscular surface – is related to sternothyroid muscle. Vascular surface – is related to carotid sheath with common carotid artery and internal jugular vein. Tubal surface – is related to two tubes: • Lower part of larynx and upper part of trachea. • Lower part of pharynx and upper part of esophagus.
..tery supply	Highly vascular thyroid gland is supplied by superior thyroid (branch of external carotid) and inferior thyroid (branch of thyrocervical trunk) arteries; occasionally by arteria thyroidea ima.

Contd...

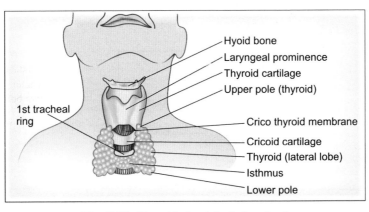

Fig. 9.33: Thyroid gland (anterior view)

Name and features	Description
Applied	• Slight enlargement of thyroid gland during puberty is known as pubertal goit Non-inflammatory; non-neoplastic growth of thyroid gland is known as goite Cancer of thyroid is also common.
Anatomical position	• Hold the butterfly shaped gland in such a way that tapering upper pole shou above. • Flat superficial surface laterally.

Brain

The human brain is like a computer. The brain controls all the functions of our body. It is well-protected within cranial cavity by bones, meninges and cerebrospinal fluid. The fresh brain is pinkish grey tissue and is extremely soft and specimens used in Anatomy are hardened by formalin. average adult male brain weights 1.6 kg and of a woman averages 1.45 kg. In terms of b weight per kg body weight, however, males females have equivalent brain size.

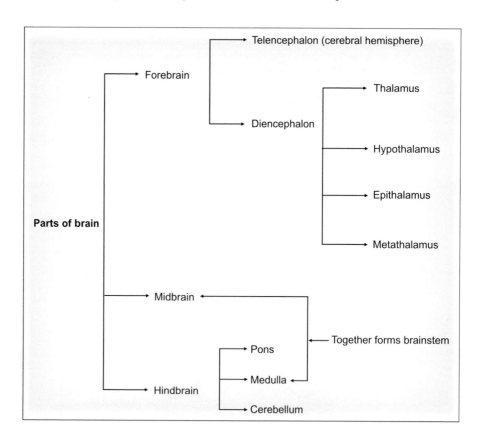

e and presenting parts	*Description*
ebral hemispheres 9.34A)	It is the most superior part of brain. The two hemispheres are separated by a longitudinal fissure into which flax cerebri (a process of dura mater) projects. Almost entire surface of cerebral hemisphere is marked by elevated ridges of tissue called gyri, separated by shallow groove, the sulci. The gyri and sulci increase the surface area of brain.
as three surfaces and e borders	Each cerabral hemisphere has three surfaces (Figs 9.34A to C): (1) convex superolateral surface, (2) the flat medial surface, (3) inferior surface which consists of anterior orbital and posterior tentorial parts. Borders are: (1) Superomedial border separates convex superolateral surface from flat medial surface. (2) Inferolateral border, which presents a notch (preoccipital notch) and it separates superolateral surface from inferior surface. (3) Inferomedial border – separates inferior surface from medial surface and is divided into anterior medial orbital borders and posterior medial occipital borders.
es/important sulci gyri on superolateral ace (Fig. 9.34A)	Three important sulci (central, lateral, parieto-occipital) and two imaginary line divides the cerebrum into four lobes: frontal, temporal, parietal and occipital. The important sulci on superolateral surfaces are central sulcus, pre-central sulci, post-central sulcus, posterior rami (branch) of lateral sulcus and parieto-occipital sulcus (extends only about ½ cm in this surface).
Central sulcus 9.34A)	The central sulcus is located 1 cm behind the half way between frontal and occipital pole and descends downwards and forwards and ends just above the posterior rami of lateral sulcus. The surface topography of this sulcus is parallel and two fingers away of coronal sulcus. This important sulcus is often difficult to identify. Pre-central sulcus lies in front and almost parallel to it. Similarly, post-central sulcus lies behind it. The gyri lies in front of central sulcus and limited by pre-frontal sulci is pre-central gyri (known as Broadman area 4) located at front lobe. This region of brain mainly controls all the motor activity of the contralateral body along with pre-motor cortex and frontal eye field (area 6). The entire body is represented in the primary motor cortex upside down; the head lies at the inferolateral part of prefrontal gyrus and toes at the superomedial part. The gyrus lies behind the crntral sulcus is post-central gyrus. It is the sensory cortex (areas 3,1,2), located in parietal lobe of brain. This area primarily concerned with conscious awareness of sensation. Recent studies show both the motor and sensory areas are not wholly motor or sensory. Some sensory fibers are located in motor area, and some motor fibers are seen in sensory area (although very scanty in number). So now-a-days, a new name is given sensory-motor cortex – where motor fiber is dominant (as in motor area) Ms1 is named, where sensory fibers dominant Sm1 (sensory) is named (capital M indicates Motor fiber predominate, capital S indicates sensory fiber predominate). Similarly, here, body is represented upside down. The motor speech area of broca (anterior) is on inferior frontal gyrus of left side. The posterior speech area of Wernicke is in the posterior part of superior and middle temporal gyrus.
ateral sulcus 9.34A)	The complicated lateral sulcus starts from inferior surface (from valleculla) of cerebral hemisphere. It has a stem and three rami, anterior horizontal, anterior ascending and posterior (largest) rami. The auditory area (areas 41, 42) is mostly lies in the floor of lateral sulcus.
ortant sulci and gyri areas on medial ace (Figs 9.34B and 5A)	The flat medial surface is connected by corpus callosum (commissural fibers). The fibers of the brain act like electric wiring for connection, integration and execution of different activities. In this surface lies callosal sulcus (just above the comma-shaped corpus

Contd...

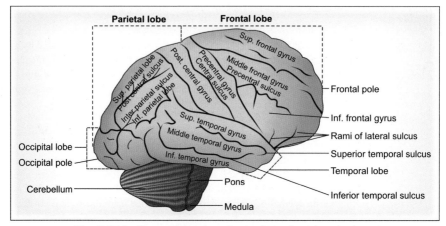

Fig. 9.34A: Superolateral surface of cerebral hemisphere

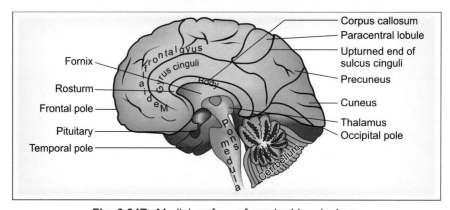

Fig. 9.34B: Medial surface of cerebral hemisphere

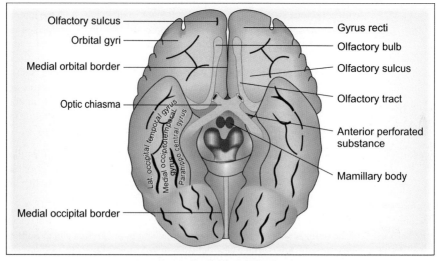

Fig. 9.34C: Inferior surface of cerebral hemisphere

e and presenting parts	*Description*

callosum). During examination, corpus callosum is divided and the cerebral hemispheres are separated. One finger breadth above the callosal sulcus lies cingulated sulcus. It ends behind the paracentral lobule. In between two sulci lies cingulated gyrus and above cingulated sulcus lies below medial frontal gyrus. The cingulated gyrus (anterior part) is the part of limbic system (concerned with our emotions). In this surface, there is oblique parieto-occipital sulcus (which extends up to superomedial border) separates parietal lobe from occipital lobe. Another deep sulcus lies in posterior part of medial surface – the calcarine sulcus. These two deep sulci converge anteriorly and meet behind the posterior part (splenium) of corpus callosum. In between parieto-occipital and calcarine sulcus, the wedge shaped tissue is known as cuneus. In front of cuneus lies precuneus (limited in front by paracentral lobule). Paracentral lobule is the area brain tissue around upper part of central sulcus. Both the motor and sensory area of lower limb, perineum is located here. Along the lips of posterior part of calcarine sulcus, visual area (17) is situated. The cortex is adjacent to area 17 on the medial and lateral surfaces of cerebral hemisphere from the visual association area. This cortex receives visual information from retina.

portant sulci, gyri on
rior surface
g. 9.34C)

Inferior surface is divided by stem of lateral sulcus into anterior orbital and posterior tentorial part. From orbital surface a medial straight sulcus strips of brain tissue and formed gyri recti. Rest of the brain tissue is divided by irregular H-shaped sulci into anterior, posterior, medial and lateral orbital gyri. The tentorial part is marked by some anteroposteriorly oriented sulci named colateral sulcus (begins from the occipital pole and extends anteriorly parallel to calcarine sulcus) and occipitotemporal sulcus (parallel to collateral sulcus and lies lateral to it). The gyrus between collateral and calcarine is lingual gyrus. The hook-shaped area in front of collateral sulcus is uncus. Medial to collateral sulcus is parahippocampal gyrus. Uncus and parahippocampal gyrus is concerned with emotions (belongs to limbic system).

tery supply
g 9.35B)

The two vertebral and two internal carotid arteries supplies the whole brain. The superolateral surface of cerebral hemisphere is mainly supplied by middle cerebral artery,

Contd...

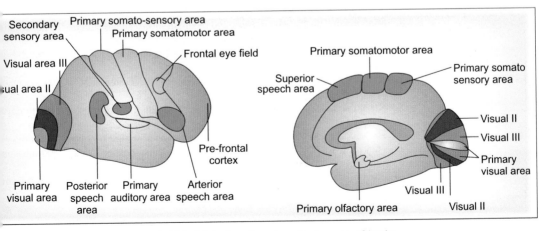

Fig. 9.35A: Main functional cortical areas of brain

Name and presenting parts	*Description*

branch of internal carotid. The medial surface is mainly supplied by anterior cerebral (branch of internal carotid) and main artery supplies the inferior surface is posterior cerebral (branch of basilar).

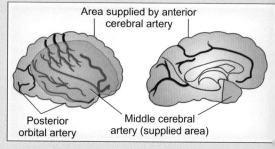

Fig. 9.35B: Blood supply of brain

Applied

- Microcephaly—It is a congenital (present from birth) condition characterised by reduced skull size and the child is mentally and physically retarded.
- Cerebrovascular accident (CVA)—It is very common, commonly known as stroke results from lack of blood supply (e.g. atherosclerosis). If the person survives developed paralysis usually of one side of body.
- Head injuries—There may be subdural and subarachnoid hemorrhage. It is treated by surgery. Other types of injuries include contusion which results in much tissue destruction.
- Alzheimer's disease—It is a progressive degenerative disease of brain which results in dementia (forgetfulness).
- Encephalitis—Inflammation of brain tissue by virus or bacteria.
- Psychoses—It is a type of functional brain disorder where the affected individual is detached away from reality and exhibits odd behaviour.
- Cerebral palsy—Temporary lack of oxygen (as in difficult delivery) may lead to cerebral palsy. It is a neuromuscular disability where muscles are poorly controlled or paralysed.

Basal nuclei
(Fig. 9.36) caudate
nucleus putamen globus
pallidus

1. Basal nuclei or corpus striatum includes the caudate nucleus, putamen and globus pallidus.
2. These structures are primarily concerned with the control of posture and movements. In clinical practice, it is known as extra-pyramidal motor system.
3. Tropographically, the putamen and globus pallidus constitute the lentiform nucleus (lens like).
4. Functionally, the caudate nucleus and putamen form a single entity – the neostriatum (striatus), while the globus pallidus forms the paleostriatum or pallidum.
5. The caudate nucleus lies in the wall of lateral ventricle. It has a globular head, body and tail.
6. The curved tapering tail of the caudate nucleus follows the curvature of lateral ventricle into temporal lobe.
7. The putamen and globus pallidus lies lateral to the internal capsule deep to cortex and insula.
8. The caudate nucleus and the putamen are the input regions of corpus striatum.
9. They receive afferents from cerebral cortex, intralaminar thalamic nuclei and substantia nigra.
10. Efferent fibers are directed to the globus pallidus and parts reticulata of substantia nigra.
11. The globus pallidus consists of two segments – medial and lateral.
12. The medial segment shares many similarities with the parts reticulata of substantia nigra, these two structures are regarded as output regions of corpus striatum.

Contd

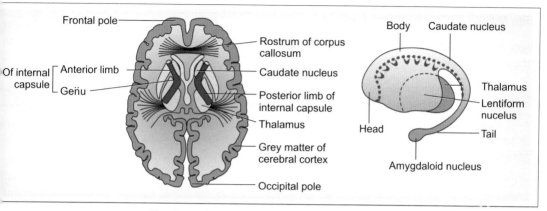

Fig. 9.36: Basal ganglia (horizontal section)

me and presenting parts	Description
	13. The globus pallidus receives afferent fibers from the stratum and the subthalamic nucleus.
	14. The medial part of globus pallidus projects primarily to the thalamus.
	15. The thalamus in turn sends fibers to the motor areas of frontal lobe.
plied g. 9.37)	• Unilateral basal ganglia lesions produce their effects on opposite sides of the body. Basal ganglia dysfunction does not cause paralysis, sensory loss or ataxia but leads to abnormal motor control, alteration of muscular tone, and there are abnormal, involuntary movements (dyskinesias).
	• Parkinson's disease is a neurodegenerative disease (dopaminergic neurone is degenerated) of substantia nigra, usually elderly group is affected of unknown cause. It is characterized by short, suffling gait, a hypokinesia (less movement), tremor, and rigidity of muscle.
	• Hepatolenticular degeneration (Wilson's disease)—It is an inherited disease of copper metabolism. Basal ganglion changes to abnormal movement and progressive dementia in childhood and youth.

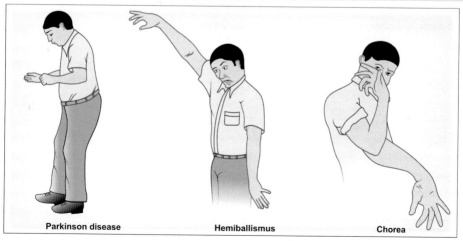

Fig. 9.37: Disorder of basal ganglia

White Matter of Cerebral Hemisphere

Fibers are classified on the basis of origin and termination. These fibers are like electric wires which connects the brain and spinal cord┃ cerebral hemisphere receives and gives inform┃ to different regions of spinal cord through ┃ fibers.

Name and features	Description
Association fibers Short Long	These fibers link cortial region within the same hemisphere. Important fiber bu┃ are superior longitudinal fasciculus, arcuate fasciculus, inferior longitudinal fasci┃ and uncinate fasciculus.
Applied	Carbon monoxide posisoning destroys the inferior longitudinal fasciculus bilater┃ In this case, the vision remains normal but cannot identify the individual faces o┃ nature of object.
Commissural fibers	These fibers connect the corresponding region of the two hemispheres. The ┃ commissural fibers are the corpus callosum, the anterior commissure and┃ hippocampal commissures.
Corpus callosum (Figs 9.38A and B)	Largest commissure, 10 cm in length. Anterior end is 4 cm away from frontal pole┃ posterior end is 6 cm away from occipital pole. It is divided into four parts; ┃ anterior to posterior aspect they are rostrum, genu, body and splenium. As the co┃ callosum is shorter than cerebral hemisphere, the callosal fibers linking the frontal┃ occipital poles curve forwards and backwards, and form forceps minor and m┃ respectively. As the splenium interconnects the occipital cortex, it is concerned ┃ visual functions.
Artery supply	By anterior and posterior cerebral artery, artery of Heubner
Applied	Destruction of splenium of corpus callosum by stroke or tumor leads to poste┃ disconnections syndrome. Such individuals can speak and write but cannot unders┃ written material. Chronic epilepsy (fit) patients may be treated by section of co┃ callosum to control the fit. But the drawback is that the person cannot name obje┃

Con┃

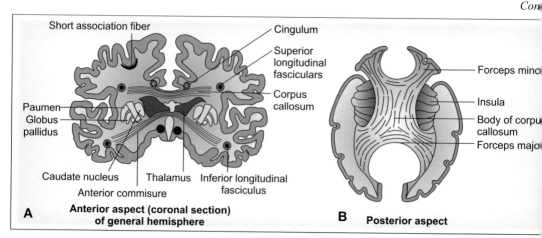

Figs 9.38A and B: Corpus callosum and its different parts

and features	Description
ction fibers	These fibers connect between the cerebral cortex and various subcortical areas. These fibers pass through corona radiata and internal capsule.
nal capsule 9.36)	• It is the important projection fiber. Corona radiata fibers become concentrated in a narrow area, and form internal capsule between thalamus and caudate nucleus medially and the lentiform nucleus laterally. The internal capsule is angulated like boomerang and has got anterior limb, genu, posterior limb, retrolentiform and sublentiform part. Through anterior limb passes fiber from thalamus to prefrontal cortex, also fibers from frontal cortex to pontine nucleus (pons). The posterior limb contains corticobulbar and corticospinal motor fibers and thalamo cortical fiber to somatosensory cortex. Through retrolenticular part passes optic radiation fiber to visual cortex through submiddle cerebral.
ry supply	By lenticulostriate arteries – branch of anterior and middle cerebral artery. One of them is large and known as charcoat artery, supply the lower limb region is frequently ruptured. It is known as artery of cerebral hemorrhage.
n stem 9.39)	Brain stem comprises of midbrain, pons and medulla from above downwards. Each segment is roughly one inch in length. Out of 12 pairs of cranial nerves, 10 pairs (except first and second) arise from brainstem. It controls automatic centers for our survival (like heart beat, respiration, GI reflex).

Contd...

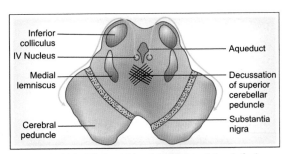

Fig. 9.40A: The mid-brain—level of the inferior colliculus and decussation of the superior cerebellar peduncle

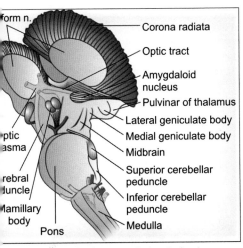

Fig. 9.39: Brain stem (lateral view)

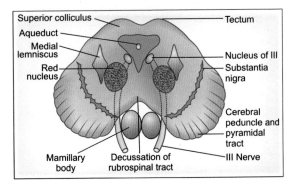

ig. 9.40B: The mid brain—level of the superior colliculus and the red nucleus

Name and features	Description
Mid brain (Figs 9.40A and B)	• It lies between diencephalons and pons. A hollow tunnel (cerebral aqueduct) p.. through it. An imaginary line passes through the aqueduct, divides the midbrain ventral cerebral peduncle (stalk) and dorsal tectum (roof).
Tectum	• Tectum consists of two pairs of elevated masses, superior and inferior colliculi. are the reflex center. The superior colliculi is receives fibers from optic tract and inf colliculi receives fibers of auditory pathway (lateral lemniscus).
Cerebral peduncle	• The ventral cerebral peduncle is divided by substantia nigra (dark pigmented . into three parts; from ventral to dorsal aspect lies crus cerebri, substantia nigra tegmentum. The middle third of crus consists of pyramidal fibers (descending tr.
Substantia nigra	• It is a dark pigmented area visible in necked eyes (section of midbrain). The subst. nigra has both afferent and efferent connection with basal nuclei (corpus striatum is associated with extra-pyramidal system.
Tegmentum	• It consist of ascending fibers (medial and lateral lemnisci) and discrete grey m. Third nerve nucleus lies in grey matter (ventral to aqueduct) at the level of sup. colliculi. At this level lies red nucleus (important motor nucleus of extrapyram system), fourth nerve nucleus lies ventral to aqueduct at the level of inferior colli Through out the tegmentum lies scattered masses of grey matter known as reti. formation.
Applied	Parkinson's disease—It is characterized by tremor (involuntary fine movement of fing rigidity (stiffness) due to degeneration of dopamine, (a neurotransmitter) producing of substantia nigra.
PONS – means bridge (Figs 9.41A and B)	It is a bridge between midbrain above and medulla oblongata below. The fifth, s seventh and eighth cranial nerves are attached to it. It is situated in posterior cranial f over the clivus. Functionally it is a conduction pathway between higher and lower b centers. It respiratory (pneumotaxic) nuclei, in addition with, medullary respiratory ce

Cor

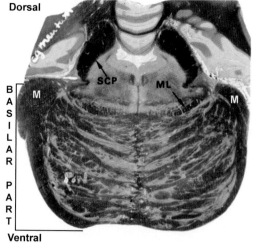

Dorsal

B
A
S
I
L
A
R

P
A
R
T

Ventral

Fig. 9.41A: Cross section of pons (middle part)
Abbreviations: SCP—Superior cerebellar peduncle,
M—Middle cerebellar peduncle, PN—Pontine nuclei

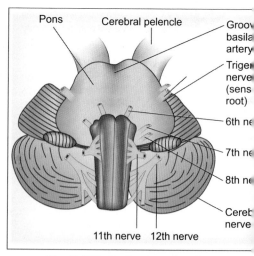

Pons   Cerebral pelencle   Groo.
basila
artery

Trige.
nerve
(sens.
root)

6th ne

7th ne

8th ne

Cere.
nerve

11th nerve   12th nerve

Fig. 9.41B: Brain stem showing pons
(anterior surface)

ame and features	*Description*
	control rate and depth of respirations. A cross section of pons shows ventral basilar part and dorsal tegmental part. Through the basilor part transversely running ponto cerebellar fibre pass to opposite middle cerebellar peduncle. Also there are vertically running pyramidal fiber scattered within these fibres are groups of pontine nuclei. The teg mentum contain 5th, 6th, 7th, 8th nerve nuclei. There is a special bluish color locus ceruleus nucleus.
Medulla oblongata (Fig. 9.42)	It is 2.5 cm long; broad above, and narrow below. Four cranial nerves, ninth, tenth, eleventh, twelveth cranial nerves are attached to it. The medulla ends below the foramen magnum—where the first cervical nerve is attached. The lower part of pons and upper part of medulla form ventral part of fourth ventricle. The dorsal wall of ventricle is formed by thin capillary riched membrane—the choroids plexus. The medulla has several externally visible landmarks. On the ventral aspects just by the side of anterior median sulcus lies pyramidal (formed by large pyramidal tract) and by the side of pyramid, in the upper part, lies oval shaped olive (formed by inferior olivary nucleus). In the mid line, we can see the cross over of pyramidal fibers (75%) known as decussation of pyramid. The inferior cerebellar peduncles are visible on dorso-lateral aspect of olive. The rootless of hypoglossal nerve (twelveth cranial nerve) emerge between pyramid and olive. Inspite of its small size, and apart from important nuclei and tracts, it also controls autonomic reflex involved in maintaining the body homeostasis. They are the cardiovascular center, respiratory center, vomiting and coughing centers.
Applied	• As the vital centers situated in medulla, a lesion is usually fatal. • Damaged to paramedian region produced medial medullary syndrome characterized by paralysis of tongue on the same side, hemiplegia (paralysis of one-half of body) to opposite side with the loss of touch and kinesthetic sense on opposite side.

Contd...

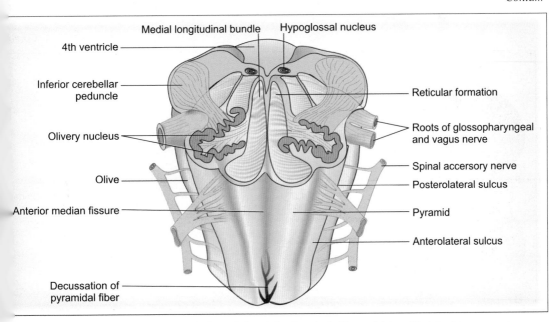

Fig. 9.42: Section (transverse) of medulla at the level of 4th ventricle with intact lower part

Name and features	Description
	• Damage to dorsolateral aspect give rise to lateral medullary syndrome. It is character by dysphonia (difficulty in speaking), dysphagia (difficulty in swallowing) du paralysis of laryngeal and palatal muscles on the same side. Loss of pain and tempera sensation on the same side of the face, and opposite side of body. Involvemen vestibular nuclei causes vertigo and nystagmus with nausea and vomiting.
Cerebellum situation (Figs 9.43A to C)	• The cauliflower like cerebellum is the largest part of hind brain; situated in poste cranial fossa, overlapping mid brain. It lies below the tentorium cerebelli (a proces dura matter). Its weight is 150 gms in adult. It forms 1/8th part of cerebrum in ad and 1/20th part of cerebrum in children. Cerebellum comprises of two cerebe hemisphere connected by vermis – superior and inferior vermis.
Parts	• It is composed two surfaces, two borders, two fissures and two notches. It is connec to brain stem by superior, middle and inferior cerebellar peduncles. The cerebe surface shows fine, parallel, plate like gyri known as folia. Deep fissures (like fiss prima, horizontal fissure) subdivide each hemisphere into anterior, posterior flocculonodular lobes. The cerebellum processes and interpretes impulses from m cortex and sensory pathways. It co-ordinates motor activity so that smooth and w timed movement can occur.
Blood supply	• Superior surface by superior cerebellar artery. Inferior surface, in anterior part anteroinferior cerebellar artery and posterior part by posterior inferior cerebellar art branch of vertebral artery.
Applied	The lesion of cerebellum gives rise to following: 1. Hypotonia—Less tone of muscles. 2. Cerebellar ataxia—Sway gait. 3. Intention tremors—Tremor (fine involuntary movement) occur at the beginning any action.

Con.

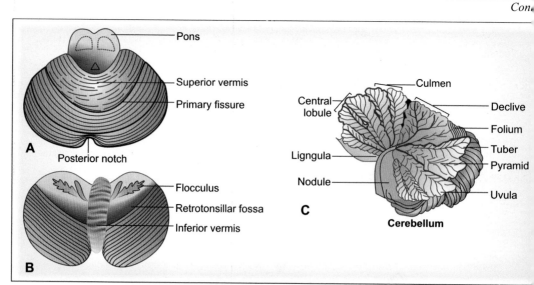

Figs 9.43A to C: (A) Superior surface (B) Inferior surface (C) Mid sagittal section through vermis

e and features	Description
	4. Dysarthria—Difficulty in articulating speech.
	5. Nystagmus—Jerky movements of the eyeball while looking at one side.
tomical position	• Hold the cerebellum in such a way that superior vermis (elevated in the middle) should be above.
	• Inferior vermis (identified by a projection between two sulci) should be placed antero-inferiorly.
	• If pons and medulla is attached, it should lie on anterior aspect.
	• If only cerebellum is present anterior aspect will be identified by presence of a large notch.
nal cord introduction (s 9.44 to 9.47)	The spinal cord lies within the vertebral canal and bears the 31 pairs of spinal nerves through which it receives fibers from periphery and again sends fibers to periphery.
gth and extension	It is 45 cm in length, cylindrical in shape. It begins at the upper border of first cervical vertebra and ends at the lower border of first lumbar vertebra. In children, it extends up to third lumbar vertebra. Lower part of spinal cord tapers out and forms conus medullaris. It has an anterior longitudinal fissure and in posterior surface a shallow post median sulcus. The cord is dialated in two regions, cervical and lumbar. Near the cord, spinal nerve divides to form dorsal and ventral roots. The spinal cord consists of a central core of grey matter containing nerve cell bodies and outer layer of white matter or nerve fibers. Within the white matter run a number of ascending and descending tracts, which link the spinal

Contd...

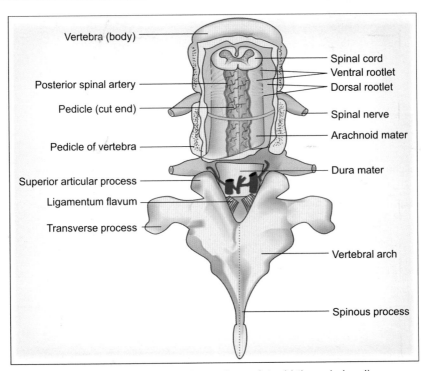

Fig. 9.44: Spinal cord with meninges (at mid thoracic level)

Name and features	Description
	cord with the brain like electric wires. The principal ascending tracts are the spinothala~~ and spinocerebellar tracts. The corticospinal tract is an important descending tract.
Blood supply	By one anterior and two posterior spinal arteries. Also supped by radicular artery.
Applied	• Lumbar puncture – withdrawal of cerebrospinal fluid from the subarachnoid spac~~ the level of L2 and L3 or L3 and L4 vertebral junction, is known as lumbar punct~~ It is used as diagnostic purpose as also for therapeautic purpose.
	• The acute (sudden onset) injury of spinal cord due to accident, is catastrophic, and individual is permanently disabled.
	• Chronic compression of cord includes herniated intervertebral disc, infectio~~ vertebrae with TB and due to tumor in vertebrae. In both the cases, the earliest si~~ pain and it is made worse by sneezing and coughing.
Anatomical position	Hold the spinal cord vertically so that: 1. Conical lower end with branches of spinal nerves should be placed inferiorly. 2. Prominent anterior median fissure should be placed anteriorly. 3. On upper end in naked eye, the rounded anterior horn is well-marked. That is ~~ another point of identification of upper end from lower end.

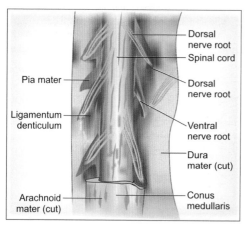

Fig. 9.45: Spinal cord with its membrane (posterior view)

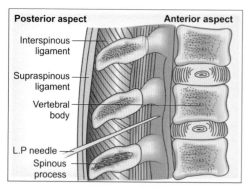

Fig. 9.46: Layers pierced by lumbar puncture (LP) needle

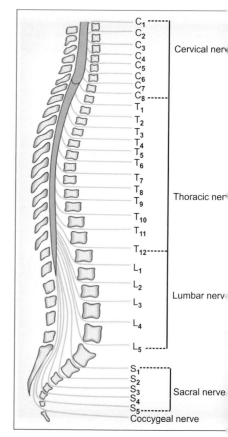

Fig. 9.47: Relationship of spinal cord, s~~ nerves and vertebral co~~

all (Figs 9.48 to 9.51)

Name	*Description*
ball . 9.48)	The eyeball or bulbus oculi is an organ of sight and its mechanism is like that of a camera.
ation pe, Size . 9.49)	It is situated in the anterior part of the orbit, not exactly spherical in size, enclosed by fascial sheath. By thin facial sheath, it is separated from orbital muscle and fat. It is about 2.5 cm in size.
ers or Coats . 9.48)	It has three coates—(1) Outer sclera; fibrous coat and cornea (2) Middle vascular layer or uveal tract (i.e. choroids, ciliary's body and iris) (3) Inner nervous tissue layer
Sclera	It is the outer whitish coat covering the posterior 5/6th of eyeball and anterior 1/6th of it is the transparent cornea (avascular). Outer coat maintains the shape of the eye and gives attachment to the extraocular muscle. The optic nerve pierces the sclera at posterior part 3 mm. to the nasal side. At the junction of sclera and cornea, a minute canal present (canal of shelmn) known as sinus venous sclere and it encircles the cornea. Sclera and inner surface of eyelid are covered by the thin epithelial layer known as conjunctiva.

Contd...

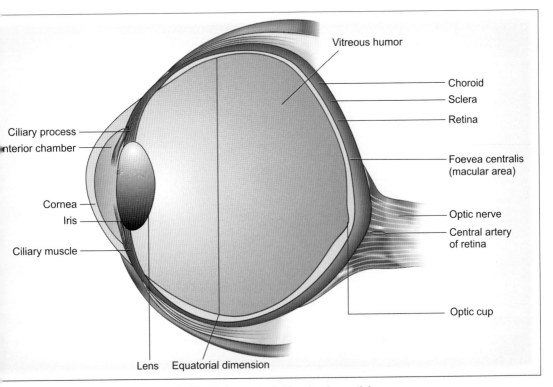

Fig. 9.48: Right eyeball (Semi schematic)

Name	Description
2. Uveal Tract	It is the vascular coat situated between sclera and retina. It consists of, from beh forwards, choroids, ciliary body and iris. The ciliary body is divided into an external the ciliary muscles and internal ciliary ridges. The ciliary body controls the curvatur the lens. The iris is a perforated diaphragm of various colors (racial variation). The like perforated area is known as pupil and its diameter is regulated by two musc sphincter pupillae, dilator pupillae.
3. Retina	Inner photosensitive coat is retina. When it is traced towards anterior aspect it end saw-edged border ; the ora serrata. An instrument, opthalmoscope, can examine the in surface of the retina. It shows (i) a yellow spot the macula lutea; (ii) a depression i (fovea centralis), and (iii) optic disc or blind spot, about 2 mm. medial to yellow spo
Interior of Eye	The space between the cornea and lens is incompletely divided into anterior and poste chamber by lens. Anterior chamber filled with a transparent fluid aqueous humour, secre by cilliary glands. This fluid gives nutrition to transparent structure like cornea, lens removes waste product from them. Behind the lens, the cavity of the eye is filled up the transparent jelly-like substance vitreous humour.
Ocular Muscles (Figs 9.49 and 9.50)	They are six in number and voluntary in nature, are known as extrinsic muscles of eye. They are connected with the movements of the eyeball; medially, laterally, upwa and downwards; and so on.

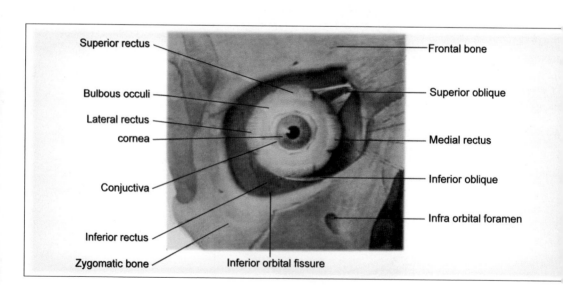

Fig. 9.49: Boundary of right orbit

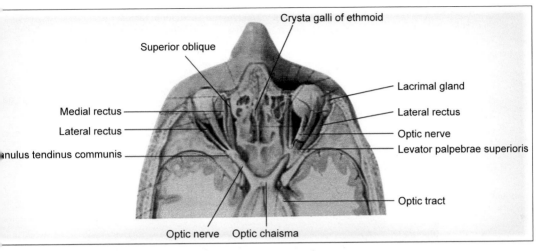

Fig. 9.50: Muscles of eye superior aspect (horizontal section)

re are Four Rectus or Straight Muscles
Two Oblique (Figs 9.50 and 9.51)

me of the muscles	Origin	Insertion	Action	Nerve supply
perior rectus	Annulus tendinus communis of zinn.	6 mm away from aclerocorneal junction	Elevation of the eyeball (rotates it upwards).	Oculomotor (3rd cranial)
erior rectus	Annulus tendinus communis of zinn.	6.5 mm away from aclerocorneal junction	Depression of the eyeball (rotates it downwards)	Oculomotor (3rd cranial)
teral rectus	Annulus tendinus communis of zinn.	7 mm away from aclerocorneal junction	Rotates the eyeball outwards	Abducent (6th cranial)
dial rectus	Annulus tendinus communis of zinn.	5.5 mm away from aclerocorneal junction	Rotates the eyeball inwards	Oculomotor (3rd cranial)
perior oblique	Roof of orbit, antero-medial to optic canal.	Upper and outer part of sclera behind the equator.	Rotates the eyeball downwards and outwards.	4th cranial nerve (trochlear).
erior oblique	Orbital surface of maxilla.		Rotates the eyeball upwards and outwards	Oculomotor (3rd cranial)

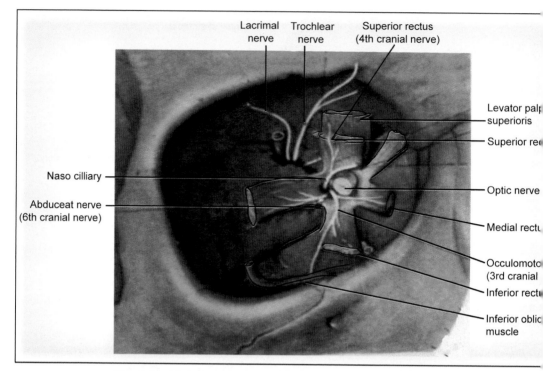

Fig. 9.51: Muscles and nerves of right eye (after removal of eyeball)

Name	Description

Applied	• Inflammation of conjunctiva due to virus, allergen or due to welding spark is known as conjunctivitis (which is very common). It produces redness of
	 • Due to vitamin A deficiency, there may be dryness of conjunctiva and prod corneal ulcer and opacity.
	 • Corneal graft—Cornea of the one person (from freshly donated dead body) be placed on the eye of another person with corneal opacity. In common lang it is called eye donation.
	 • Rise in the intraocular pressure (Glaucoma)—It is due to rise of the pressu aqueous humour due to blockage of circulation.
	 • Retinal detachment—It is the condition where nervous layer (2 to 10) is deta from pigmented layer due to developmental cause.
	 • Cataract—Opacity in lens is known as cataract. It may be present from birt develop in elderly.
	 • Defect of vision—
	  (a) Myopia or short sightedness—Image form, in front of retina due to exces growth of eyeball in the childhood. Corrected by biconcave lens (m power).
	  (b) Hypermetropia—Far sightedness- Image form, beyond retina. Correcte covex lens (plus power).
	  (c) Presbyopia—It develops in 36 to 40 age group, due to loss of elasticit lens. Convex (plus) lens are used for correction.
	  (d) Squint—It is a condition when one eye deviates always from a fixation p corrected by surgery.

Embryology

nenclature Used in Embryology

Albicans (L) – white.

Albugenia (L) – whitish

Allantois (G) – elongated diverticulum (sausage shaped).

Annulus (L) – ring.

Branchial (L) – pertaining to gills

Caudal (L) – tail.

Cephalic – head.

Chorion (G) – skin or covering

Cloaca (L) – drain.

Diverticulum – an offshoot from main tube

Ectopic (G) – out of place

Fetus – unborn offspring

Gamete (G) – spouse.

Gonad (G) – seed; hence the sex glands

Gubernaculums – a rudder.

Infundibulum – a funnelshaped passage

Lanugo – fine soft hair

Notochord (G) – the cord of the back

Palcode (G) – thickened plate of ectoderm

Proctodeum (G) – anus

Stomodum (G) – mouth

Tunica (L) – a coat

Urachus (G) – a urine container

Vas (L) – a vessel

Vitelline – related to yolk sac.

Stages of General Embryology (Figs 10.1A to D)

- Fertilization (male + female gamete) takes place in the ampullary part of uterine tube.
- The haploid gamete unites to form diploid zygote (contain 46 chromosome).
- The large zygote cell divide by cleavage division to form morula (mass of cells), which travel from uterine tube to body of uterus.
- Fluid enters into morula and there are separation of cells. Morula is now called blastocyst. The cells arrange in outer layer, known as trophoblast and inner layer form the inner cell mass.
- Cells of blastocyst continue to divide and the trophoblast implants the blastocyst in the uterine wall at 6 to 7 days after fertilazation. This is interstitial (within) implantation.
- The inner cell mass multiplies rapidly and form circular embryonic disc. The division of labor takes place in the inner cell mass. The outer aspect of the disc, form ectoderm and the inner side form entoderm.
- Two cavities appear, one on ectodermal side, known as amniotic cavity and another on the entodermal side, known as yolk sac cavity.
- The bilaminar disc become trilaminar due to the growth of cells from primitive streak, at on day 15. The primitive streak develop in the caudal aspect of entoderm. It is the primary organizer and initiates the formation of notochord and intraembryonic mesoderm (in between ecto- derm and endoderm). The disc shaped

Development of human being at a glance

Approximation of Male gamete + Female gamete
↓
Fertilization (At ampullary part of uterine tube)
↓
Formation of Zygote
↓
Morula (12 to 16 cell stage)
↓
Blastocyst
↓
(Normal implantation-junction of fundus and body of uterus. Abnormal implantation uterine tube)
↓
Blastocyst presents
↓

Inner cell mass (form embryo)   Outer cell mass (from placenta)

Ectoderm   Mesoderm   Entoderm

Syncytiotrophoblast   Cytotrophoblast

Together with primary extra embryonic mesoderm form chorion (two varieties)

Chorion laevae ultimately   Chorion frondosum (Frondosum + Maternal ba
form part of fetal membrane   zone of endometrium form placenta)

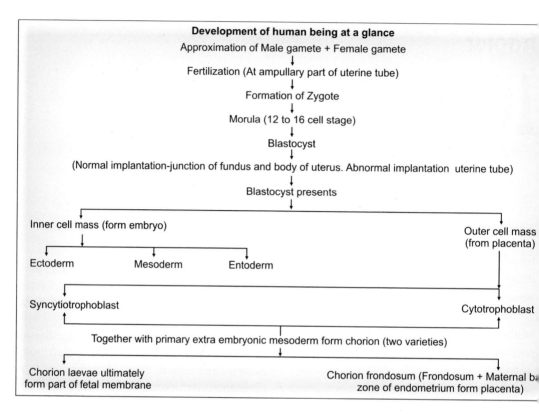

A — Fertilisation and achorage of blastocyst in uterine body

B — Blastocyst

C — Blastocyst with bilaminar embryo

D — Trilaminar ge disc

E — Development of connecting stalk

F

G — Developing fetus in the uterus

Fig. 10.1A: Development of human being

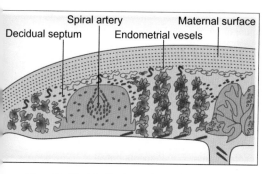

Fig. 10.1C: Vertical section of placenta

embryonic area become pyriform in shape on day 19. The mesoderm does not insinuate in the cephalic region known as, procordal plate, later, form the buccopharyngeal membrane; and in caudal aspect, bilaminer disc remain as cloacal membrane.

- The cells of primitive streak multiply and form rounded primitive node. Multiplication of cells of primitive node gives rise to cells, which migrate in the mid line to form a rod like structure — the notochord.
- Most of the notochord disappear. Its remnant in adult is nucleus pulpous of inter vertebral disc.

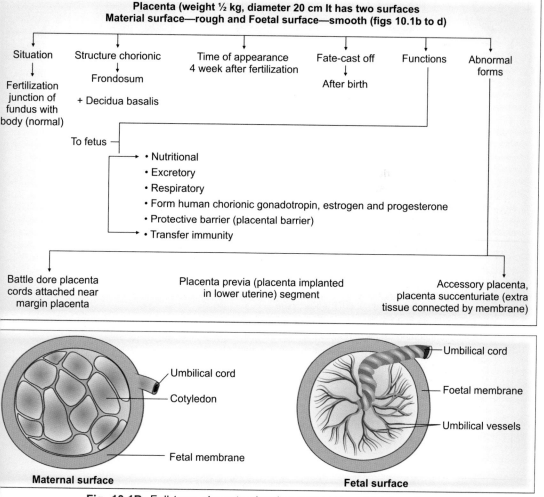

Fig. 10.1B: Full term placenta showing maternal and fetal surface

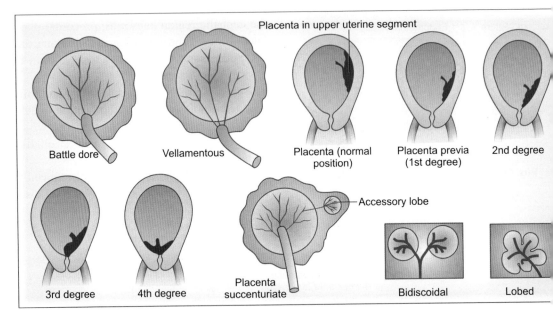

Fig. 10.1D: Anomalies of placenta

EMBRYO BLAST (inner cell mass) DERIVATIVES

Ectoderm gives rise to
- Central nervous system
- Peripheral nervous system
- Sensory epithelium of eye, ear and nose
- Skin (includes hair and nails)
- Pituitary, mammary and sweat glands
- Enamel of teeth

Mesoderm gives rise to
- Dermis of skin and subcutaneous tissue
- Cartilage and bones
- All supporting tissue of body
- Vascular system (arteries, veins, lymphatic channel)
- Urogenital system (except U.bladder)
- Spleen, cortex of suprarenal glands

Entoderm gives rise to
- Epithelial lining of GI tract, respiratory tract and urinary bladder, tympanic cavity, auditory tube
- Parenchyma of thyroid, parathyroid, liver and pancreas

wide plate of ectoderm in the midline lies over the notochord thickened, and form neural plate. groove appear in the middle of neural plate on y 21, and subsequent closure of the groove oduces neural tube. From here whole of the ntral nervous system develop.

Concomitant to ectodermal development, **intraembryonic mesoderm** shows three subdivision by the appearance of a groove on the medial aspect. The part medial to the groove, mesoderm is cubical, known as paraxial mesoderm — later, forms somite. Age of the embryo can be determined as presomite stage, somite stage and post somite stage. The somite divides into: (i) *sclerotome*. ventromedially, forms, vertebrae and ribs. (ii) the *dermomyotome* or the muscle plate dorso laterally. It produces the muscles of body wall and the dermis of skin.

The mesoderm in the lateral part of embryonic disc is called lateral plate mesoderm. Due to rapid growth there is development of small cavities which unite and form a single cavity – the intra embryonic coelome or body caivity. It splits the mesoderm into two layers—*splancho- nopleure* lies in contact of entoderm and, *somatopleure*, which lies in contact with ectoderm. Intraembrynic coelome later form the pericardial, pleural and peritoneal cavities. The intermediate cell group is known as intermediate cell mass. It project ventrally between the other two strips. From lateral side of intermediate cell mass, develop urinary system. Its medial portion, give rise to genital system and cortex of suprarenal gland.

Folding of embryo: As a result of more rapid growth of the embryonic area, the trilaminar embryo under goes folding. The original yolk ac is reduced, due to incorporation of yolk sac s gut. The cranial end folds and incorporate part of the yolk sac as foregut; the caudal end olds and incorporate the hind gut; two lateral fold coverge and incorporate midgut. The gut is closed cranially, by prochoradal plate (converted into buccopharyngeal membrane), and caudally limited by cloacal membrane.

- *The limb bud* develop from lateral plate mesoderm.

- The *septum transversum,* consists of mass of mesoderm lying on the cranial aspect of pericardial cavity. Fibrous pericardium and diaphragm develop from it.

- *Development of placenta*: Placenta develops from two sources — partly from embryo and partly from uterine wall known as decidua. Its function is to transport the nutrients, oxygen, to fetus and for, removal of waste products.

- Before implantation of blastocyst, there is formation of trophoblast, which gradually differentiate into inner cellular *cytotrophoblast* and outer *syncitiotrophoblast* (no define cellular outline). The trophoblast, first form villi (finger like projection); the *primary villi.* They are made up of, central core of cytotrophoblast, covered by syncytio-trophoblast. This is converted into secondary villi, by insinuation (going inside) of mesoderm. Next, tertiary villi is formed when mesoderm in changed into blood vessels. Villi are surrounded *intervillous space,* which contain maternal blood. As the placenta enlarges septa grows within the intervillous space and form placental lobes. The mature placenta is about 6 inches in diameter; 500 gm in weight and fetal surface is shinny where as maternal surface is rough.

Applied

Trophoblast secretes human chorionic gonadotro- phin which is responsible for positive pregnancy test in first week, after the missed period. It is known as pregnancy test or Gravindex test.

Short Note on General Embryology

- *Spermatogenesis*—It is a series of process by which spermatogonia are changed to spermatozoa (sperms) (Figs 10.2A and B). The spermatogenesis is divided into three phases— Spermatocytosis, Meiosis and Spermiogenesis. Primordial germ cells divide by mitosis repeatedly to provide a continuous reserve of sperm cells. Some of the spermatogonia are specialised and form type B spermatogonia, from where primary spermatocyte (contains diploid chromosome) is derived by mitosis division (spermatocytosis). The large primary spermatocyte undergoes first meiotic division and forms secondary spermatocyte with haploid number of chromosome. After completion of meiosis, one secondary spermatocyte gives rise to four equal sized spermatids; out of which, two bear the X chromosome and two bear the Y chromosome. The change over of spermatids to mature spermatozoa is known as spermiogenesis. These changes include (1) shadding of excess cytoplasm (which is engulfed by Sertoli cells) (2) condensation of nucleus (3) formation of acrosomes at the head, which contains a number of important enzymes (4) formation of neck, middle piece and tail. In

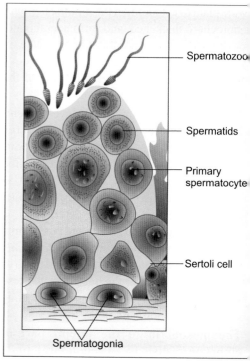

Fig. 10.2A: Transverse section of seminiferous tu showing different stages of maturation of male g cells

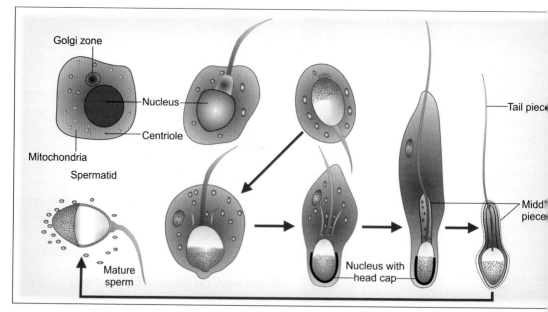

Fig. 10.2B: Spermiogenesis

mans the time required for a spermatogonium develop into a mature spermatozoon is proximately 64 days. In males, differentiation primordial germ cells begins at puberty.

ogenesis—In female, the maturation of imitive germ cells to mature gamete is known oogenesis (Fig. 10.3). Oogenesis starts in enatal life. It includes three processes:

Repeated mitosis – produces a number of oogonia

Specialisation of some oogonia into primary oocyte (with diploid number of chromosome).

Meiotic division starts before birth of baby and completed (formation of secondary oocyte), if there is fertilisation.

ne oocyte with follicular cells surrounding em is known as primordial follicle. The imary oocyte does not complete their first eiotic division and remains in diplotene stage ntil puberty. With the onset of puberty, a imber of follicles begin to mature, with each varian cycle, but only one of them reaches ll maturity. During the process, one primary ocyte gives rise to one ovum (instead of four) d three polar bodies. Mature ovum with its llicular cells is known as graafian follicle, hich lies at the surface of the ovary and can e examined by laparoscope.

lastocyst—It is derived from morula by ccumulation of fluid inside it. It has two parts one is trophoblast and other embryoblast.

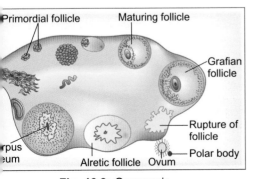

Fig. 10.3: Oogenesis

Implantation on blastocyst in uterine body takes place on sixth or seventh day after fertilisation. Implantation anywhere in the upper of uterine cavity is considered as normal. Sometimes blastocyst is embedded in abnormal situation which may be extrauterine and intrauterine. If blastocyst is implanted in lower uterine segment, it gives rise to placenta praevia; and if occurs in uterine tube, it is known as tubual pregnancy.

- *Notochord*—It is the forerunner of vertebral column and extends from prochordal plate upto primitive tail end of embryo. It is formed by differentiation of head process. The notochordal process undergo different changes that convert it first into a canal and finally back into rodlike solid structure. Most of the notochord disappears. In adults remnants persist as apical ligament of odontoid process and nucleus pulposus of intervertebral disc.

- *Chorion*—Literally chorion means skin (outer covering) (Fig. 10.4)**.** It is an important membrane, which surrounds embryo. It is formed by parietal layer of extra embryonic mesoderm and the trophoblast. The chorion plays an important role in child birth. It appears in 24 days of development. It consists of chorion frondosum and chorion laeve.Chorionic frondosum forms placenta and gives nutrition to developing embryo. Abnormal growth of chorion is known as hydatidiform mole with non-development of embryo.

- *Allantois*—It lies first within the body stalk and later within umbilical cord. It is diverticulum from developing hindgut. It appears on fifteenth day of development. Vascularisation of embryo starts first in this region. Allantois is vestigial organ in human. Its remnant is known as urachus. It's abnormalities are, patent urachus, urachal cyst and urachal fistula.

- *Placental barrier*—Placental barrier is the membrane that separates fetal blood from maternal blood. (Fig. 10.6) It is made up of endothelium of fetal blood vessels, surrounding mesoderm, syncyto-trophoblast and cytotropho-

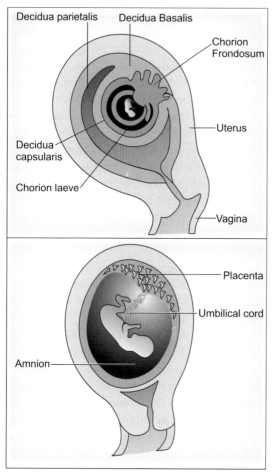

Fig. 10.4: End of the second month

blast. Interchanges of oxygen, nutri
respiration and waste product takes p
through this membrane. Maternal anti
passes to fetus which protects the fetus
certain infections. However, certain drug
thalidomide, tetracycline, etc. can pass thr
the barrier and can damage the fetal tissu
one should take precaution about
administration during pregnancy.

* *Umbilical cord*—It connects abdominal w
fetus with the fetal side of placenta (Fig.
At full term, it measures about 50 cm in le
and 2 cm in breadth. The cord is twisted
presents false knots. Umbilical cord is fo
from body stalk (Fig. 10.5). It appears as
week of intrauterine life and is a vasc
pathway between fetus with placent
consists of two umbilical arteries and a ve
is cut off after birth. Too short cord or too
cord may produce difficulty during birth of

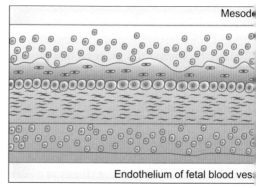

Fig. 10.6: Placental barrier (membrane)

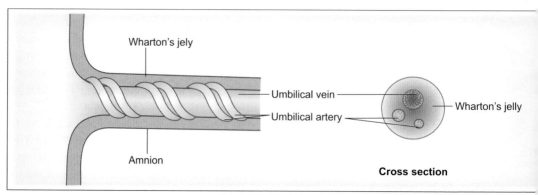

Fig. 10.5: Umbilical cord

Amnion—Encloses embryo and umbilical cord. Amniotic sac is membranous sac, filled with amniotic fluid. It appears at the beginning of second week. The membrane is known as amnion, the cavity it encloses is called amniotic cavity – the fluid inside it is, amniotic fluid. With the floding of embryo, amniotic cavity enlarges and encroaches on all aspects of embryo. The amniotic fluid is secreted first by amniogenic cells, the fetal urine and slight secretion from fetal tracheobronchial tree are added in its volume. At the full term, the amniotic fluid measures about 1,500 to 2,000 cc. The amniotic fluid more than 2,000 cc is known as hydramnios and less than 1.000 cc is known as oligohydramnios (oligo means scanty). Obstetrician terminology of amnion is 'the bag of waters'– which helps fetus maintaining a constant hydrostatic environment and dilates cervix during the child birth.

- *Mackel's diverticulum*—The extra embryonic part of yolk sac is connected with the midgut by vitelo intestinal duct. This part normally disappears. But when it is present, the condition is known as Mackel's diverticulum. It is present in 2% of cases, 2 inch in length, attached 2 feet away from ileiocaecal junction at antimesenteric border. It is the site of development of peptic ulcer.
- *Twining*—(Figs 10.7A and B) Usually, human gives birth normally one offspring at a time. Simultaneous development of two or more embryos is known as twining or multiple birth. It occurs 1 in 80 birth (approximately). Twins are of different varieties, e.g. uniovular or monozygotic, binovular or dizygotic and conjoint twins. Monozygotic twin runs in family (hereditary character) and the two twins are of same sex, and appearance. Dizygotic twin results from fertilization of two ova by two separate sperms. The twins are usually not of same sex and their appearance and character is different. Conjoint twins are those monozygotic twins which are joined with each other to a small or large extent.

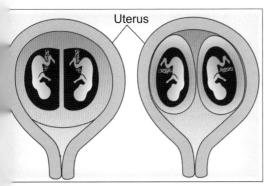

Fig. 10.7A: Twining

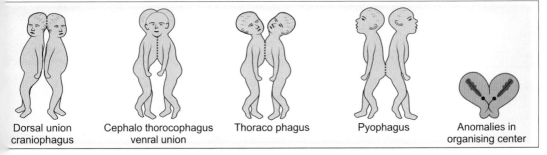

| Dorsal union craniophagus | Cephalo thorocophagus venral union | Thoraco phagus | Pyophagus | Anomalies in organising center |

Fig. 10.7B: Conjoint twins

DEVELOPMENT OF CERTAIN IMPORTANT ORGANS (SPECIAL EMBRYOLOGY)

Development of Heart

Heart is a hollow muscular organ, which pumps blood continuously throughout the body, till death. The development of heart takes place in cardiogenic area below the stomodeum. Primitive angioblastic tissues fuse together to form two paramedian heart tube (Fig. 10.8). Two tubes fuse to form a single heart tube. Single heart tube undergoes enormous expansion and five chambered heart is formed. From caudal to cranial aspect, they are; sinus venosus, primitive atrium, primitive ventricle, bulbus cordis and truncus arteriosus. Further growth within this limited area (pericardial cavity)

produces bending of heart tube. As a result bending, the venous end is carried dorsally and cephalic position. The bulbus cordis tends to lo its identity and to merge with ventricle on one ha and truncus arteriosus on other hand. The comm atrium is partitioned into primitive right and le atria by means of intra-atrial septum, and primiti ventricle is divided by development interventricular septum (Fig. 10.9).

DEVELOPMENT OF INTERATRIAL SEPTUM (FIG. 10.10)

It is developed from three sources – septu primum, septum intermedium and septu secondum. Atrium communicates with primiti

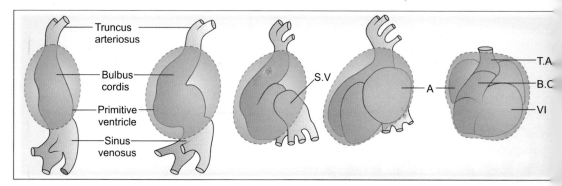

Fig. 10.8: The bending of heart tube within pericardial cavity

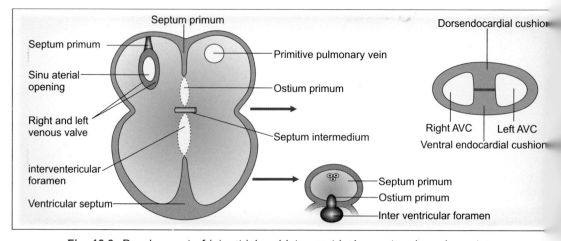

Fig. 10.9: Development of interatrial and inter ventricular septum in various stages

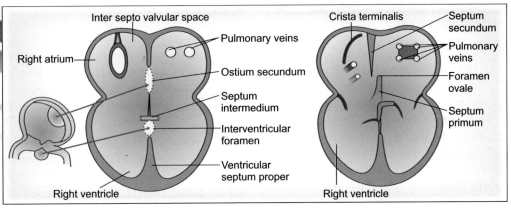

Fig. 10.10: Stages of development of inter atrial septum

icle through atrioventricular opening. There velopment of two swelling from the dorsal ventral aspect of atrioventricular orifice known entral and dorsal endocardial cushion. The ion fuses to form a broad anteroposterior tion– the septum intermedium. During the time from the roof and dorsal wall of primitive m septum primum (an endocardial fold) lops and it grows caudally. Its lower margin e and concave. The two ends of the septum to the anterior and posterior ends of septum medium and a foramen exists in the middle— ed ostium primum. Gradually, there is closure tium primum. As the function of fetal lung is here is disintegration of upper and posterior of septum primum and formation of ostium ndum. In the later part of fetal life, ostium ndum is guarded by a flap valve due to growth nother fold – the septum spurium. Ostium

secundum then is known as foramen ovale. After birth of baby, when the lungs begins to function, the pressure of left atrium increases and forces the primary septum against side of the secondary septum. They fuse and form the complete interatrial septum. The fossa ovalis is developed from septum primum and the limbous fossa ovalis developed from septum secundum.

Applied

- Common type of malformation is atrial septal defect (ASD) (Fig. 10.11). In 25% of individuals small opening exists, known as probe patency of foramen ovale. It is insignificant clinically.
- When the defect is large, the left atrial blood passes to right atrium and 50% cases die. If the right atrial blood passes to the left, there is cyanosis (bluish discoloration).

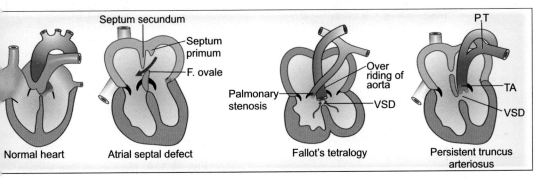

Fig. 10.11: Various anomalies of heart

DEVELOPMENT OF INTERVENTRICULAR SEPTUM (FIG. 10.12)

It is developed from three sources:
1. Ventricular septum proper—Develops from floor and ventral wall of primitive ventricle. It forms muscular part of interventricular septum. It does not grow as far as septum intermedium. A foramen exists in between them.
2. Proximal bulbar septum—This septum partially closes the upper part of ventricular foramen.
3. Septum intermedium—The area between ventricular septum proper and proximal bulbar septum is closed by growth of right edge of septum intermedium.

Applied

Persistent interventricular foramen– It is d the defect in development of membra part. It may be associated with other ca defect. Blood flow from left to right. S opening is asymptomatic. Large defect can sh life.

Fallot's tetrology (Fig. 10.11) – Here four ca anomalies are seen– (1) Pulmonary stenosi. Displacement of aortic orifice, (3) Ventri septal defect (VSD), (4) Hypertrophy of ventricle.

ALIMENTARY SYSTEM (FIGS 10.13A an

The alimentary system is developed from ento of definitive yolk sac during folding of eml The part within the head fold of embryo foregut, within the tail fold is the hindgu between two lateral folds forms midgut (10.13A and B). The mucous mem-brane is fo from entoderm, muscle coat and outer co formed by invading mesoderm. The glan accessory organs (liver, pancreas, salivary g and gallbladder) are formed from outpocketi foregut entoderm.

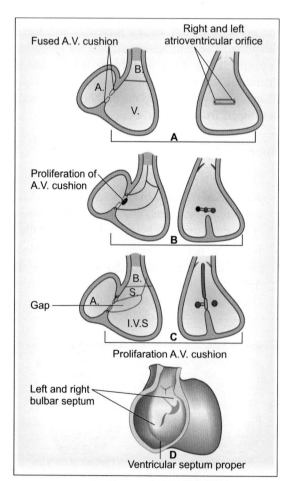

Fig. 10.12: Formation of intra ventricular septum

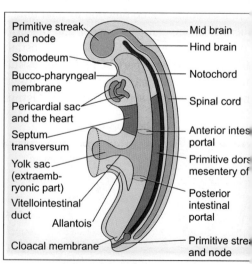

Fig. 10.13A: Median sagittal section of the embryo (Early stage)

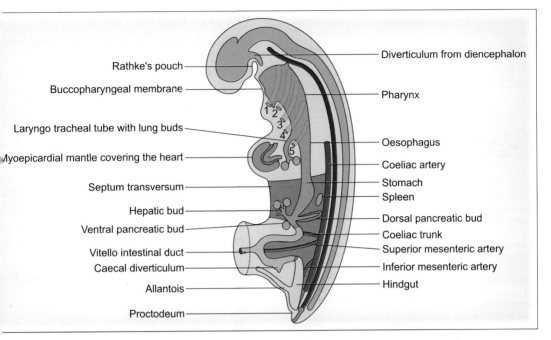

Fig. 10.13B: Median sagittal section of the embryo (More advanced stage)

DEVELOPMENT OF FACE
(FIGS 10.13C and D)

Face is developed as a result of changes around the stomodeum (oral) aperture. In the fifth week of IUL, the stomodeum is deepened by the appearance of 5 processes around it – the process or elevations are the frontonasal process above, the right and left maxillary process (arising from first arch) from sides, and right and left mandibular process below. Within the frontonasal process, two swellings (olfactory) appear which divide the process into one median nasal and two lateral nasal processes. Median nasal process gives rise to philtrum of upper lip, premaxilla with four incisor teeth and nasal septum. The right and left mandibular processes meet in the midline and form lower lip and lower jaw. Fusion of frontonasal process with right and laft maxillary process forms upper lip. The cheeks are formed by fusion of the posterior part of maxillary and mandibular process.

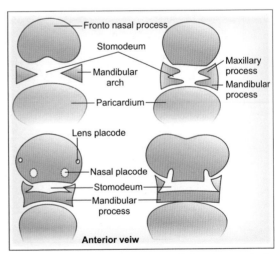

Fig. 10.13C: Different stages of development of face (earlier stage)

Applied

Failure of fusion completely leads to various forms of hare lip.

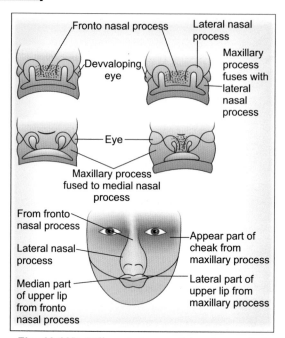

Fig. 10.13D: Different stages of development of face (anterior view) (in late stage)

DEVELOPMENT OF PALATE (FIG. 10.14

Palate is developed by fusion of right and left s like palatine process which arises from maxil processes with premaxilla (developed f frontonasal process). The two palatal proce unite with each other and with nasal septum f before backwards. Deficiency in fusion lead various forms of cleft palate. It may be parti complete. Arrest in union varies from uvula to g In the later case, the cleft runs between la incisor and canine teeth. Complete cleft pa produces nasal regurgitation of milk and needs repair. The cleft palate is due to administratio teratogen during seventh to eighth week of IU

BRANCHIAL (PHARYNGEAL) ARCHES AND ITS DERIVATIVES

The secondary mesoderm of the neck reg consists of only paraxial and lateral p mesoderm. There is no intermediate mesode

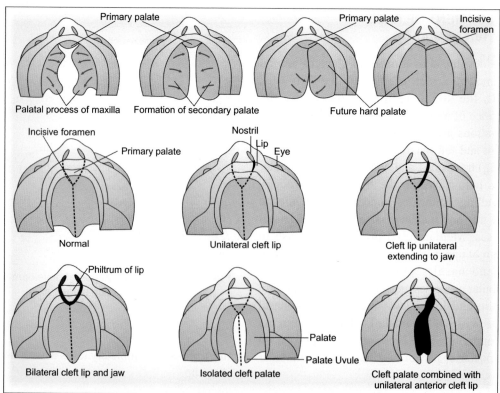

Fig. 10.14: Development of gum, lip and nose and their anomalies (ventral view)

ivatives (Fate) of 6 Branchial Arches (Fig. 10.15)

Nerves	Skeletal derivative	Muscular derivative	Nerve	Artery
st arch	Meckel's cartilage – from which incus and malleus is developed. Anterior ligament of malleus, sphenomandibular ligament, body of mandible and maxilla also developed	Muscles of mastication, e.g. mylohyoid, anterior belly of digastric, tensor veli palatine, tensor, tympani.	1. Mandibular 2. Chorda tympani	Maxillary
plied	Unilateral agenesis of mandible shows weakness of muscle of mastication and there is facial assemetry.			
ond arch	Stapes, styloid process, stylohyoid ligament lesser cornu and superior part of hyoid bone.	Muscles of facial expression, stapedius, stylohyoid, posterior belly of digastric.	Facial	Stapedial artery
rd arch	Greater cornu and inferior parts of body of hyoid bone	Stylopharyngeous muscle	Glossopharyngeal	Common carotid and proximal part of internal carotid.
urth arch	Thyroid cartilage	Cricothyroid muscle	Superior laryngeal	Left fourth arch forms part of arch of atorta and right fourth arch form part of right subclavian artery
th arch	Disappear	No important remnant		
th arch	Cricoid, epiglottics and arytenoids cartilage.	All intrinsic muscles of larynx except cricothyroid.	Recurrent laryngeal.	Ventral part both side of right and left form pulmonary artery. Dorsal part form ligamentum arteriosum. Dorsal part of right disappear.

eral plate mesoderm has no cavity. A series of densed mesoderm forms six pairs of arches ed branchial arches which pushes the peri-lial cavity downwards. In between the arches, e are gaps which have got only ectodermal ng outside and entodermal lining within. Due rowth of mesodermal arches, 5 cleft develop rnally known as branchial cleft (one on each e), while entodermal furrows on the inner ect forms 5 pairs of pharyngeal pouches. Each nchial arch gives rise to skeletal element, otome, nerve of the arch, artery of the arch.

DERIVATIVES OF PHARYNGEAL POUCHES

There are five pharyngeal pouches on each side. Except for the first, each pouch has got ventral and dorsal positions:

DEVELOPMENT OF TONGUE (FIG. 10.16)

Tongue has composite origin. It is formed by different element which do not appear simultaneously. Ventral end of first branchial arch are swollen and form the lingual swelling. Another swelling called tuberculum impar appears in the

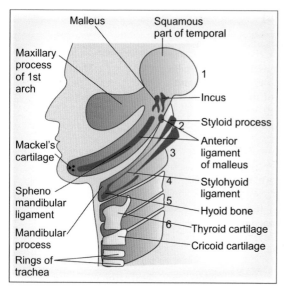

Fig. 10.15: Fate of skeletal derivatives (bones + cartilage) of branchial arches

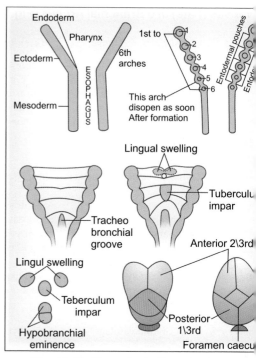

Fig. 10.16: Floor of primitive pharynx and development of tongue (coronal section)

floor of first pharyngeal pouch. These lingual swelling and tuberculum impar fuse to form anterior 2/3rd of tongue. The posterior 1/3rd of tongue develops from a cranial part median swelling called hypobranchial eminence (which is formed by fusion of mesederm of ventral ends of second, third, and part of fourth branchial arches). At first, the regions of tongue, teeth, and lip are not demarcated from each other. Soon tongue

forms a big mass, which is separated from res the mandibular process by formation of ling gingival sulcus. Gradually, this sulcus deepens makes the inferior surface free from floor of mo in anterior part. Muscles are developed fr

Name of pouch	Derivatives
First–ventral Dorsal form	Atrophy Tubotympanic recess forming auditory tube, middle ear, mucous lining of tympan membrane.
Second–ventral Dorsal form	Atropy Palatine tonsil and along with first pouch form part of tubotympanic recess
Third–ventral Dorsal form	Thymus Parathyroid (lower)
Fourth–ventral Dorsal form	Lateral lobe of thyroid Parathyroid (upper).
Fifth–ventral	Ultimobranchial body – forms parafollicular cells of thyroid.

ated occipital myotome, but some embryo- say muscles are developed from regional derm. Taste buds are developed from nerve ngs.

ied

nkyloglossia or tongue tie – It is due to ficiency in formation of alveolingual groove. ere frenulum is short. There may be certain difficulty in speech according to the degree of tie.

- Bifid tongue – A split in the anterior 2/3rd due to failure of fusion of two lingual swellings.
- Macroglossia – Large tongue, due to enlarge plexuses and tissue spaces. In all these cases, there is difficulty in speech.

Development of Individual Organ in Short (Special Embryology)

Name	Description
phagus	It is developed from the part of foregut between pharynx and stomach. It is elongated during the formation of neck and caudal migration of septum transversum. Upper 1/3rd musculature is developed from musculature of branchial apparatus. That why upper 1/3rd musculature is for voluntary type; rest are involuntary.
plied	• Tracheo esophageal fistula – It communicate with trachea due to failure of caudal growth of tracheo esophgeal septum. • Cardiospasm (achalasia)—It is due to neuromascular in coordination at cardio-esophageal junction. As a result proximal part dialates and distal part narrows down.
mach	It is developed from fusiform dilatation from lower part of foregut during fourth or fifth week. It lies initially in the median plane. There is rapid growth of dorsal border which forms the greater curvature. Due to differential growth, there is alteration in size and shape of stomach. The original ventral border face upwards and to the left and becomes the antero superior surface and left surface becomes the posteroinferior surface.
plied	Congenital hypertrophic pyloric stenosis. It is more common in male. Here the circular muscular coat undergoes hypertrophy and there is also neuromuscular in coordination. The child suffers from progressive vomiting. A mass is felt in the transpyloric line 1 cm right to mid line.
odenum	The part of duodenum above the orifice of bile duct is developed from foregut. The part below it is developed from proximal part of midgut.
unum and ilium	Midgut loop has got two segment. Above the superior mesenteric artery is known as pre arterial segment and below the artery is known as postarterial segment. The whole of jejunum and most of the ilium have developed from pre arterial segment. The terminal part is developed from postarterial segment near the caecal bud.
ecum and pendix	Developed from caecal bud which is developed from postarterial segment of midgut within fifth to tenth week. In order to reach the right iliac fossa caecum and appendix undergoes 210° rotation. Within the abdomen caecum and appendix pass successively through the left iliac fossa, umbilical, subhepatic, right lumbar and finally reach the right iliac fossa.

Contd...

Name	Description
Applied (Fig. 10.17)	• According to shape adult caecum are of four types (1) Fetal type (2%) – caecum is conical and appendix. (2) Infantile type (3%) – The two saccules of caecum are of equal in sizes, develops from each side of base of appendix. (3) Adult or normal type.- In this case the right saccules enlarges more that left one and appendix is located 2 cm below the ileocaecal junction. (4) Exaggrated type – In this case the right saccules enlarges and the left saccules atrophies. The appendix lies close to ileocaecal junction. • According to position (due to defect in the rotation of gut) - The caecum with appendix may be in the following position (1) in the left hypochondrium, below the right lobe of liver and right iliac fossa due to reverse rotation of the gut. 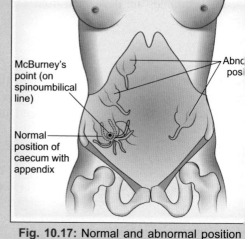 Fig. 10.17: Normal and abnormal position caecum with appendix
Transverse colon *Right 2/3rd of transverse colon*	It is developed from two sources. Right 2/3rd from caudal part of midgut loop and left 1/. from proximal part of hind gut loop. Endothelium of mucous membrane including the glands is developed from entoderm of midgut. Rest of the layers including the musculature is developed from splanchic mesode
Left 1/3rd of transverse colon up to pelvic colon.	Endothelium is developed from entoderm of hind gut. Rest of the layers including musculature are developed from splanchinic mesoderm.
Rectum	The caudal part of the gut is dialated to form the entodermal cloaca. The mesoderm betwe gut and allantois in vaginated the wall of entodermal cloaca and divides into two parts Dorsal part forming rectum and anal canal, (2) ventral part with allantois. The preallant. part gives rise to rectum above the third Houston valve. Rest part of rectum including musculature are developed from the postallantoic part.
Anal canal	1. Part of the anal canal above pectinate line is developed from caudal part of dorsal porti of the endodermal cloaca. Rest of the layers develop from splanchic mesoderm. So inter and spincter is involuntary and supplied by the autonomic nerve. 2. It is developed from ectodermal cloaca. So lining membrane is skin (i.e. stratified squamou The rest of the layer including musculature is developed from somatic mesoderm. sphincter ani externus is innervated from the somatic nerve.
Applied	• Agenesis of rectum and anal canal. • Imperforate anus – Failure of rupture of colacal membrane, which is known as anal sept in the fetal stage, leads to impertorate anus.

Conte

Name	Description
Liver	The liver is developed from two sources: 1. An entodermal diverticulum grows within the mesoderm of ventral mesogastrium, at the junction of foregut and midgut. This form the parenchyma of liver. 2. The fibrous architecture of liver is developed from the mesenchyme of the septum transversum.
Pancreas	It develops in two parts: 1. Ventral pancreatic diverticulum—It develops from bile duct diverticulum. It forms the lower part of head of pancreas and uncinate process. 2. Dorsal pancreatic diverticulum—It extends within dorsal mesentery of the gut from bile duct diverticulum. This diverticulum form upper part of the head, whole of the neck, body and tail of the pancreas.
Applied	The original structure of ventral pancreatic bud sometimes failed to fuse to form single mass. In this condition two lobes develop in opposite directions. Accessory pancreatic tissue—Heterotrophic modules of pancreatic tissue may be found in the deodenum, gallbladder and in Mackel's diverticulum.
Kidney *(Fig. 10.18)*	Three different sets of kidneys develop from intermediate cell mass. During the fourth week of development pronephros appear (first tubular system). It degenerates gradually after the development of second set. It is never functional and disappear completely by the sixth week. The pronephric duct persist. It is utilised by second duct system that is mesonephros. It utilizes the pronephric duct and now, known as mesonephric duct. The mesonephric kidney disappear once again and finally third set; metanephros develops. It persists as adult kidney along with ureteric bud. The ureteric buds push superiorly from the mesonephric duct. The distal end of the bud produce renal pelvis collecting tubules; their unexpanded

Contd...

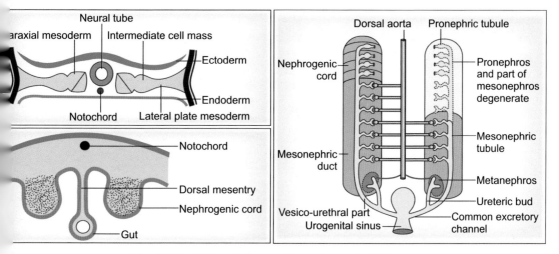

Fig. 10.18: Different stages of development of kidney

Name	*Description*
	proximal part become the ureter. As the kidneys develop in the pelvis it has to ascends to reach their final position in abdomen. This metanephric kidney excreates urine by the third month of development.
Applied	• Horse shoe shaped kidney—When kidney ascends from pelvis, if the kidneys are very close together, the lower pole fuse together in the midline forming a single horse shaped kidney. This condition is usually asymptomatic. • Polycistic kidney—It is inherited disease where the kidneys have many urine filled cyst. It results from failure of communication of collecting tubule. • Pelvic kidney—When the kidney fail to ascend. It remains in pelvis with normal functions.

Window Dissections that Come in Examination

re you start dissection you have to notice the wing structures:—-

n

It has: two parts—epidermis (responsible for different coloration of skin) and

dermis (collagen fiber in it, is responsible for cleavege lines);

two glands—sebaceous gland (secretes oily substance), and sweat gland

two appendages—nail and hair follicle

two thickenings—in palm and sole.

In the cadaver the skin feels more thick due preservative material.

perficial fascia (subcutaneous tissue)—Lies low skin, adherent to dermis. Vessles, nerves into it. Fat is deposited here in obese person ar abdomen, hip, waist). In non obese person, s maximally found in palm and sole.

ep fascia—Lies deep to superficial fascia. It present in limbs, neck; absent in face and domen. Beneath these one can get all the uctures like muscles, bones, vessels and rves.

The instruments require for dissection are:
1. Forceps ⟶ Tooth
   Forceps ⟶ Untooth
2. Scalpel ⟶ Handle with changeable blade.
3. Scissors ⟶ Long pointed.
   Scissors ⟶ Blunt.
4. Chain with hook.

The cadaver (you dissect) is the best textbook of anatomy and always try to demonstrate structures as clearly as possible.

Skin first applied (skin)

- Boil—Infection hair follicle.
- Curbuncle—Infection of several hair follicles.
- Paronychia—Infection beneath the nail fold.
- Sebaceous cyst—It is a cystic swelling found largely in head and neck and it is developed collection of sebum due to blockage of hair pores.
- Line of cleavage—Surgical incision along this langerhans line produces minimal scar.
- Burn—The depth of burn is the criterion of skin healing. Superficial burn heals quickly but that extends deeper the sweat gland, heals slowly.

NB—Tissues heal faster and leave less scar in young, than in aged

CLAVI PECTORAL FASCIA

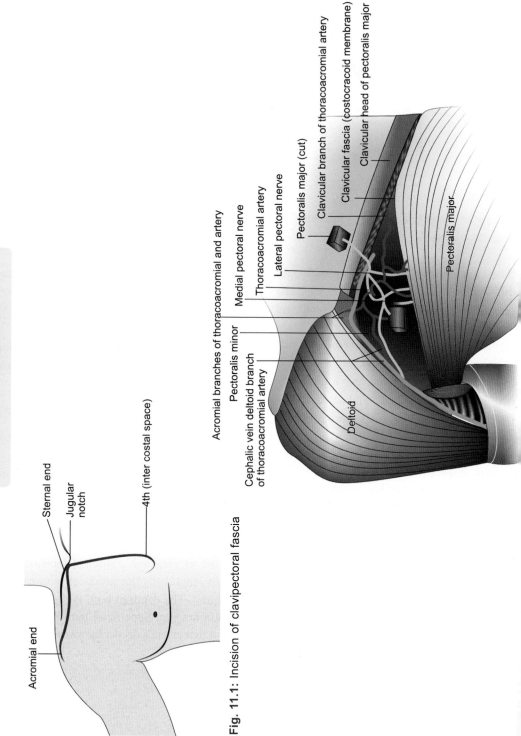

Fig. 11.1: Incision of clavipectoral fascia

Acromial end

Sternal end

Jugular notch

4th (inter costal space)

Acromial branches of thoracoacromial and artery

Medial pectoral nerve

Thoracoacromial artery

Lateral pectoral nerve

Pectoralis minor

Cephalic vein deltoid branch of thoracoacromial artery

Pectoralis major (cut)

Clavicular branch of thoracoacromial artery

Clavicular fascia (costocracoid membrane)

Clavicular head of pectoralis major

Pectoralis major

Deltoid

NAME OF THE DISSECTION–CLAVI PECTORAL FASCIA

POSITION OF BODY–SUPINE, WITH UPPER LIMB IS AT RIGHT ANGLE TO THE BODY

Incision (Fig. 11.1)	*Comment*	*Identification*	*(Applied Anatomy)*
• A transverse incision from sternal notch along the clavicle upto its acromial end.	It is a strong fascia, situated deep to clavicular head of pectoralis major, and extends from lower part of subclavius to upper border of pectoralis minor. Above it splits to enclose the subclavius, below it splits again and cover the pectoralis minor. It is then it blends with axillary fascia. Medially extends upto 1st rib. Laterally extends upto coracoid process and coraco clavicular ligament.	Clavipectoral fascia and structure piercing it, i.e.	• Cephalic vein catheterisation
• A vertical incision from sternoclavicular joint upto 4th costal cartilage. Triangular flap of skin reflected lateraly and downward.		• Branches of Thoraco acromial artery a branch of 2nd part of axillary artery.	• Placement of space –maker in infraclavicular fossa.
• Superficial fascia (Containing fat) is exposed with cutaneous branches of supraclavicular nerves (lateral, intermediate and medial division). It is reflected by similar incision.		• Caphalic vein drain the lateral side of hand.	• Developmental anomalies of breast.
		• lateral pectoral nerve—Branch of lateral cord.	• Drainage of breast abscess.
• Upper part of pectoralis major is exposed.		• Muscles–Pectoralis major (Fig. 11.2)	
• Calvicular head of pectoralis major is cut and reflected downwards laterally.			
• Clavipectoral fasica is exposed.			

AXILLA

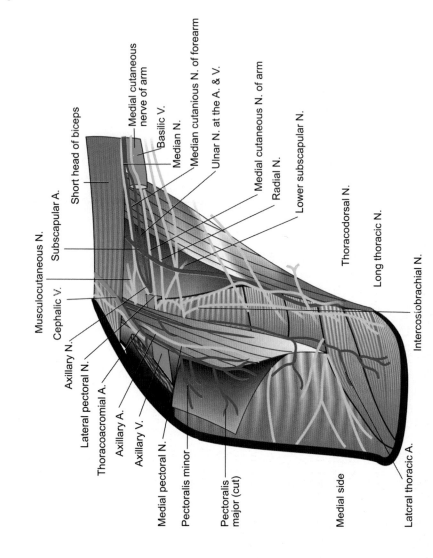

Musculocutaneous N.
Subscapular A.
Short head of biceps
Medial cutaneous nerve of arm
Basilic V.
Median N.
Median cutanious N. of forearm
Ulnar N. at the A. & V.
Medial cutaneous N. of arm
Radial N.
Lower subscapular N.
Thoracodorsal N.
Long thoracic N.
Cephalic V.
Axillary N.
Lateral pectoral N.
Thoracoacromial A.
Axillary A.
Axillary V.
Medial pectoral N.
Pectoralis minor
Pectoralis major (cut)
Medial side
Lateral thoracic A.
Intercostiobrachial N.

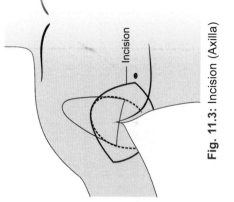

Incision

Fig. 11.3: Incision (Axilla)

NAME OF THE DISSECTION–AXILLA

POSITION OF BODY–SUPINE, WITH UPPER LIMB IS AT RIGHT ANGLE TO THE BODY

Incision (Fig. 11.3)	*Comment*	*Identification (Fig. 11.4)*	*(Applied Anatomy)*

• A curved incision along the anterior border axilla from the 4th space (ICS) extending upto junction of upper ¼th of and lower ¾th of arm.
• Two transverse incisions are given from the ends of curved incision upto the table
• Skin with superficial fascia is exposed.
In it lies the intercostobrachial nerve. (branch of 2nd Throracic NV.)
• Remove fat and lymph node carefully
All the structures of the axilla is exposed.
	Axilla is a pyramidal space between lateral side of chest and arm. It has a apex directed upwards and medically, a base—directed downwards. Anterior wall, is formed by pectoralis major, minor, and subscapularis post wall—latissimus dorsi and Teres major. Medial wall—Serratus anterior in upper space, lateral wall—upper ¼th of humerus.	Contents of axilla
		1. Medial wall –
		  • long thoracic nerve.
		  • lateral thoracic vessels.
		2. Lateral wall–from Medial to lateral.
		  • Medial cutaneous nerve of arm.
		  • Axillary vein.
		  • Medial cutaneous nerve of forearm.
		  • Ulnar nerve.
		  • Axillary artery (3rd part)
		  • Medial root of median nerve crosses in front of axillary artery.
		  • Median nerve.
		  • Musculocutaneous nerve. – it pierces the muscle-coraco brachialis.
		3. In posterior wall–Subscapular vessels (branch of 3rd part of axillary artery)
		  • Posterior-circumflex humoral vessel
		  • Axillary nerve accompanied by posterior humeral circumflex artery.
		  • Upper and lower subscapular nerve.
		  • Thoracodorsal nerve.
		4. Axillary pad of fat.
			• Paralysis of long thoracic nerve from its origin produces winging of scapula.
			• Cervical rib syndrome
			• Erb's palsy.
			• Klumke's palsy
			• Saturday night palsy
			• Crutch paralysis.
			• Carcinoma of breast.
			# Surgical neck–Produces axillary nerve paralysis.

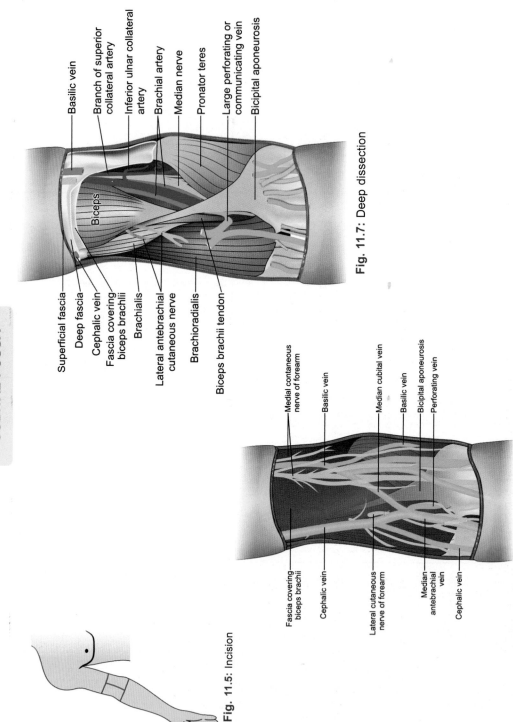

Fig. 11.5: Incision

Fig. 11.7: Deep dissection

Superficial fascia

Deep fascia

Cephalic vein

Fascia covering biceps brachlii

Brachialis

Lateral antebrachial cutaneous nerve

Brachioradialis

Biceps brachii tendon

Basilic vein

Branch of superior collateral artery

Inferior ulnar collateral artery

Brachial artery

Median nerve

Pronator teres

Large perforating or communicating vein

Bicipital aponeurosis

Biceps

Medial contaneous nerve of forearm

Basilic vein

Median cubital vein

Basilic vein

Bicipital aponeurosis

Perforating vein

Fascia covering biceps brachii

Cephalic vein

Lateral cutaneous nerve of forearm

Median antebrachial vein

Cephalic vein

NAME OF THE DISSECTION–CUBITAL FOSSA

POSITION OF BODY–SUPINE, WITH UPPER LIMB IS AT RIGHT ANGLE TO THE BODY

Incision (Fig. 11.5)	Comment	Identification (Figs 11.6 and 11.7)	(Applied Anatomy)
• Transverse incision one finger above the two epicondyles	• It is a fossa in the front of arm forearm junction. It is bounded	1. Cephalic veins	• Blood pressure is measured.
• Transverse incision at the junction of upper 1/3rd to lower 2/3rd of the front of forearm.	• laterally–medial border of brachioradialis	2. Median cubital vein.	• Intravenous injection is given in medial cubital Vein
• Vertical incision from the mid point of proximal to mid point of distal incision	• Medially–lateral border of pronator teres	3. Bicipital aponeurosis.	• Cubital tunnel syndrome, Pronator syndromes.
• It is cut and reflected with skin. Deep fascia is exposed.	• apex–by meeting of brachioradialis and pronator teres.	4. Brachioradialis.	
• It is cut in same way and muscles and vessels and exposed.	• Base–Imaginary like joining the two epicondyles of humerus.	5. Pronator teres,	
• Reflect the skin flap side ways.	Floor–by supinator and brachialis.	6. Supinator,	
• Preserve the superficial vein (cephalic and, basilic and median cubital vein		7. Brachialis	
• Superficial fascia is cut like skin and reflected		8. Tendon of biceps brachii	
• Deep fascia is exposed.		9. Brachial artery and vein	
• It is cut and reflected like skins.		10. Radial blood vessels	
• Boundaries and contents of cubital fossa is exposed.		11. Ulnar artery and vein	
		12. Superficial and deep division of radial nerve.	
		13. NV to pronator teres.	

FRONT OF ARM

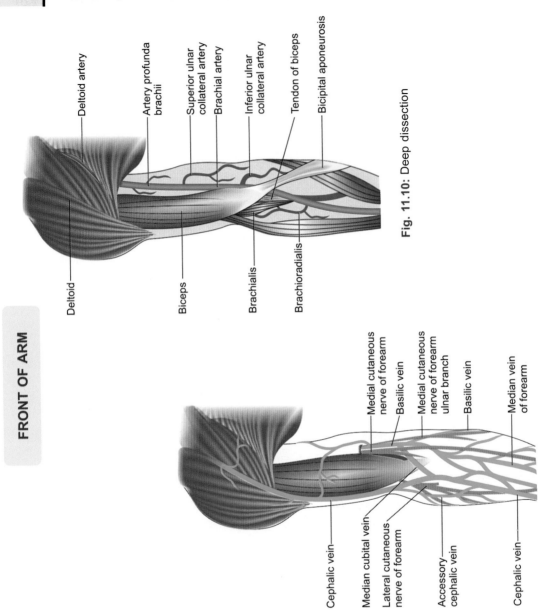

Deltoid artery

Artery profunda brachii

Superior ulnar collateral artery

Brachial artery

Inferior ulnar collateral artery

Tendon of biceps

Bicipital aponeurosis

Deltoid

Biceps

Brachialis

Brachioradialis

Fig. 11.10: Deep dissection

Medial cutaneous nerve of forearm

Basilic vein

Medial cutaneous nerve of forearm ulnar branch

Basilic vein

Median vein of forearm

Cephalic vein

Median cubital vein

Lateral cutaneous nerve of forearm

Accessory cephalic vein

Cephalic vein

Fig. 11.8: Incision

POSITION OF BODY–SUPINE, WITH UPPER LIMB IS AT RIGHT ANGLE TO THE BODY

Incision (Fig. 11.8)	Comment	Identification (Figs 11.9 and 11.10)	(Applied Anatomy)
• One transverse incision at the junction of upper ¼th to lower ¾th of arm • Another Transverse incision at the point of epicondyles of humerus. • A longitudinal incision along the midpoint of two transverse incisions. • Skin flaps is reflected. • Superficial fascia is exposed	Muscles forming the fleshy belly (biceps) actually acts upon the forearm as flexor of elbow joint and supinator of forearm. You all familiar to show this buldge to your friends. Deep to biceps lies another important flexor of forearm is brachialis.	• Cephalic vein in delto pectoral groove. • Basilic vein on medial side of the arm unites with brachial vein in the upper ¼th of arm and form axillary vein. • Biceps brachii (long head and short head) • Coraco brachialis • Brachialis • Brachial artery • Musculocutaneous nerve—continuation of lateral cord of brachial plexus. • Median nerve • Ulnar nerve–continuation of medial cord of brachial plexus • Radial nerve along with arterial profunda brachialis.	• Nerve injuries. • Supracondylar fracture. • Auto mobile accident. • Amputation.

FRONT OF FOREARM

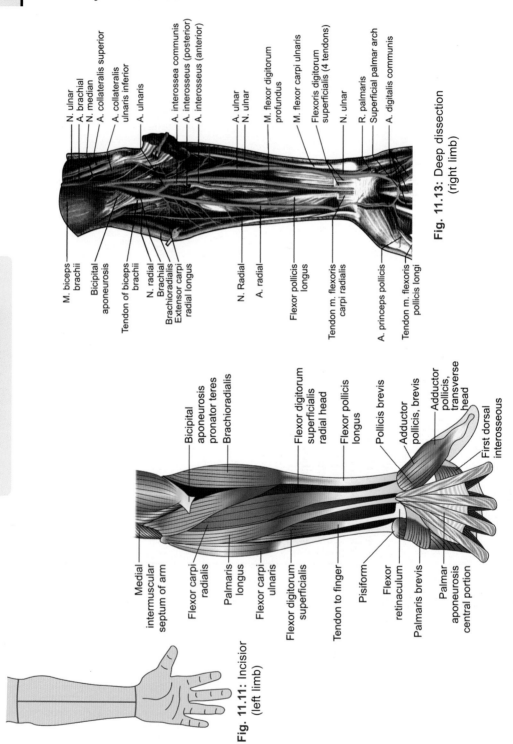

M. biceps brachii
Bicipital aponeurosis
Tendon of biceps brachii
N. radial
Brachial
Brachioradialis
Extensor carpi radial longus

N. Radial
A. radial

Flexor pollicis longus

Tendon m. flexoris carpi radialis

A. princeps pollicis

Tendon m. flexoris pollicis longi

N. ulnar
A. brachial
N. median
A. collateralis superior
A. collateralis ulnaris inferior
A. ulnaris

A. interossea communis
A. interosseus (posterior)
A. interosseus (anterior)

A. ulnar
N. ulnar
M. flexor digitorum profundus
M. flexor carpi ulnaris
Flexoris digitorum superficialis (4 tendons)
N. ulnar
R. palmaris
Superficial palmar arch
A. digitalis communis

Fig. 11.13: Deep dissection (right limb)

Medial intermuscular septum of arm
Flexor carpi radialis
Palmaris longus
Flexor carpi ulnaris
Flexor digitorum superficialis
Tendon to finger
Pisiform
Flexor retinaculum
Palmaris brevis
Palmar aponeurosis central portion

Bicipital aponeurosis
pronator teres
Brachioradialis

Flexor digitorum superficialis radial head

Flexor pollicis longus

Pollicis brevis

Adductor pollicis, brevis

Adductor pollicis, transverse head

First dorsal interosseous

Fig. 11.11: Incisior (left limb)

SOME OF THE DISSECTION—FRONT OF FOREARM

POSITION OF BODY-SUPINE, WITH UPPER LIMB IS AT RIGHT ANGLE TO THE BODY

Incision (Fig. 11.11)	Comment	Identification (Figs 11.12 and 11.13)	(Applied Anatomy)
• Transverse incision at the of elbow. • Transverse incision at the wrist from ulnar styloid process to radial styloid process. • Mid line vertical incision from proximal to distal part. Reflect skin sideways.	The extremities possess deep fascia. So in front of forearm there is superficial fascia. Deep fascia, preserving the important veins like median cubital veins in the middle, basilic vein on the medial side of forearm. Superficial fascia is reflected like skin. Deep fascia is exposed. It look like a tracing paper. It is incised like skin and muscles of forearm and neurovascular structures are exposed. • Mind that all muscles of forearm-are supplied by median nerve in forearm except flexor carpi ulnaris—supplied by ulner nerve.	• Median cubital vein • Cephalic vein on lateral side. • Basilic vein in the medial side. • Medial cutaneous NV of forearm. • Pronator teres. • Flexor carpi radialis • Flexor digitorum super-ficialis • Palmaris longus. • Flexor carpi ulnaris. • Flexor digitorum profun-dus • Supinator • Ulnar artery are separated from ulnar nerve by deep head of pronator teres • Ulner nerve are separated by deep head of pronator teres • Radial artery • Radial nerve • Median nerve is plastered under flexor digitorum superficialis.	• Carpal tunnel syndrome • Effect of nerve injury • Space of parona.

PALM

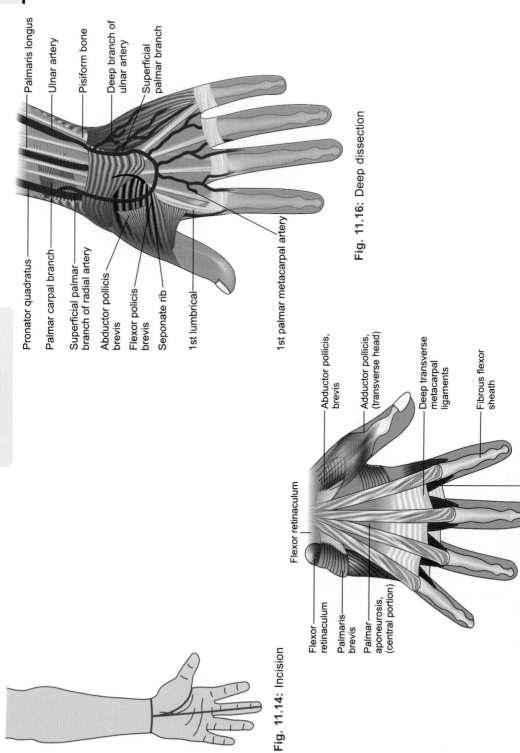

Palmaris longus
Ulnar artery
Pisiform bone
Deep branch of ulnar artery
Superficial palmar branch

Pronator quadratus
Palmar carpal branch
Superficial palmar branch of radial artery
Abductor pollicis brevis
Flexor pollicis brevis
Seponate rib
1st lumbrical

1st palmar metacarpal artery

Fig. 11.16: Deep dissection

Abductor pollicis, brevis
Adductor pollicis, (transverse head)
Deep transverse metacarpal ligaments
Fibrous flexor sheath

Flexor retinaculum

Flexor retinaculum
Palmaris brevis
Palmar aponeurosis, (central portion)

Fig. 11.14: Incision

POSITION OF BODY–SUPINE, WITH UPPER LIMB IS AT RIGHT ANGLE TO THE BODY

Incision (Fig. 11.14)	Comment	Identification (Figs 11.15 and 11.16)	(Applied Anatomy)
• Transverse incision (proximal incision) from radial styloid process to ulnar stylod process.	The skin of the palm and sole are thick and known as glabrous skin. It is devoid of hair follicle, Sebaceous gland. Palm of hand is very important. Lateral 3½ digit are innervated by median nerve medical 1½ digit are innervated by ulnar nerve.	• Palmar cutaneous branch of median and ulnar nerve	• Claw hand
• Transverse incision along the distal part along the webs of the finger.		• Palmaris brevis, which increases the power of grip.	• Ape hand
• Vertical incision from mid point of tip of middle finger upto middle of (1st proximal) incision		• Palmar aponeurosis	• Mid palmer space and thenar space infection.
• Another longitudinal incision from the mid point of proximal incision upto base of thumb.		• Muscles of thenar eminence, i.e. Abductor pollicis brevis. Flexor pollcis and oppoens pollicis	• Ulnar tunnel syndrome
• Skin flaps are reflected. Superficial fascia with cutaneous nerve and only subcutaneous muscle palmaris brevis is exposed.	Superficial fascia is reflected like skins. Palmar aponeurosis (shiny deep fascia) is exposed.	• Adductor pollicis	• Infection of pulp space of finger
		• Muscle of hypothenar eminence.	• Dupuytren's contracture.
		• Abductor digiti minimi	
		• Flexor digiti minimi	
		• Opponens digiti minimi	
		• Superficial palmar arch—formed mainly by superficial branch of ulnar artery.	

TRIANGULAR AND QUADRANGULAR SPACE

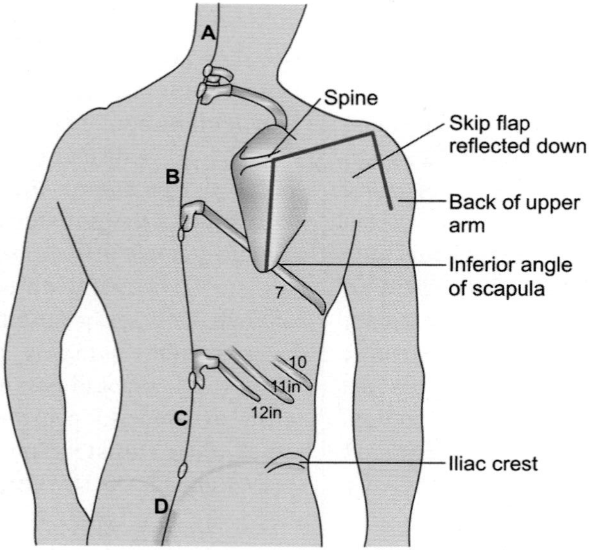

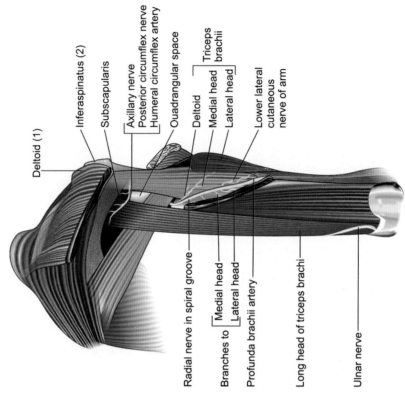

Deltoid (1)

Inferaspinatus (2)

Subscapularis

Axillary nerve
Posterior circumflex nerve
Humeral circumflex artery

Quadrangular space

Deltoid

Medial head
Lateral head] Triceps brachii

Lower lateral
cutaneous
nerve of arm

Radial nerve in spiral groove

Branches to [Medial head
Lateral head]

Profunda brachii artery

Long head of triceps brachi

Ulnar nerve

Fig. 11.18: Deep dissection

Spine

Skip flap
reflected down

Back of upper
arm

Inferior angle
of scapula

Iliac crest

10
11in
12in

7

A

B

C

D

Fig. 11.17: Incisions (triangular; quadrangular space)

NAME OF THE DISSECTION–TRIANGULAR AND QUADRANGULAR SPACE

POSITION OF BODY–PRONE WITH ARM AT RIGHT ANGLE TO THE BODY

Incision (Fig. 11.17)	Comment (Fig. 11.18)	Identification (Fig. 11.18)	(Applied Anatomy)
• Feel the spine of scapula. • From the midpoint of spine a vertical incision extend upto inferior angle of scapula. • Oblique incision extends from above incision along the back of the spine upto acromion and the upper part of arm. From it extends downwards towards the table. • Oblique incision from inferior angle of scapula upwords and laterally upto posterior axillary fold.	• The lower border of teres minor is separated by a gap from the upper border of major. This gap is divided and long head of triceps into medial quadrangular and lateral triangular space. Boundary of quadrangular space. • Above–teres minor below – Teres major medially–long-head of triceps. Laterally–surgical neck of humerus • Contents: axillary nerve, posterior humeral circum-flex artery. • Triangular space—upper by teres minor. Lower–upper border of teres major. Laterally–By long head of triceps.	• Muscles, teres minor, long head of triceps. • Vessels • Posterior humeral circum-flex vessels, circumflex, Scapular vessels, and • Nerves—axillary nerve and its branches pseudo ganglion over the nerve to teres minor.	• Nailing of humeral surgical neck done through this space; care should be taken during nailing, as it may damage the axillary nerve.

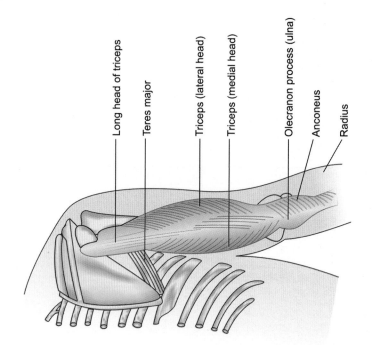

Long head of triceps

Teres major

Triceps (lateral head)

Triceps (medial head)

Olecranon process (ulna)

Anconeus

Radius

Fig. 11.19B: Muscles of back of arm

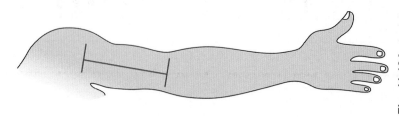

Fig. 11.19A: Incision

NAME OF THE DISSECTION–BACK OF ARM

POSITION OF BODY–PRONE WITH ARM REST OVER THE WOODEN SHEET AT RIGHT ANGLE TO BODY

Incision (Fig. 11.19A)	Comment (Fig. 11.19B)	Identification (Fig. 11.19B)	(Applied Anatomy)
• Transverse incision at the upper ¼th of arm. • Transverse incision from medial epicondyle to lateral epicondyle. • Midline vertical incision extends from upper to lower incision.	There is only one large fleshy muscle in the back, which cover the structures of radial groove. The muscle is triceps brachii which is a powerful forearm extensor. Out of three heads, long and lateral head lies superficial to medial head.	• long, lateral and medial head of triceps. • Insertion of triceps • Radial nerve. • Arteria profuna brachii	Injury to radial nerve in spiral groove. • Saturday night palsy • Crutch paralysis • Wrist drop.

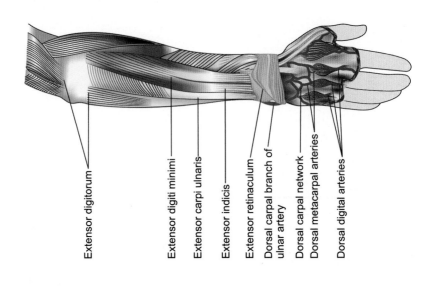

Extensor digitorum

Extensor digiti minimi

Extensor carpi ulnaris

Extensor indicis

Extensor retinaculum

Dorsal carpal branch of ulnar artery

Dorsal carpal network

Dorsal metacarpal arteries

Dorsal digital arteries

Fig. 11.22: Deep dissection

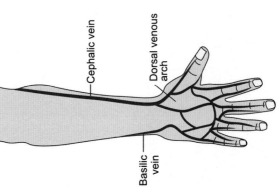

Cephalic vein

Dorsal venous arch

Basilic vein

Fig. 11.21: Superficial dissection

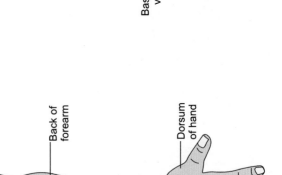

Back of forearm

Dorsum of hand

Fig. 11.20: Incision

POSITION OF BODY (PRONE WITH FOREARM FULLY PRONATED)

Incision (Fig. 11.20)	Comment (Fig. 11.21)	Identification (Fig. 11.22)	(Applied Anatomy)
Back of forearm • Transverse incisions from medial epicondyle to lateral epicondyle. • Transverse incision extends from radial styloid process to ulnar styloid process • Midline vertical incision connecting of the two transverse incision.	• Superficial fascia with cephalic vein on lateral side and basilic vein on medial side is exposed. • Remove superficial fasica (preserving the vein) and deep fascia like similar incision as skin. • Muscles are exposed all the extension group arises from a common tendons from the post surface of lateral condyle of humerus.	• Extensor retinaculum • Abductor pollicis longus and abductor pollicis brevis—out cropping muscles. • Extensor pollicis longus • 4 tendons of extensor digitorum. • Extensor carpi radialis longus and brevis. • Extensor indicis • Extensor digiti minimi • Extensor carpi ulnaris.	• Wrist drop • Mallet finger
Dorsum of Hand • Transverse incisions from ulnar styloid process to radial styloid process. • Transverse incision along the roots of finger • Vertical incision extendes from proximal incision upto nail to middle finger.	The skin here is so thin that you can visualise the superficial veins. Not only that you will get here Anatomical snuffbox (Bounded laterlly by abductor pollicis longus and extensor pollicis brevis Medially by extensor pollicis longus. Base formed by scaphoid, trapezium and base 1st (metacarpal) Realise all the tendon present in dorsum by producing its movement.	• Dorsal venous arch • Tendon of extensor pollicies brevis • Tendons of extensor pollicis longus • 4 tendons of extensor digitorum. • Extensor indicis • Extensor digiti minimi • Extersor digitorum brevis • Cutaneous branches of radial and ulnar nerve.	• Synovial cyst. • Digital block • Paresthesia

FEMORAL TRIANGLE

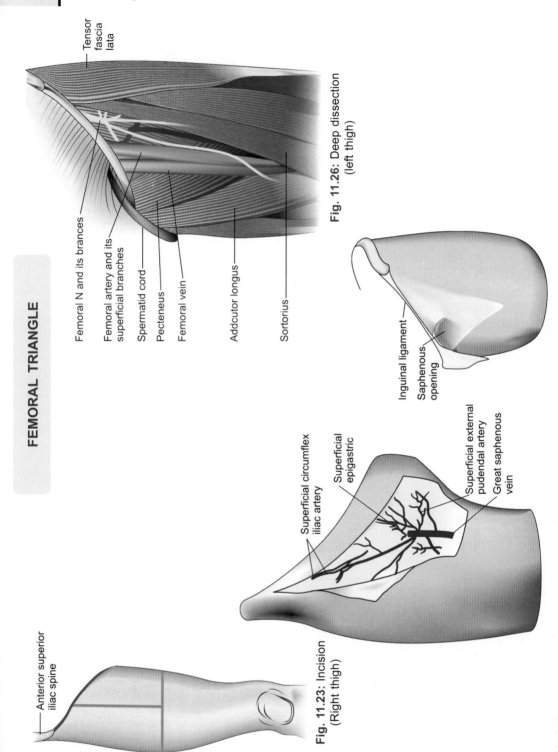

Tensor fascia lata

Femoral N and its brances

Femoral artery and its superficial branches

Spermatid cord

Pecteneus

Femoral vein

Addcutor longus

Sortorius

Fig. 11.26: Deep dissection (left thigh)

Inguinal ligament

Saphenous opening

Superficial circumflex iliac artery

Superficial epigastric

Superficial external pudendal artery

Great saphenous vein

Anterior superior iliac spine

Fig. 11.23: Incision (Right thigh)

NAME OF THE DISSECTION–FEMORAL TRIANGLE
POSITION OF BODY–BODY SUPINE WITH THIGH ABDUCTED LATERALLY

Incision (Fig. 11.23)	Comment (Fig. 11.26)	Identification (Figs 11.24 to 11.26)	(Applied Anatomy)
• One oblique incision from anterior superior iliac spine to pubic tubercle along the inguinal ligament. • One transverse incision at the junction of upper 1/3rd and lower 2/3rd of front of thigh. Which extends below anterior superior iliac spine. No need of extension of transverse incision away from this level. • A midline vertical incision extending from mid inguinal point to lower transverse incision.	The triangle is situated in front of the upper 3rd of thigh. Base (above) formed by inguinal ligament. Apex (below) meeting of Sartorius and adductor longus Medial border–by medial border of adductor longus. lateral border–by sartorius. Floor–From lateral to medial–Iliacus, psoas, pectineus, abductor longus muscles.	• Inguinal ligament. • Great saphenous vein • Femoral sheath (contents–Femoral artery, femoral vein, femoral canal) • Femoral nerve in ilio psoas groove • Lateral femoral cutaneous nerve, below anterior superior iliac spine. • Inguinal lymph nodes. • Adductor longus • Pectineus • Iliacus. • Psoas	• Swelling of inguinal lymph nodes. • Psoas abscess • Femoral hernia more common in female. • Varicose veins. • Meralgia paresthetica. • Repair of femoral hernia. • Spastic paralysis • Riders bone • Venous graft in caronary surgery.

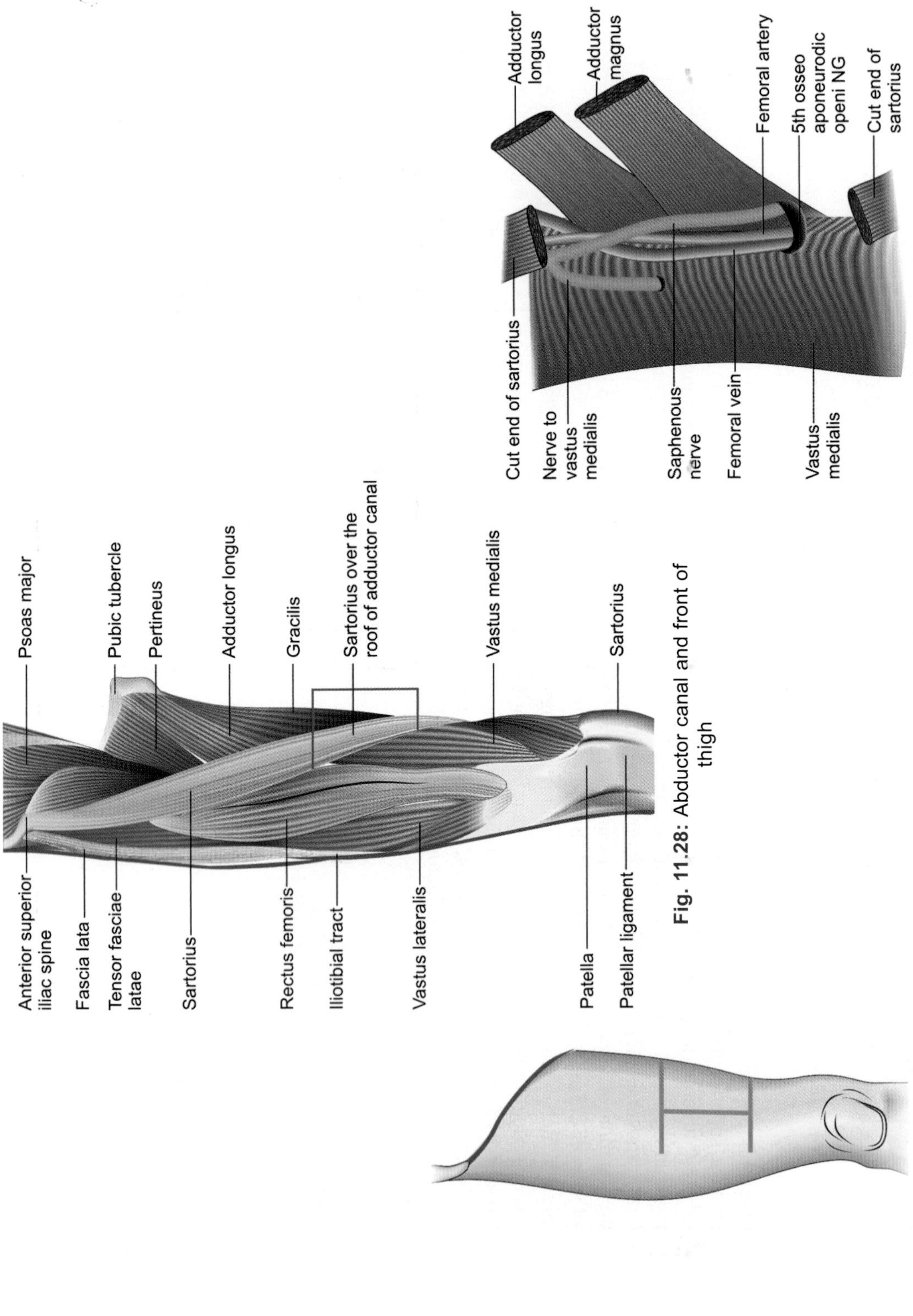
Adductor longus
Adductor magnus
Femoral artery
5th osseo aponeurodic openi NG
Cut end of sartorius
Cut end of sartorius
Nerve to vastus medialis
Saphenous nerve
Femoral vein
Vastus medialis
Psoas major
Pubic tubercle
Pertineus
Adductor longus
Gracilis
Sartorius over the roof of adductor canal
Vastus medialis
Sartorius
Anterior superior iliac spine
Fascia lata
Tensor fasciae latae
Sartorius
Rectus femoris
Iliotibial tract
Vastus lateralis
Patella
Patellar ligament

Fig. 11.28: Abductor canal and front of thigh

POSITION OF BODY (SUPINE WITH THIGH EXTENDED, AND ROTATED LATERALLY)

Incision (Fig. 11.27)	Comment (Fig. 11.28)	Identification (Figs 11.28 and 11.29)	(Applied Anatomy)
• One transverse incision at the front of the lower 2/3rd of the front of thigh (extends upto the level of anterior superior iliac spine) • Another transverse incision at the level of lower 1/3rd of thigh. • A midline vertical incision from midpoint of proximal and distal incisions	Adductor canal or Hunter's canal is exposed after removal of deep fascia. Boundary—laterally—by medialis border of vastus medialis; medially—above by adductor longus; below by adductor magnus. roof—Formed by deep fascia.	• lateral and medial circumflex femoral artery. • Deep division of femoral nerve and its muscular branches. • Saphenous nerve (only cutaneous branch of posteior division of femoral nerve) • Nerve to vastus medialis • Vasti and adductor longus, adductor brevis muscles.	• ligature of femoral artery done in this canal during popliteal artery aneurysm • Stab injuries of thigh injuries the structures of adductor canal.

NAME OF THE DISSECTION–FRONT OF THIGH
POSITION OF BODY–BODY SUPINE AND KNEE EXTENDED

Incision	Comment	Identification (Fig. 11.28)	(Applied Anatomy)
One transverse incision from head of fibula to tibia (upper end) Other incision is given before.	Reflect the skins laterally and medially	• The vastus medialis, lateralis, rectus femoris and vastus intermedius	• Quadriceps weakness. (due to constant wearing of high heel shoes and also in persons having long standing duties

ANTERO LATERAL COMPARTMENT

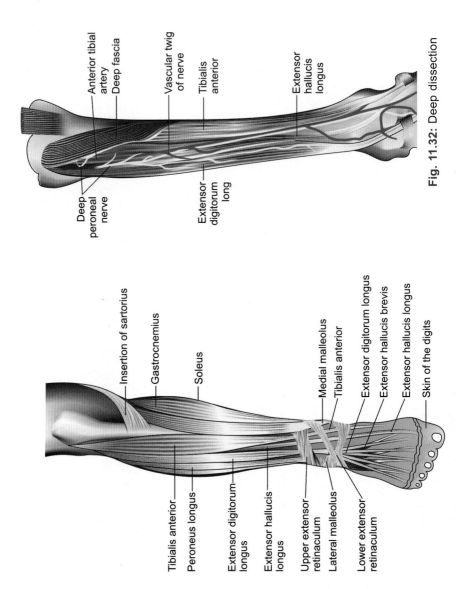

Anterior tibial artery
Deep fascia
Vascular twig of nerve
Tibialis anterior
Extensor hallucis longus
Deep peroneal nerve
Extensor digitorum long

Fig. 11.32: Deep dissection

Insertion of sartorius
Gastrocnemius
Soleus
Medial malleolus
Tibialis anterior
Extensor digitorum longus
Extensor hallucis brevis
Extensor hallucis longus
Skin of the digits

Tibialis anterior
Peroneus longus
Extensor digitorum longus
Extensor hallucis longus
Upper extensor retinaculum
Lateral malleolus
Lower extensor retinaculum

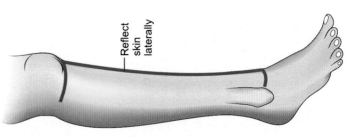

Reflect skin laterally

Fig. 11.30: Incision

(ANTERIOR COMPARTMENT OF LEG)

POSITION OF BODY–SUPINE WITH THIGH ABDUCTED LATERALLY

Incision (Fig. 11.30)	Comment (Fig. 11.31)	Identification (Figs 11.31 and 11.32)	(Applied Anatomy)
• Transverse incision from tibial tuberosity to head of fibula (proximal incision) • Distal in incision from mid point between two malleoli upto lateral malleolus. • Vertical incisions from tibial tubersity to distal incision. • Reflect superficial and deep fascia laterally	Anterior compartment of leg is exposed. Boundary–Medially by antero lateral surface of shaft of tibia laterally–by anterior inter-muscular, septum. Anteriorly by deep fascia of leg (fascia cruris) Posteriorly–by interosseous membrane	• Tibialis anterior • Anterior tibial veins • Deep peroneal nerve in between tibialis anterior and extensor digitorum longus. • Extensor hallucis longus. • Peroneous tertious	• Anterior compartment of leg syndrome • Infiltration common pero-neal nerve producing anes-thesia.

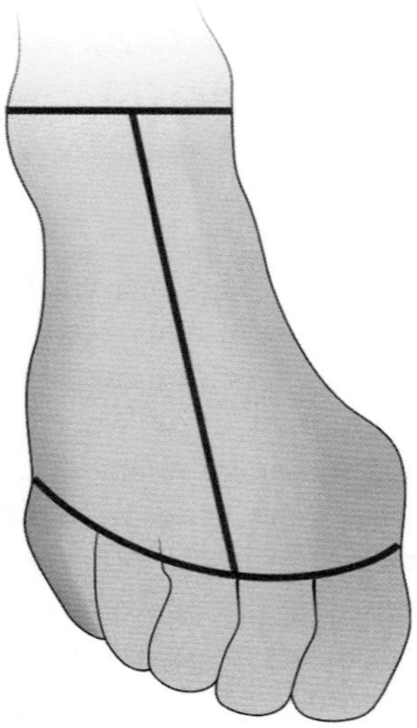

DORSUM OF FOOT

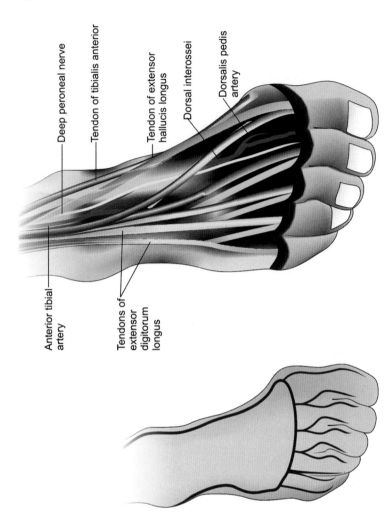

Deep peroneal nerve

Tendon of tibialis anterior

Tendon of extensor hallucis longus

Dorsal interossei

Dorsalis pedis artery

Anterior tibial artery

Tendons of extensor digitorum longus

Fig. 11.35: Deep dissection

Fig. 11.34: Dorsal venous network

Fig. 11.33: Incision

POSITION OF BODY (Supine with Slight Planter Flexion of Foot)

Incision (Fig. 11.33)	Comment	Identification (Figs 11.34 and 11.35)	(Applied Anatomy)
• Proximal transverse incision from medial malleoli to lateral malleoli. • Distal curved incision along the roots of the toes.	The skin is thin, with minimum amount of subcutaneous tissue so during movents of toes all the tendons can visible through skins.	• Dorsal venous network, lies dorsal to tendons of extensor muscles. • Tendon of extensor hallucis longus. • 4 tendons of extensor digitorum longus. • Peroneus tertius. • Dorsalis pedis artery and deep peroneal nerve in between tendon of hallucis and digitorum longus.	Palpation of • dorsalis pedis pulse. • Buerger disease. • Venae section. • Varicose vein • Football ankle.

GLUTEAL REGION

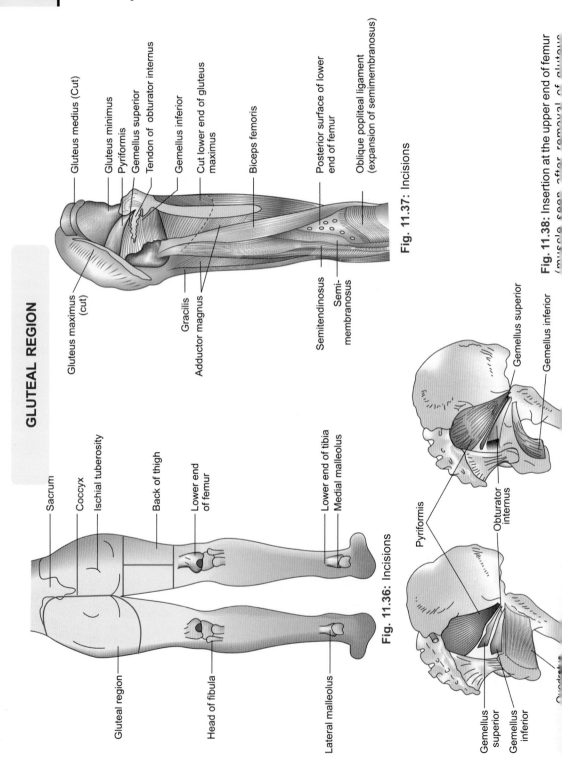

Fig. 11.36: Incisions

- Sacrum
- Coccyx
- Ischial tuberosity
- Back of thigh
- Lower end of femur
- Lower end of tibia
- Medial malleolus
- Gluteal region
- Head of fibula
- Lateral malleolus

Fig. 11.37: Incisions

- Gluteus medius (Cut)
- Gluteus minimus
- Pyriformis
- Gemellus superior
- Tendon of obturator internus
- Gemellus inferior
- Cut lower end of gluteus maximus
- Biceps femoris
- Posterior surface of lower end of femur
- Oblique popliteal ligament (expansion of semimembranosus)
- Gluteus maximus (cut)
- Gracilis
- Adductor magnus
- Semitendinosus
- Semi-membranosus

Fig. 11.38: Insertion at the upper end of femur (muscle seen after removal of gluteus

- Pyriformis
- Gemellus superior
- Gemellus inferior
- Obturator internus
- Gemellus superior
- Gemellus inferior

NAME OF THE DISSECTION–GLUTEAL REGION
POSITION OF BODY–Prone

Incision (Fig. 11.36)	Comment	Identification (Figs 11.37 and 11.38)	(Applied Anatomy)

• Curved incision from posterior superior iliac spine along the iliac crest towards anterior superior iliac spine (as far as body will permit)
 • From posterior superior iliac spine downwards and medially upto coccyx.
 • From coccyx a curved incision downwards and laterally upto the junction of upper one fourth and lower 3/4th of back of the thigh (below the gluteal fold)
 • Skin with superfical fascia is reflected laterally and downwards.
	It is an extensive region covered with plenty of fat. The region extends above upto iliac crest, below limited by gluteal fold. Anteriorly it extends upto a line from anterior superior iliac spine upto greater trochanter, posterior limit is natal fold.	• Gluteus maximus (coarse fiber)
		 • Gluteal aponeurosis.
		 • Structures under the gluteus maximus.
		  a. gluteus medius.
		  b. pyriformis
		 • **Above the pyriformis :**
		  c. Superior gluteal vessels and nerve.
		 • **Below the pyriformis**
		  d. Inferior gluteal vessels and nerve.
		  e. Sciatic nerve (widest nerve in the body)
		  f. Posterior femoral cutaneous nerve.
		  g. Structures over ischial spine
		   • Internal pudendal vessels and nerve.
		   • Nerve to obturator internus
			• Intramuscular injection
			 • Muscle transplant
			 • Weavers bottom
			 • muscle weakness and paralysis

POPLITEAL FOSSA

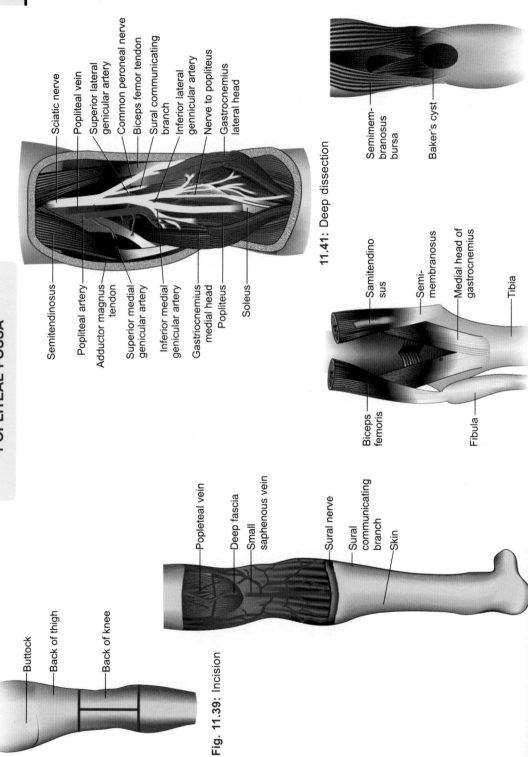

Sciatic nerve

Popliteal vein

Superior lateral genicular artery

Common peroneal nerve

Biceps femor tendon

Sural communicating branch

Inferior lateral genicular artery

Nerve to popliteus

Gastrocnemius lateral head

Semitendinosus

Popliteal artery

Adductor magnus tendon

Superior medial genicular artery

Inferior medial genicular artery

Gastriocnemius medial head

Popliteus

Soleus

11.41: Deep dissection

Semimem-branosus bursa

Baker's cyst

Samitendino sus

Semi-membranosus

Medial head of gastrocnemius

Tibia

Biceps femoris

Fibula

Popleteal vein

Deep fascia

Small saphenous vein

Sural nerve

Sural communicating branch

Skin

Buttock

Back of thigh

Back of knee

Fig. 11.39: Incision

POSITION OF BODY–PRONE WITH EXTENDED KNEE

Incision *(Fig. 11.39)*	*Comment* *(Fig. 11.42)*	*Identification* *(Figs 11.40 to 11.42)*	*(Applied Anatomy)* *(Fig. 11.43)*
• Transverse incision at the junction of upper 2/3rd and lower 1/3rd of back of thigh. Another vertical incision connecting the mid point of the proximal and distal incision. • Transverse incision at the back of leg at the junction of upper 1/3rd and lower 2/3rd.	This fossa is situated at the back of knee bounded above and medially by semimembranosus, semitendinosus below and medially by medial head of gastrocnemius. Above and laterally by biceps femoris. Below and laterally by lateral head of gastrocnemius and plantaris floor of the fossa formed by (From above downwards) Popliteal surface of femur, oblique pepliteal ligament, popliteus muscle. Roof by deep fascia which is pierced by small saphenous vein.	• The muscles : both head of gastrocnemius • Plantaris. • Semimembranosus • Semitedinosus • Popliteus. Vessels–popliteal artery with genicular and muscular branches. Popliteal vein with its tributaries. Behind the middle of knee the relation of three structures are (from superficial to deep) tibial nerve, popliteal vein and artery. **Nerves**–Tibial nerve with its muscular branches and a cutaneous branch in the middle of the fossa. • Common peroneal nerve with its branches at the medial border of biceps femoris.	• Popliteal cyst. • Backer cyst. • Popliteal artery aneurysm.

BACK OF THIGH

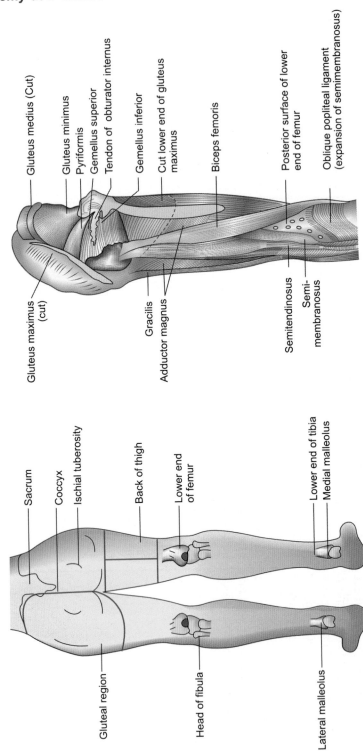

Gluteus medius (Cut)
Gluteus minimus
Pyriformis
Gemellus superior
Tendon of obturator internus
Gemellus inferior
Cut lower end of gluteus maximus
Biceps femoris
Posterior surface of lower end of femur
Oblique popliteal ligament (expansion of semimembranosus)

Gluteus maximus (cut)

Gracilis
Adductor magnus

Semitendinosus
Semi-membranosus

Fig. 11.45: Incisions

Sacrum
Coccyx
Ischial tuberosity

Back of thigh

Lower end of femur

Lower end of tibia
Medial malleolus

Gluteal region

Head of fibula

Lateral malleolus

Fig. 11.44: Incisions

POSITION OF BODY–PRONE WITH EXTENDED KNEE

Incision (see Fig. 11.44)	Comment	Identification (see Fig 11.45)	(Applied Anatomy)
• Transverse incision in the back of thigh at the level of upper 2/3rd and lower 1/3rd. (Proximal) • Transverse incision at the back of leg at the level of upper 1/3 (distal) and lower 2/3rd of the back of leg. • Vertical incision joining the mid point of the two.	Hamstring muscles are visible clearly. Criteria of this muscles are : • They must arise from ischial tuberosity • Inserted in the bone beyond femurs. • Must be supplied by tibial component of sciatic nerve. • Flexors of knee and extensor of hip.	Muscles are : Semitendinosus, semimem-branosus, Ischial fibers of adductor magnus and long head of biceps femoris. **Vessels are:** Perforating vessels. **Nerves :** • Sciatic • Posterior femoral cutaneous nerve.	• Sciatica • Safe site of injection • Hamstrig Strain (Seen in athlet).

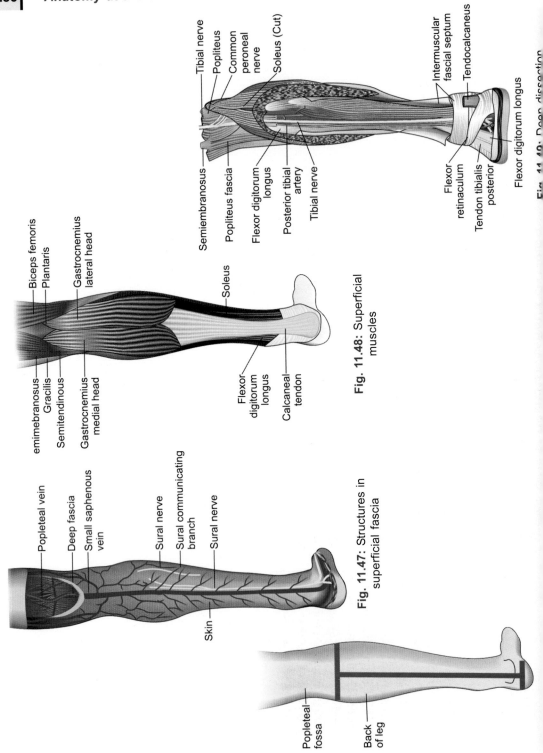

Fig. 11.47: Structures in superficial fascia

Fig. 11.48: Superficial muscles

Fig. 11.49: Deep dissection

NAME OF THE DISSECTION—BACK OF LEG

POSITION OF BODY (Prone with Extended Knee)

Incision *(Fig. 11.46)*	*Comment*	*Identification* *(Figs 11.47 to 11.49)*	*(Applied Anatomy)*
• Proximal–Transrverse incision at the level of fibular head. • Distal–between two malleal at the back of ankle joint. • Midline vertical incision from proximal to distal incisions. • Superficial fascia is exposed and short saphenous vein is seen along with sural nerve.	This region is known as posterior compartment of leg. The leg is divided into anterior, lateral and posterior compartments by anterior and posterior intermuscular septum again the posterior compartment of leg is divided into superficial, middle and deep part by superficial and deep transverse fascia.	• Muscles : – Lateral and medial head of gastrocnemius. – Soleus. – Tendocalcaneus. – Plantaris. – Popliteus – Flexor digitorum longus on medial side. – Flexor hallucis longus. on the lateral side (more bulkier than digitorum) – Tibialis posterior lies in between digitorum and hallucis longus tendon. • Vessels – Posterior tibial art–branch of popliteal artery. – Venae comitantes along the artery. • Nerve – Tibial nerve in leg.	• Foot drop • Tarsal tunnel syndrome.

SOLE

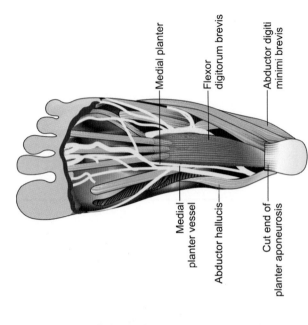

Medial planter

Flexor digitorum brevis

Abductor digiti minimi brevis

Medial planter vessel

Abductor hallucis

Cut end of planter aponeurosis

Fig. 11.52: Muscles of 1st layer

Digital vessels and nerves

Medial plantar artery

Adbuctor hallucis

Central part of plantar aponeurosis

Abductor minimi digiti

Lateral calcanean vessels

Madial calcanean vessels

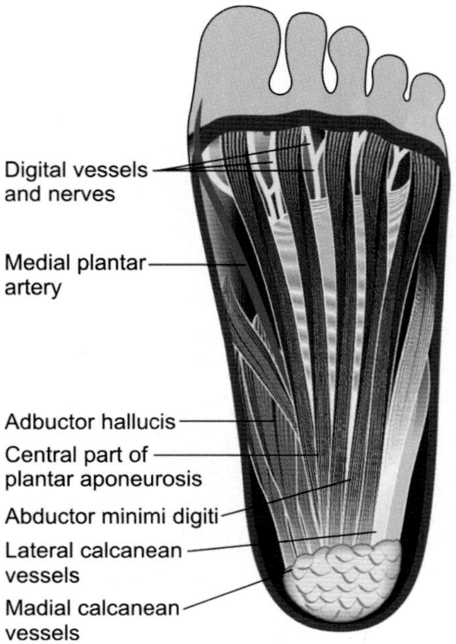

Fig. 11.51: Planter aponeurosis

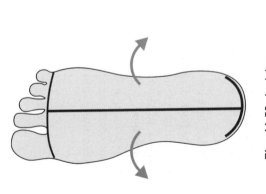

Fig. 11.50: Incision

NAME OF THE DISSECTION–SOLE
POSITION OF BODY–PRONE OR LITHOTOMY POSITION

Incision (Fig. 11.50)	*Comment*	*Identification* (Figs 11.51 and 11.52)	*(Applied Anatomy)*
• Proximal–a curved incision along the heel. • Distal–curved incision at the ball of the toes. • Mid line vertical incision from the tip of 2nd toe upto the midpoint of heel. • Skin is reflected medially and laterally.	Superficial fascia is exposed. It is very much thickened with fat particularly in the weight bearing areas. This type of skin is known as glabrous skin (It is devoid of hairs). Muscles are in four layers but for examination purpose only two superficial layer is important.	• Subcutaneous thick faulty tissue which form the cushion of heel. • Planter aponeurosis (Medial part). Planter aponeurosis (Central part) Planter aponeurosis (lateral part) After cutting planter aponeurosis from proximal aspect 1st layer muscles are exposed. • Medial side–Abductor hallucis • Central–Flexor digitorum brevis. • Lateral side–Abductor digiti minimi. After cutting the flexor digitorum, 2nd layer structures are exposed. • Flexor digitorum accessorius muscle • Lumbicales arises from tendon of flexor digitorum longus.	• Planter fasciitis. • Different variety of club foot. • Police man heel • Bunion.

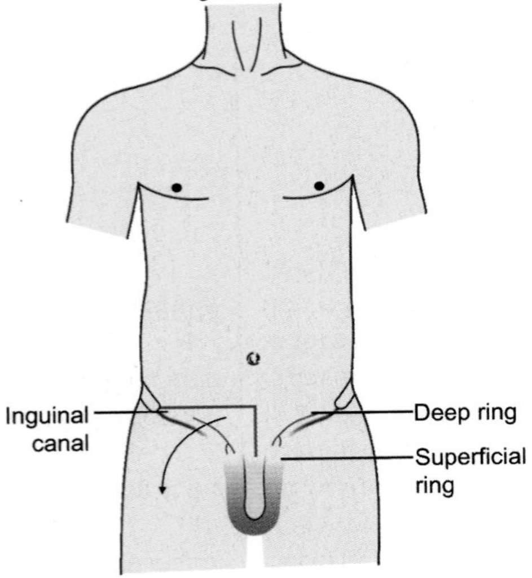

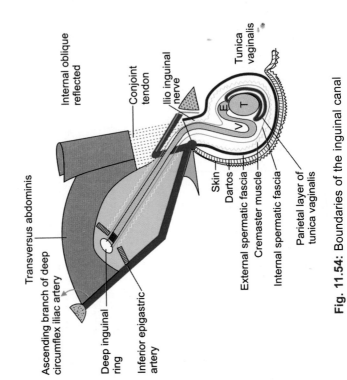

Internal oblique reflected

Conjoint tendon

Ilio inguinal nerve

Tunica vaginalis

Transversus abdominis

Skin
Dartos
External spermatic fascia
Cremaster muscle
Internal spermatic fascia
Parietal layer of tunica vaginalis

Ascending branch of deep circumflex iliac artery

Deep inguinal ring

Inferior epigastric artery

Fig. 11.54: Boundaries of the inguinal canal

Inguinal canal

Deep ring
Superficial ring

Inguinal canal

Fig. 11.53: Incision

NAME OF THE DISSECTION-INGUINAL CANAL
POSITION OF BODY (SUPINE WITH THIGH EXTENDED)

Incision (Fig. 11.53)	Comment (Fig. 11.54)	Identification (Fig. 11.54)	(Applied Anatomy)
• Transverse incision from anterior superior iliac spine upto midline. • Vertical incision from the midline upto pubic tubercle. Reflect the skin and superficial fascia downwards and laterals.	This canal is 4 cm long and extends from deep ring to superficial inguinal ring. Anterior wall– • Throughout its whole extent formed by external oblique aponeurosis. • Anterolaterally re-emforced by internal oblique and transverses abdominis. Post wall–Throughout its whole extent it is formed by fasica transversalis. Medial part of this wall is reinforced by conjoint tendon. Roof–formed by arched fibers of internal oblique and transversus abdominis Floor–inguinal ligament.	• Inguinal ligament. • External oblique muscle and aponeurosis. • Arched fibers of internal oblique and transversus abdominis. • Deep inguinal ring • Ilio inguinal nerve. • Spermatic cord in male and round ligament of uterus in female.	• Hernia direct • Hernia indirect • Extravasation of urine between two layers of superficial fascia during ruptured urethra.

RECTUS SHEATH

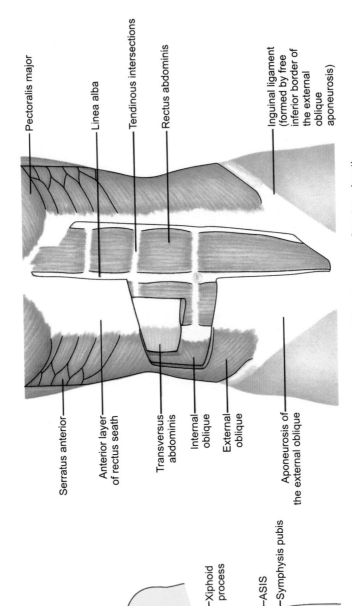

Pectoralis major

Linea alba

Tendinous intersections

Rectus abdominis

Inguinal ligament (formed by free inferior border of the external oblique aponeurosis)

Serratus anterior

Anterior layer of rectus seath

Transversus abdominis

Internal oblique

External oblique

Aponeurosis of the external oblique

Fig. 11.56: Exposure of rectus sheath

Rectus sheath

Xiphoid process

ASIS

Symphysis pubis

Fig. 11.55: Incision
ASIS—Anterior superior iliac spine

POSITION OF BODY (Supine with Thigh Extended)

Incision *(Fig. 11.55)*	*Comment* *(Fig. 11.56)*	*Identification* *(Fig. 11.56)*	*(Applied Anatomy)*
• Transverse incision from xiploid process upto 4½" (10 cm) laterally. • Another oblique incision from anterior superior iliac spine upto pubic tubercle. • Midline vertical incision extending from the mid points of these two incisions. • Skin along with superficial fascia is exposed and reflected sideways. Anterior layer of rectus sheath is exposed.	It is an aponeurotic sheath that is present almost wholly around the rectus abdominis muscle. Lower 1/3rd, it is deficient, where arcuate line is formed. Middle 2/3rd it is aponeurotic and complete. After removing the anterior wall of sheath we can see the transverse intersections.	• Rectus abdonimis muscle. • Pyramidalis, if present • lower 7th to 12th thoracic nerve and iliohypogastric and ilioinguinal nerve enters the muscle towards its lateral aspect. • Free posterior part of sheath.	• Hematoma within the muscle due to injury. • Divertication of recti. • Incisional hernia.

KIDNEY FROM BACK

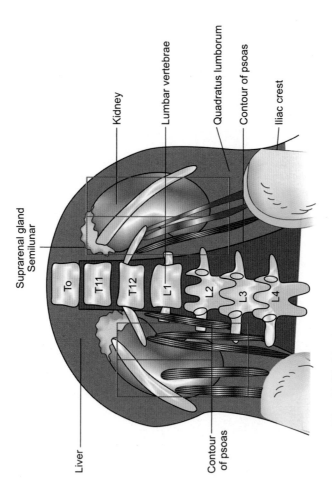

Suprarenal gland
Semilunar

Kidney

Lumbar vertebrae

Quadratus lumborum

Contour of psoas

Iliac crest

To
T11
T12
L1
L2
L3
L4

Liver

Contour
of psoas

Fig. 11.57: Morris paralleogram (Dissection of kidney from back)

POSITION OF BODY (PRONE)

Incision (Fig. 11.57)	*Comment*	*Identification (Fig. 11.57)*	*(Applied Anatomy)*

• Transverse incision extends 1" away from the level of T-11 spine laterally upto 4"
 • Another transverse incision 1" away from L3 spine upto 4" laterally
 • Connect this by vertical incision closer to spine.
	The lower part of kidney is easily found from this dissection. After skin incisions reflect superficial fascia laterally, erector spinae muscle is exposed. All muscles should be retracted medially and fascia should be retracted laterally. Retracted medially posterior layer of thoracolumbar fascia is exposed. Retract the fascia laterally. Quadratus lumborum is exposed. It is retracted medially. Middle layer of thoracolumbar fascia is seen. It is retracted laterally. Lower pole is exposed. This way is safer to expose as it kidney does not posses the peritoneum.	• Erector spinae.
		 • Quadratus lumborum.
		 • Thoracolumbar fascia
		 • Nerves subcostal
		   – Iliohypogastric
		   – Ilioinguinal
		 • Lumbar triangle
		 • Lower pole of kidney
			• Renal angle.
			 • Nephrectomy in the lower pole.
			 • Bimanual palpation of kidney.
			 • Lumbar hernia through triangle.

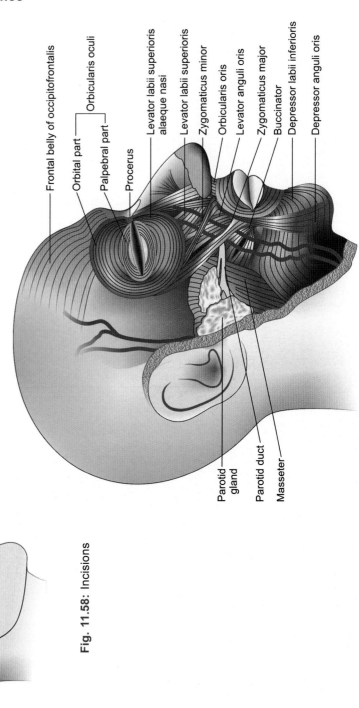

Fig. 11.58: Incisions

NAME OF THE DISSECTION–FACE
POSITION OF BODY–SUPINE

Incision (Fig. 11.58)	Comment	Identification (Fig. 11.59)	(Applied Anatomy)

• Vertical incision extents from nasion to chin; It must encircle the eyes, nostrils and orifice of mouth.
• Transverse incision from outer angle of eye to the upper part of tragus.
• Transverse incision from the angle of the mouth to the lower part of tragus.
• Transverse incision from chin to angle of mandible.
	It is the anterior part of head, extents from one ear to other transversly; vertical extension from scalp to chin.
	It is contributed by facial bones whose architecture produce the shape of face. This shape is also variable by muscles of facial expression muscles have got no bony origin but they are inserted in the skin. They produce facial expression, nonverbal communication.
	They lift the eyebrows, close and open the eyes, flare the nostinal, open and close the mouth. Its importance is very much observed when the muscles are paralysed.
		• Muscles of facial expression particularly.
		  - Orbicularis occuli.
		  - Zygomaticus major and minor
		  - Levator anguli oris.
		  - Orbicularis oris.
		  - Buccinator
		  - Masseter
		• Vessels
		  - Facial artery (tortuous) facial vein (Straight) and lies posterior to artery.
		• Branches of facial nerve.
		• Parotid duct–cord like structure lies between upper buccal and lower buccal nerve.
		• Superficial temporal. vessels and auriculo-temporal nerve.
			• Danger area of face
			• Bells palsy
			• Stone in porotid duct.
			• Accessory parotid gland.

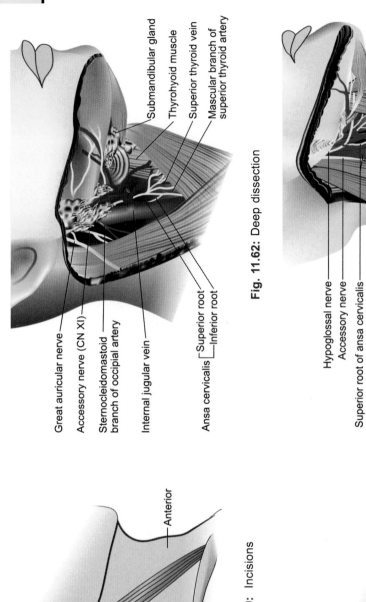

Great auricular nerve

Accessory nerve (CN XI)

Sternocleidomastoid branch of occipial artery

Internal jugular vein

Ansa cervicalis ⌈Superior root
              ⌊Inferior root

Submandibular gland

Thyrohyoid muscle

Superior thyroid vein

Mascular branch of superior thyroid artery

Fig. 11.62: Deep dissection

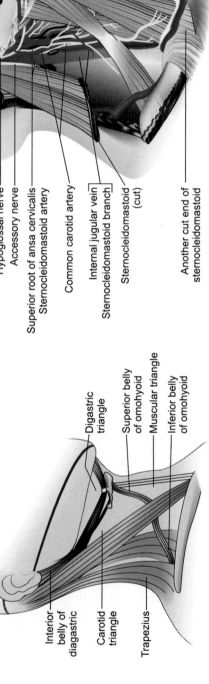

Hypoglossal nerve

Accessory nerve

Superior root of ansa cervicalis

Sternocleidomastoid artery

Common carotid artery

Internal jugular vein
Sternocleidomastoid branch

Sternocleidomastoid (cut)

Another cut end of sternocleidomastoid

Anterior

Posterior

Fig. 11.60: Incisions

Interior belly of diagastric

Carotid triangle

Trapezius

Digastric triangle

Superior belly of omohyoid

Muscular triangle

Inferior belly of omohyoid

POSITION OF BODY (SUPINE WITH NECK EXTENDED)

Incision *(Fig. 11.60)*	*Comment*	*Identification* *(Figs 11.61 to 11.63)*	*(Applied Anatomy)*
• Midline vertical incision from symphysis menti upto the jugular notch of sternum. • Transverse incision extends from symphysis menti along the base of mandible, upto the angle and then upto the mastoid process. • Flap of skin reflected downwards laterally	The anterior triangle is bounded anteriorly by arterior midline of neck, behind by anterior border of sternocleidomastoid. Base is above forms by mandible and apex is directed below towards jugular notch. It is subdivided into different triangles by two bellies of diagastric and superior bolly of omohyoid.	Muscles : • Platysma • Sternocleidomastoid • Anterior belly of diagastric • Posterior belly of diagastric • Sternohyoid • Sternothyroid • Omohyoid (Superior belly) Vessels : • Carotid sheath with its contents. • Common carotid artery, internal jugular vein. • Nerves • Vagus nerve. • Hypoglossal nerve. • External carotid artery with its superior thyroid branch, lingual, and facial branches. Thyroid gland.	• Carorid pulse • Branchial cyst. • Cannulation in internal Jugular vein. • Jugular venous pressure • Enlargement of thyroid • Stenosis of internal carotid artery. • lesion of cervical sympathetic nerve.

POSTERIOR TRIANGLE OF NECK

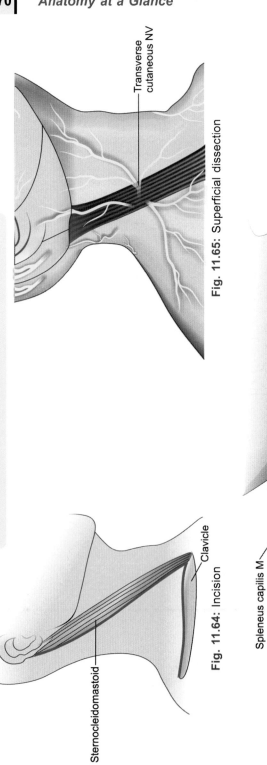

Fig. 11.64: Incision

Sternocleidomastoid

Clavicle

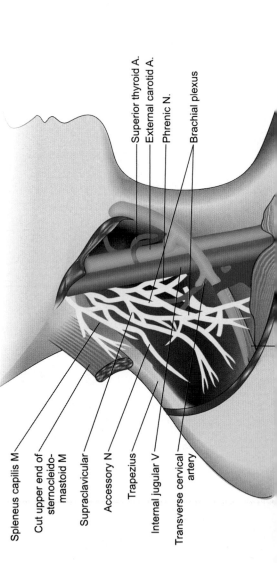

Fig. 11.65: Superficial dissection

Transverse cutaneous NV

Superior thyroid A.

External carotid A.

Phrenic N.

Brachial plexus

Spleneus capilis M

Cut upper end of sternocleido-mastoid M

Supraclavicular

Accessory N

Trapezius

Internal jugular V

Transverse cervical artery

POSITION OF BODY (SUPINE WITH NECK TURNED TOWARDS OPPOSITE SIDE)

Incision *(Fig. 11.64)*	*Comment*	*Identification* *(Figs 11.65 and 11.66)*	*(Applied Anatomy)*
• Vertical incision along the posterior border of sternocleidomastoid. • Transverse incision from angle of mandible upto a furrow behind sternocleidomastoid and mastoid process. • Another transverse incision from sternocleidomastoid (lower attachment) upto anterior margin of trapezius.	• Boundary—*Anterior* posterior border of sternomastoid. *Posterior*—by anterior border of trapezius. *Apex* of triangle directed upwards formed by meeting of trapezius and stenocleidomastoid. Base—by clavicle. Floor—by scalenus medius, Levator scapulae, Splenius capitis, semispinalis capitis.	• Supraclavicular nerve. • Transverse cutaneous nerve of neck. • Lesser occipital nerve • Accessory nerve and branches from C_2 and C_3 • Muscles like inferior belly of omohyoid. • Scalenus medius. • Levator scapulae • Splenius capitis • Semispinalis capitis • Sternocleidomastoid, trapezius. • Artery Transverse cervical artery.	• Spasmodic torticolis • Wry neck • Subclavian vein puncture. • Prominence of external Jugular. • Severance of external jugular vein. • Nerve block in posterior triangle • Injury to accessory nerve during surgery of posterior triangle. • Air embolism in external jugular vein. • Compression of subclavian artery. • Cold abscess.

Chapter 12

Histology

Histology—study of different tissues of body by microscope is known as histology.

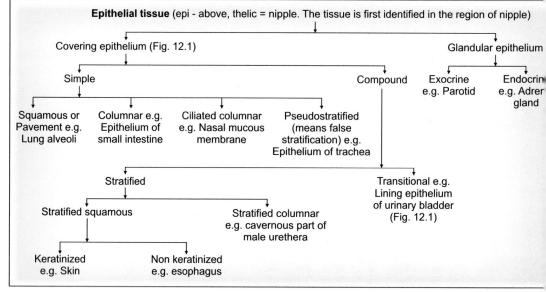

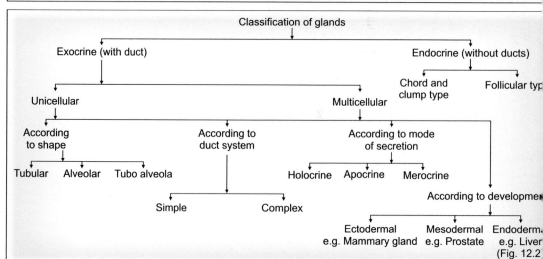

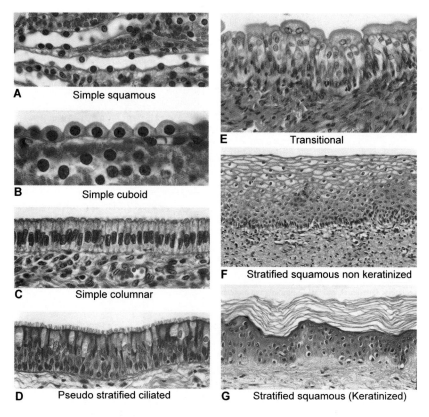

A Simple squamous

B Simple cuboid

C Simple columnar

D Pseudo stratified ciliated

E Transitional

F Stratified squamous non keratinized

G Stratified squamous (Keratinized)

Fig. 12.1: Different types of epithelia

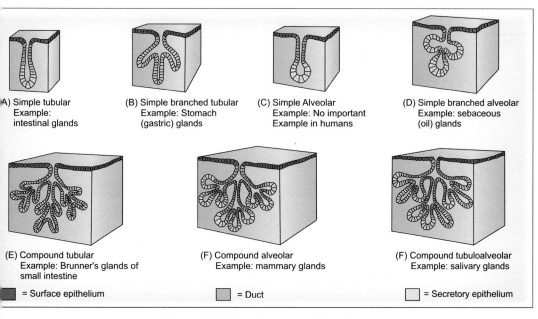

A) Simple tubular
Example:
intestinal glands

(B) Simple branched tubular
Example: Stomach
(gastric) glands

(C) Simple Alveolar
Example: No important
Example in humans

(D) Simple branched alveolar
Example: sebaceous
(oil) glands

(E) Compound tubular
Example: Brunner's glands of
small intestine

(F) Compound alveolar
Example: mammary glands

(F) Compound tubuloalveolar
Example: salivary glands

■ = Surface epithelium   □ = Duct   □ = Secretory epithelium

Fig. 12.2: Different varies of glands

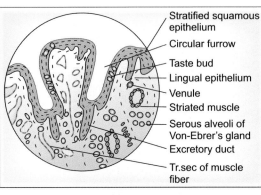

Fig. 12.3A: Fungiform papilla of tongue (HE stained)

- Stratified squamous epithelium
- Circular furrow
- Taste bud
- Lingual epithelium
- Venule
- Striated muscle
- Serous alveoli of Von-Ebrer's gland
- Excretory duct
- Tr.sec of muscle fiber

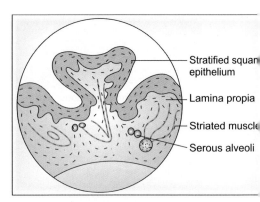

Fig. 12.3B: Circumvallate papilla of tongue (HE stained)

- Stratified squam epithelium
- Lamina propia
- Striated muscle
- Serous alveoli

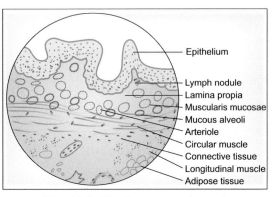

Fig. 12.4: TS of upper esophageal wall (stained with HE)

- Epithelium
- Lymph nodule
- Lamina propia
- Muscularis mucosae
- Mucous alveoli
- Arteriole
- Circular muscle
- Connective tissue
- Longitudinal muscle
- Adipose tissue

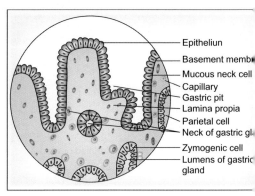

Fig. 12.5: TS of fundus of body of stomach (stained with HE)

- Epitheliun
- Basement memb
- Mucous neck cell
- Capillary
- Gastric pit
- Lamina propia
- Parietal cell
- Neck of gastric gl
- Zymogenic cell
- Lumens of gastric gland

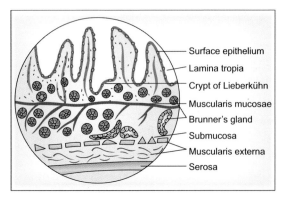

Fig. 12.6: Section of deudenum (HE stained)

- Surface epithelium
- Lamina tropia
- Crypt of Lieberkühn
- Muscularis mucosae
- Brunner's gland
- Submucosa
- Muscularis externa
- Serosa

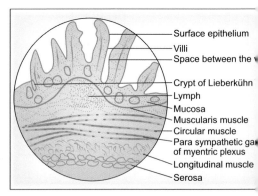

Fig. 12.7: TS of small intestine (stained with H

- Surface epithelium
- Villi
- Space between the v
- Crypt of Lieberkühn
- Lymph
- Mucosa
- Muscularis muscle
- Circular muscle
- Para sympathetic ga of myentric plexus
- Longitudinal muscle
- Serosa

**ME AND POINTS OF IDENTIFICATIONS
DER MICROSCOPE**

trointestinal System

Name	Identifying points under microscope (stained with hematoxylin and Eosin)
ongue Figs 12.3A and B)	• From outside inwards presence of stratified squamous epithelium. • Muscle coat is very thick and haphazard direction. • Papillae present (filiform and fungiform) and sometimes circumvallate
sophagus Fig. 12.4)	• From inside outwards presence of stratified squamous epithelium. • Presence of prominent muscularis mucosae. • Presence of outer longitudinal and inner circular muscle layer.
tomach Fig. 12.5)	• From inside outwards presence of columnar epithelium with gastric glands. • Presence of muscles are arranged in three layers: (a) Inner oblique (b) Middle circular (c) Outer longitudinal.
Duodenum Fig. 12.6)	• From inside outwards presence of columnar epithelium with villi. • Submucous Bruner's gland is present. • Presence of outer longitudinal and inner circular layer.
ejunum and ileum Fig. 12.7)	• From inside outwards presence of brush border columnar epithelium, with intestinal gland (crypts of Lieberikühn). • presence of finger like villi is seen. • We get serous coat, muscle arranged in outer longitudinal and inner circular; submucous coat and mucous membrane.

Contd...

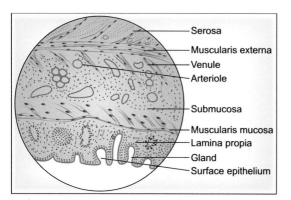

Fig. 12.8: TS of large intestine (stained with HE)

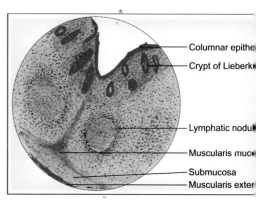

Fig. 12.9: Vermiform appendix

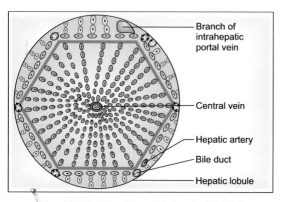

Fig. 12.10: TS of liver (stained with HE)

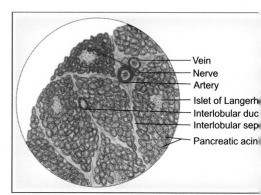

Fig. 12.11: Sectional view of pancreas

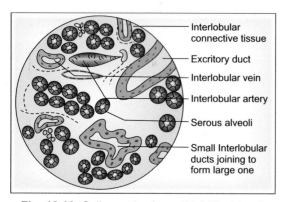

Fig. 12.12: Salivary gland parotid (HE stained)

Name	Identifying points under microscope (stained with hematoxylin and Eosin)
Large gut except appendix and anus (Fig. 12.8)	• From inside outwards, it is lined by columnar epithelium with plenty of goblet cells. • Tenae present (aggregation of longitudinal muscle fiber)
Appendix (Fig. 12.9)	• Absence of intestinal villi • Columnar epithelium with goblet cells. • Promonent lymphoid tissue in submucous coat. • Presence of gap in the muscular coat (hiatus muscularise).
Liver (Fig. 12.10)	• Presence of liver lobule (hexagonal in shape) with central vein. • Presence of portal triad at the different corner of lobule.
Pancreas (Fig. 12.11)	• Connective tissue septa divides the gland into lobules. • Darkly stained serous acini present. • Discrete lightly stained islets of Langerhan present.
Parotid gland (Fig. 12.12)	• Connective tissue septa divides it into number of small lobules containing mainly serous and mucous acini. • No islets of Langerhan. • Ducts are lined by pseudostratified columnar epithelium.

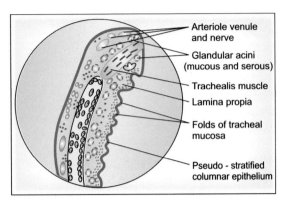

Fig. 12.13: Sectional view of trachea

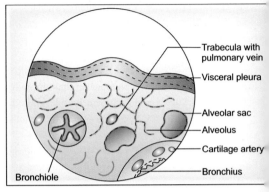

Fig. 12.14: Sectional view of lung (HE stained)

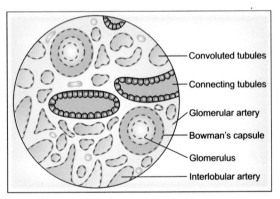

Fig. 12.15: TS of deep cortical area of kidney (stained with HE)

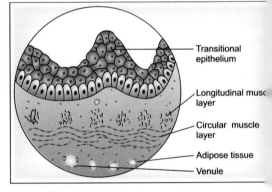

Fig. 12.16: TS of ureter (HE stained)

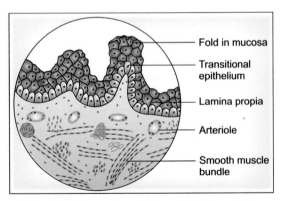

Fig. 12.17: A section of the wall of the urinary bladder (HE stained)

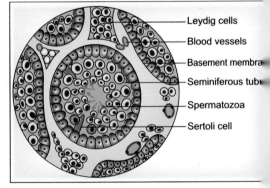

Fig. 12.18: Section of testis (HE stained)

piratory System

Name	Identifying points under microscope (stained with hematoxylin and Eosin)
rachea (Fig. 12.13)	• Lumen lined by pseudostratified columnar epithelium. • Presence of hyaline cartilage (uniform blue color with chondrocyte present in lacunae). • Presence of abundant glands and trachialis muscle.
ungs (Fig. 12.14)	Presence of innumerable alveoli lined by pavement epithelium • Presence of bronchus (identified by incomplete ring of hyaline cartilage). • Presence of bronchiole (cartilage absent) and flower like appearance.
idney (Fig. 12.15)	• Section shows plenty of Bowman's capsules with glomeruli. • Different shapes of tubules (due to cut into different planes) are present
Jreter (Fig. 12.16)	• From within outwards lined by transitional epithelium (from which outwards) • Lamina propla present • Muscular coat – inner longitudinal and outer circular • Outermost fibrous coat.
Jrinary bladder (Fig. 12.17)	• From within outwards lined by transitional epithelium • Muscles coat arragned in three layers which is indistincly differentiated
estis (Fig. 12.18)	• A number of semin, ferrous tubule is present (in different shapes). • Spermatogenic cells are arranged in different stages of maturation • Tall columnar sertoli cells are present.

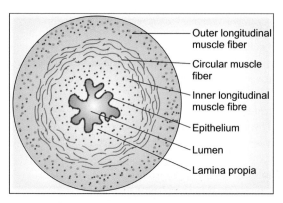

Fig. 12.19: A section of vas deferens (HE stained)

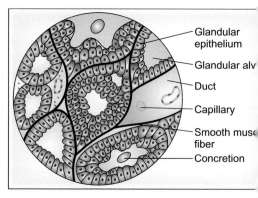

Fig. 12.20: A section of prostate (HE stained)

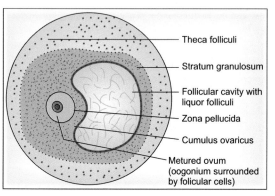

Fig. 12.21: Section of ovary showing mature follicle (high power)

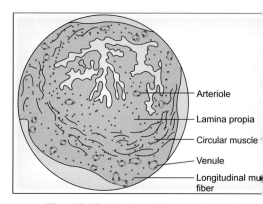

Fig. 12.22: Section of the uterine tube (HE stained)

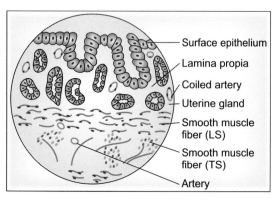

Fig. 12.23: Section of the uterus (follicular phase)

itourinary System

Name	Identifying points under microscope (stained with hematoxylin and Eosin)
as deferens (Fig. 2.19)	• From within outwards narrow irregular lumen. • Muscular layer is the thickest coat – inner longitudinal; middle circular and other longitudinal. • Outer fibrous coat.
rostate Fig. 12.20)	• Fibromuscular capsule covers the fibromusculo-glandular storma. • Amyloid bodies (prostatic concretion).
vary Fig. 12.21)	• From outside inwards covered by cubical germinal epithelium. • Outer border zone contains ovarian follicles in different state of maturation; atretic follicles also present.
terine tube Fig. 12.22)	• From inside outwards inner mucous membrane thrown into fold which branch and rebranch in such a way that rarely a lumen is visible. • Mucous folds do not anastomise. • Outer longitudinal and inner circular muscle coat is present. • Outer most serous coat (made up of mesothelium).
terus Fig. 12.23)	• From inside outwards lined by simple columnar epithelium. • Lamina propna composed of connective tissue contains uterine glands.

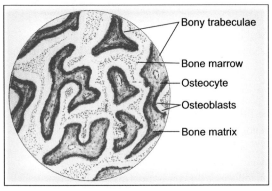

Fig. 12.24: Spongy bone

Bony trabeculae
Bone marrow
Osteocyte
Osteoblasts
Bone matrix

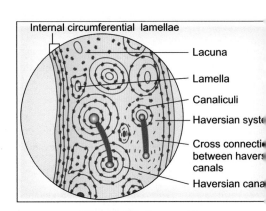

Fig. 12.25: Compact bone

Internal circumferential lamellae
Lacuna
Lamella
Canaliculi
Haversian syste
Cross connecti
between havers
canals
Haversian cana

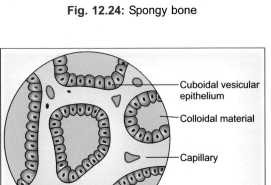

Fig. 12.26: Section of thyroid gland (HE stained)

Cuboidal vesicular epithelium
Colloidal material
Capillary

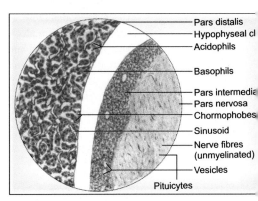

Fig. 12.27: Pituitary gland (high power)

Pars distalis
Hypophyseal cl
Acidophils
Basophils
Pars intermedia
Pars nervosa
Chormophobes
Sinusoid
Nerve fibres (unmyelinated)
Vesicles
Pituicytes

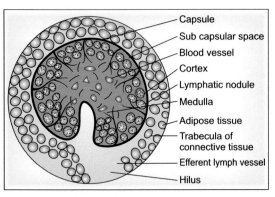

Fig. 12.28: Lymph node (Panoramic view) (HE stained)

Capsule
Sub capsular space
Blood vessel
Cortex
Lymphatic nodule
Medulla
Adipose tissue
Trabecula of connective tissue
Efferent lymph vessel
Hilus

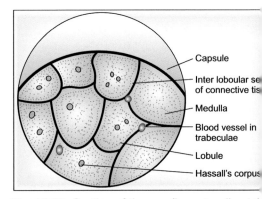

Fig. 12.29: Section of thymus (hematoxylin stai

Capsule
Inter loboular se
of connective tis
Medulla
Blood vessel in trabeculae
Lobule
Hassall's corpus

thers

Name	Identifying points under microscope (stained with hematoxylin and Eosin)
Bone (spongy) (Fig. 12.24)	• Bony trabecular, contains irregular lamillar plate. • Marrow spaces containing bone marrow.
Bone (compact) (Fig. 12.25)	• Presence of haversian system. • Lacunae contain osteocytes.
Thyroid gland (Fig. 12.26)	• A number of follicles with different shapes and sizes present. • Follicles contain homogeneous pink colored colloid.
Pituitary gland (Fig. 12.27)	• Pars anterior contains anastomising cords of chromophobe and chromophil cells. • Pars posterior contains pituicyles and large number of nerve fibers.
Lymph node (Fig. 12.28)	• From outside inwards bean shaped. • Subcapsular space is present. • Cortex contains numerous germinal epithelium.
Thymus (Fig. 12.29)	• From outside inwards outer lobulated cortex covered by thin capsule. • Cortex is dark stained. • Inner medulla contains Hassall's batch. Corpuscle.
Spleen (Fir. 12.30)	• From outside inwards presence of fibrous capsule. • Send incomplete septa from fibrous capsule. • Presence of red pulp and white pulp. • White pulp presents eccentric arteriole.

Contd...

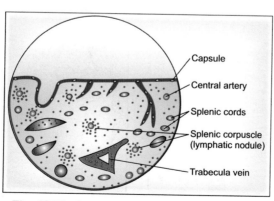

Fig. 12.30: Section of spleen (Panoramic view) (HE stained)

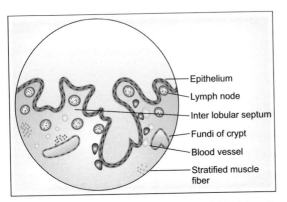

Epithelium
Lymph node
Inter lobular septum
Fundi of crypt
Blood vessel
Stratified muscle fiber

Fig. 12.31: Section of palatine tonsil (HE stained)

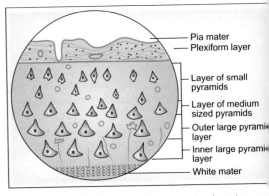

Pia mater
Plexiform layer
Layer of small pyramids
Layer of medium sized pyramids
Outer large pyramid layer
Inner large pyramid layer
White mater

Fig. 12.32: Section of the cerebral cortex

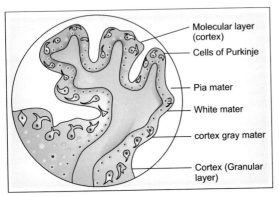

Molecular layer (cortex)
Cells of Purkinje
Pia mater
White mater
cortex gray mater
Cortex (Granular layer)

Fig. 12.33: Section of cerebellum

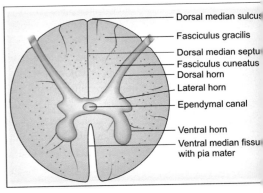

Dorsal median sulcus
Fasciculus gracilis
Dorsal median septum
Fasciculus cuneatus
Dorsal horn
Lateral horn
Ependymal canal
Ventral horn
Ventral median fissure with pia mater

Fig. 12.34: Section of the spinal cord

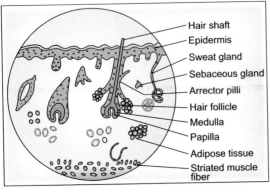

Hair shaft
Epidermis
Sweat gland
Sebaceous gland
Arrector pilli
Hair follicle
Medulla
Papilla
Adipose tissue
Striated muscle fiber

Fig. 12.35: Sectional view of scalp

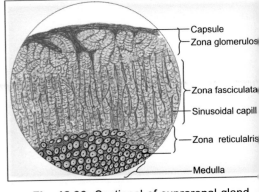

Capsule
Zona glomerulosa
Zona fasciculata
Sinusoidal capill
Zona reticulalris
Medulla

Fig. 12.36: Sectional of suprarenal gland

Name	*Identifying points under microscope (stained with hematoxylin and Eosin)*
Palatine tonsil (Fig. 12.31)	• Surface is covered by stratified squamous non keratinised epithelium. • Crypts are present. • Presence of partial capsule.
Cerebrum (Fig. 12.32)	Laminated appearance usually consists of 6 layers • Molecular layer • External granular layer • External pyramidal layer • Internal granular layer • Internal pyramidal layer • Multiform layer Very large pyramidal shaped neurons (Beta cells) are present in internal pyramidal layer.

Cerebellum (Fig. 12.33)	• From outside inwards outer grey matter divided into three zones
	   – Molecular (outer) layer.
	   – Purkinje layer (intermediate).
	   – Inner granular (dark bluish violet stain).
	• Inner white matter contains nerve fiber stained pink.

Spinal cord (Fig. 12.34)	• H shaped grey matter inside. • Outer white matter. • Anterior median fissure and posterior median sulcus present. • Anterior horn is bulbous.
Skin (Fig. 12.35)	• From superficial to deep presence of stratified squamous keratinised epithelium. • Hair follicle present.
Suprarenal gland (Fig. 12.36)	• Outer pale stained cortex which is divided into three zones – zona glomerulosa, zona faciculata, zona reticularis. • Inner dark blue medulla.

Chapter 13

Radiology (Imaging Technique)

RADIOLOGY

It is the study of structures of body by means of radiophoto.

1. **Conventional radiography** (Fig. 13.1A)—The making of X-ray picture on photo film is known as radiography. It is excellent for high contrast structures like bones and lungs. Normally soft tissue with slight thickness are not visible. So, the contrast media is used to identify soft structures. Contrast media are of two different types:

   Translucent–(air, oxygen)

   Opaque—e.g. barium sulphate, iodine compound.

   The rays when readily absorbed by a substance is known as radiolucent (like soft tissue). The tissue like bone is so dense that X-rays do not pass through it, is known as radio-opaque substance.

Advantages

1. To diagnose bony deformities and fractures.
2. To diagnose a congestion of soft tissue, or space occupying the lesion (tumor, etc).

STANDARD POSITION USED IN RADIOLOGY EXAMINATION

1. **Anteroposterior view (AP view)**—In this view the source of light is in front of the subject and the film lies behind the subject. Posterior structure is better visualized in this view, AP view of hip joint, elbow joint, etc.

2. **Posteroanterior view (PA view)** (Fig. 13.1A)—Here the source of light is behind subject and the rays passing postero anteri as the film is in front, e.g. PA view of the sk chest.

3. **Lateral view**—This view is used to assess depth of structures. The position in this view at the right angle to AP and PA.

Other Methods of Imaging Technique

1. **Angiographies**—Visualisation of vascular by introducing iodinated contrast med through catheter is known as angiography. useful in visualising tumor vascularity an assess the position of arteries.

2. **Ultrasound** (Fig. 13.1B)—It is inaudible so with frequency of more than 20, 000 cycles

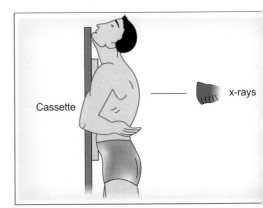

Fig. 13.1A: Technique of X-ray of PA view

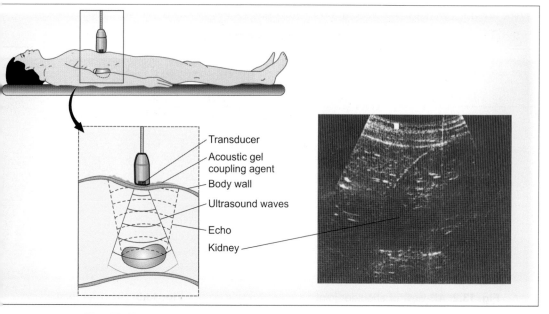

Fig. 13.1B: Technique for producing an abdominal ultrasound image

s passed to obtain the image or photograph of an organ and tissue; it is known as ultrasonography, or ultrasound in common language. Ultrasound is difficult in very obese person.

Computerized Topography (CT) (Fig. 13.1C)—It permits the study of tissue in slices, by which we can clearly localised the area of lesion and changes produced by it. The procedure is safe and quick.

4. **Magnetic Resonance Imaging (MRI)** – Here magnetic property of H-Nucleus is excited by radio frequency radiation and photograph is taken. MRI is safe and structures are more clearly visualized than CT scan.

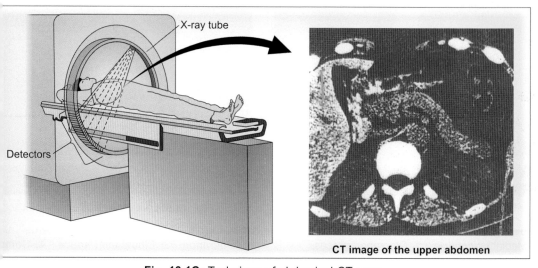

CT image of the upper abdomen

Fig. 13.1C: Technique of abdominal CT scan

Here are few conventional X-ray plates which often come in examination:

SUPERIOR EXTREMITY

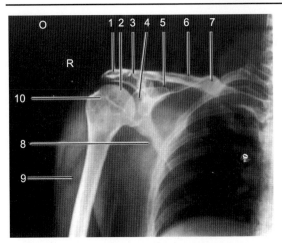

Fig. 13.2: AP view of shoulder joint

Showing: 1. Aeromian 2. Head of humerus 3. Acromio-clavicular joint space 4. Glenoid cavity 5. Coracoid process 6. Clavicle 7. Superior angle (scapula) 8. Lateral border of scapula 9. Soft tissue shadow 10. Anatomical neck of humerus

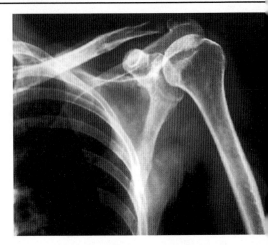

Fig. 13.3: Shoulder joint

My beloved student: Outline the different structures by probe and practise

ELBOW JOINT

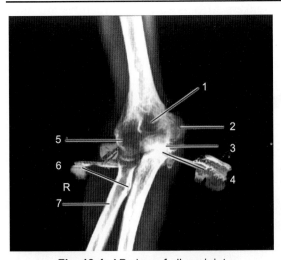

Fig. 13.4: AP view of elbow joint

Showing: 1. Olecranon and coronoid fossae 2. Medial epicondyle 3. Olecranon process 4. Elbow joint space 5. Lateral epicondyle (flatter appearance) 6. Head and tuberosity of radius 7. Soft tissue shadow

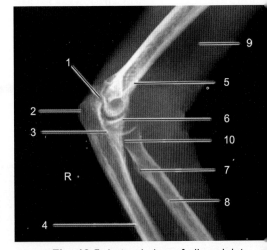

Fig. 13.5: Lateral view of elbow joint

Showing: 1. Two epicondyles of humerus 2. Olecranon 3. Elbow joint space 4. Comp bone 5. Supracondylar ridge 6. Coron process 7. Tuberosity of radius 8. Medull cavity 9. Soft tissue shadow 10. Head of radi

POSTERO-ANTERIOR VIEW OF WRIST JOINT AND HAND

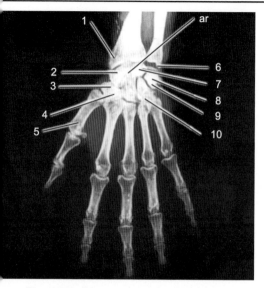

Fig. 13.6: PA view of wrist and hand

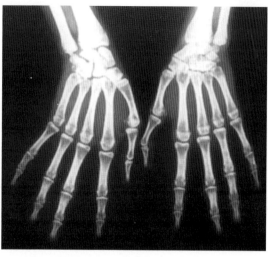

Fig. 13.7: PA of wrist and hand outline the different structures by probe and practise

owing: 1. Styloid process of radius 2. Scaphoid Trapezium 4. Trapezoid 5. 1st metacarpal Ulnar styloid process 7. Lunate 8. Triquitral and form 9. Capitate 10. Hammate with hook

CHEST

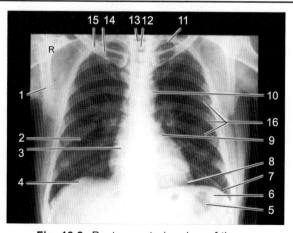

Fig. 13.8: Postero anterior view of thorax

owing: 1. Lateral border of scapula 2. Hialar shadow due to lympho-glandular vascular components Right border of mediastinal shadow 4. Right dome of diaphragm 5. Gas in fundus of stomach 6. Left ne of diaphragm 7. Costo-phrenic angle (left) 8. Cardio phrenic angle (left) 9. Left border of mediastinal dow 10. Aortic knuckle formed by arch of aorta 11. Thoracic inlet 12. Spine of vertebra visualized ugh shadow of trachea 13. Shadow of trachea 14. 1st rib 15. Clavicle 16. Ribs

ABDOMEN

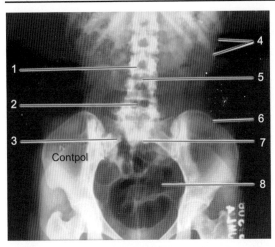

Fig. 13.9: Plain or straight X-ray of abdomen

Showing: 1. Vertebral body 2. Intervertebral disc space 3. Ala of sacrum 4. Lower ribs 5. Spine of vertebra 6. Iliac crest 7. Sacral promontory 8. Gas in large gut

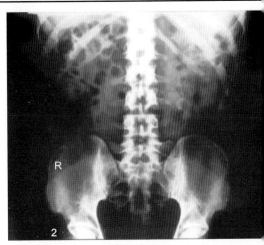

Fig. 13.10: Straight X-ray of abdomen

Please practice by probe

CONTRAST RADIOGRAPHY

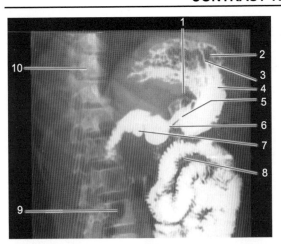

Fig. 13.11: Barium meal X-ray of stomach

Showing: 1. Lesser curvature of stomach 2. Fundic gas shadow 3. Rugae 4. Greater curvature of stomach 5. Pyloric antrum 6. Pyloric canal 7. Duodenal cap (due to barium in 1st one inch of 1st part of duodeneum) 8. Feathery intestinal mucosa 9. Gas shadow in colon 10. Shadow of pedicle

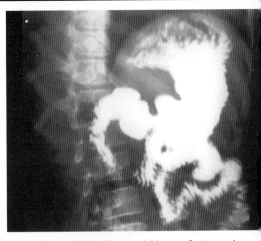

Fig. 13.12: Ba-meal X-ray of stomach

Please practice by probe

ABDOMEN

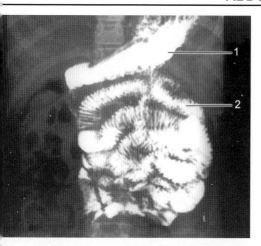

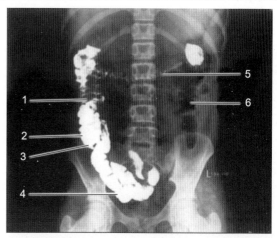

Fig. 13.13: Barium meal X-ray of stomach and follow through intestine

Showing: 1. Stomach 2. Feathery appearance of small intestine (due to barium entangle between mucous folds)

Fig. 13.14: Barium meal X-ray showing large gut

Showing: 1. Ascending colon 2. Caecum 3. Appendix 4. Small gut in pelvis 5. Transverse colon 6. Descending colon

PYLOGRAM

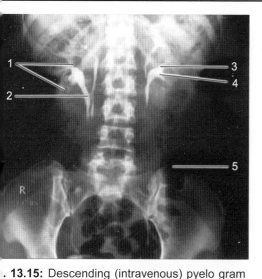

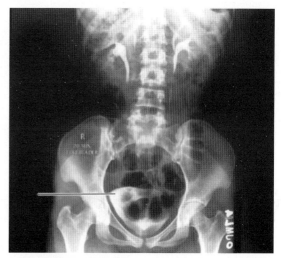

Fig. 13.15: Descending (intravenous) pyelo gram

Showing: 1. Minor calices 2. Double ureter on side 3. Major calices 4. Pelvis of ureter 5. in descending colon

Fig. 13.16: Descending pyelogram showing the dye contentrated in urinary bladder student, must outline the different shadows for practice

HEAD AND NECK

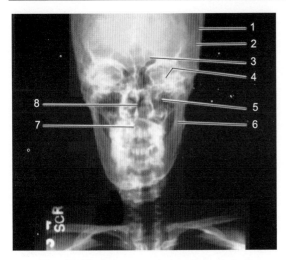

Fig. 13.17: Antero posterior view of skull

Showing: 1. Outer table 2. Inner table 3. Frontal air sinus 4. Petrous part of temporal bone 5. Maxillary air sinus 6. Ramus of mandible 7. Soft tissue shadow of tongue 8. Nasal septum and turbinate

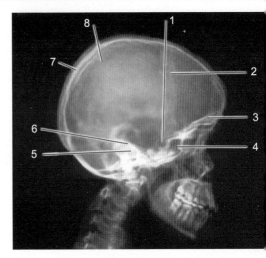

Fig. 13.18: Lateral view of skull

Showing: 1. Pituitary fossa 2. Coronal suture 3. Orbital plate of frontal bone 4. Sphenoidal sinus 5. External auditory meatus 6. Petrous of temporal bone 7. Outer table of parietal 8. Inner table of parietal

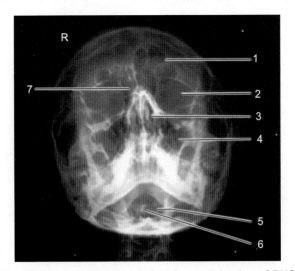

Fig. 13.19: Occipito meutal view for examination of PNS (Para-nasal air sinuses)

Showing: 1. Frontal air sinus 2. Orbital cavity 3. Nasal cavity 4. Maxillary air sinus 5. Foramen magnum 6. Axis (adontoid process) 7. Ethmoidal air cells

HEAD AND NECK *(Contd...)*

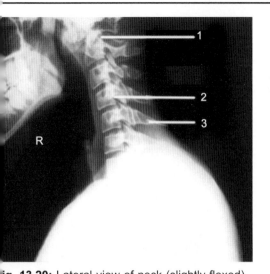

ig. 13.20: Lateral view of neck (slightly flexed)

>wing: 1. Dens (odontoid process) 2. Inter 'ebral foramen 3. Spine (cervical)

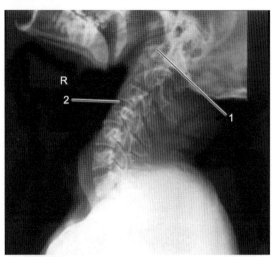

Fig. 13.21: Lateral view of neck (extended)

Showing: 1. Anterior arch of atlas 2. Disc space (intervertebral)

INFERIOR EXTREMITY

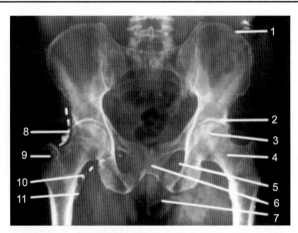

Fig. 13.22: Antero posterior (AP) view of hip joint

Showing: 1. Iliac crest 2. Acetabular magnum 3. Head of femur 4. Neck of femur 5. Obturator foramen 6. Symphysis pubis 7. Soft tissue shadow of external genitalia (by which you can identify sex) 8. Upper curved line 9. Greater trochanter of femur 10. Shenton's line 11. Lesser trochanter of femur

INFERIOR EXTREMITY *(Contd...)*

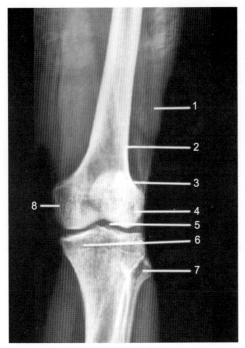

Fig. 13.23: Antero-posterior view of knee

Showing: 1. Soft tissue shadow 2. Lower end of femur 3. Outline of patella 4. Lateral condyle of femur 5. Knee joint space 6. Lateral and medial condyles of tibia 7. Head of fibula 8. Medial condyle of femur

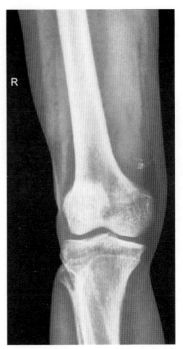

Fig. 13.24: AP view of knee
Student please practice with a probe

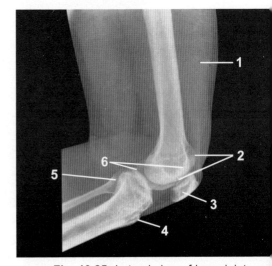

Fig. 13.25: Lateral view of knee joint

Showing: 1. Soft tissue shadow 2. Late condyle of femur 3. Patella 4. Tibial tuberosity 5. Head of fibula 6. Medial condyle of femur

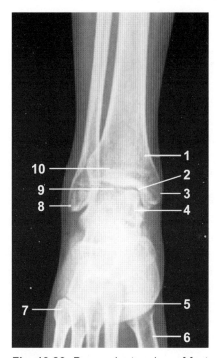

Fig. 13.26: Dorso planter view of foot

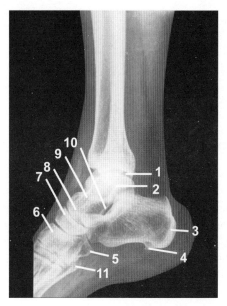

Fig. 13.27: Lateral view of foot

Showing: 1. Lower end of tibia 2. Ankle joint ~~ce~~ (line) 3. Medial malleolus 4. Talus 5. 2nd ~~atarsal~~ 6. 1st metatarsal 7. Styloid process of ~~metatarsal~~ 8. Lateral malliolus 9. Trachlear ~~ular~~ surface of talus 10. Epiphyseal line

Showing: 1. Ankle joint space 2. Medial comma like articular surface of talus 3. Calcaneum 4. Calcaneal spur 5. Cuboid 6. Medial cuneiform 7. Navicular 8. Head of talus 9. Neck of talus 10. Trochlear articular area of talus 11. Tuberosity of 5th metatarsal (at base)

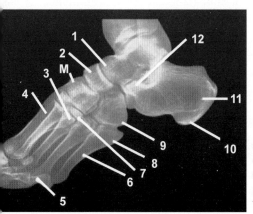

Fig. 13.28: Lateral view of foot

Showing: 1. Head of talus 2. Navicular 3. Base of 2nd metatarsal 4. 1st metatarsal 5. Phalanx 6. 5th metatarsal 7. Lateral cuneiform 8. Styloid process of 5th metatarsal 9. Cuboid 10. Calcaneal tuberosity 11. Calcaneum 12. Sinus tarsi

Chapter 14

Surface Anatomy

SURFACE ANATOMY

Study of anatomy in relation to body surface is known as Surface Anatomy. Physical examination of patient is the clinical application of surface anatomy. For this carefully selected landmark is used. There are:
1. Visible landmark
2. Palpable landmark.

Visible Landmark

Those landmarks are those which one can visible with nacked eye. Majority of them are produced by bones and cartilage, only nipple and umbilicus is soft tissue landmark identified by inspection.

Palpable Landmarks (Fig. 14.1)

These land-marks are felt through skin, muscles and tendons. Artery pulsation is felt against bone (e.g. radial pulse, femoral pulse, etc.). Nerves can be rolled against bone (e.g. ulnar nerve, termination of common peroneal nerve). Superfical tendon can be felt by making the muscle prominent. Parotid duct and vas deferens can be felt through skin. During examination it is better to use white chalk powder for points as well as for lines (because it is more prominent) as white color can be used in any type of drawings. In drawing an artery and a vein, please put a lumen inside two lines. In case of nerve one should draw a single line.

Applied Importance (Surface Anatomy)

1. Physical examination of patient is the clin application of surface anatomy.
2. Determination of peripheral pulse reduces complication of vaso occlusive dise (Buerger's disease)
3. Prominence of some veins help in diagnosis also therapeutic management of patient.
4. Determination of certain diseases by palpat nerves (e.g. thickening of ulnar nerve in lepro as well as nerve injuries due to fracture bones.

SUPERIOR EXTREMITY

Points

1. **Angle of Acromian Process** (Fig. 14.2): Fo a subcutaneous bony prominence. It can defined by following, the lateral margin acromion across the tip of the shoulder.
2. **Pisiform Bone**: Felt at the medial part of base of the hypothenar eminence.
3. **Head of the Radius**: It lies in the depress below the lateral epicondyle and latera olecranon process, which is felt dur pronation and supination.
4. **Head of the Ulna**: The wrist is flexed forearm pronated - the head is seen and felt as a swelling.
5. **Tip of Coracoid Process**: 2 cm below junction of lateral 1/4th and medial 3/4th of

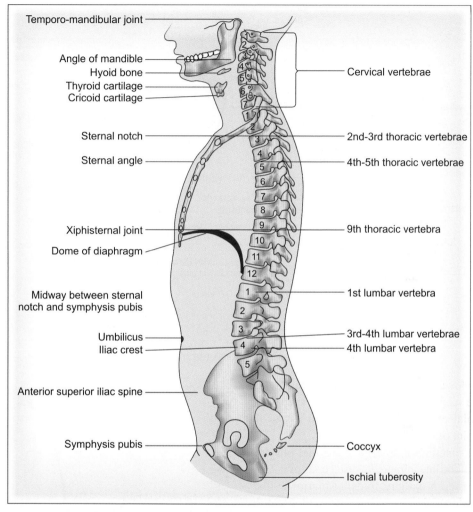

Fig. 14.1: Important visible points and palpable bony prominences used in surface marking

clavicle. It lives deep to anterior fibres of deltoid and felt by deep palpation.

Styloid Process of Radius: It is traced from the lower end of anterior border of radius. Tip is felt in the floor of anatomical snuff box. It lies 1.5 cm. below the ulnar styloid process.

Styloid Process of Ulna: It is felt in the posteromedial aspect of wrist just the line of wrist joint, 1.2 cm. above the level of styloid process of radius.

Lines

Bifurcation of Brachial Artery or Beginning of Radial Artery (Fig. 14.3): 1.25 cm below the mid point of the line joining two epicondyles of humerus, medial to the tendon of biceps brachii. It moves upward in the middle of cubical fossa when the elbow is flexed.

Left Axillary Artery (Fig. 14.3): Arm is abducted at right angles to the body. The points are:

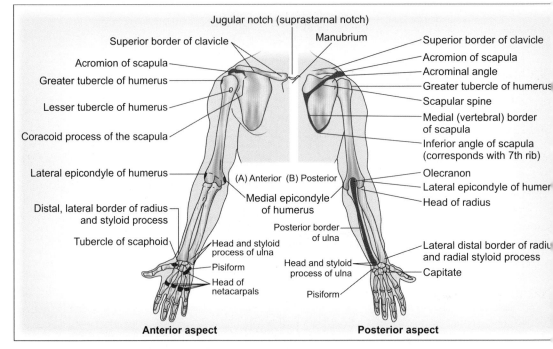

Fig. 14.2: Dark area palpable features of superior extremity

i. At the lower border of midpoint of the clavicle. Please identify the sternal end and then stress acromial end of clavicle and then assess the midpoint of clavicle.

ii. At the junction of anterior 2/3rd and posterior 1/3rd of the line joining the distal ends of anterior and posterior axillary folds. (Anterior axillary fold is formed by pectoralis major and later by teres major and latissimus dorsi).

2 parallel lines joining the above points represents the axillary artery.

Brachial Artery (Fig. 14.3)

1. At the junction of anterior 2/3rd and posterior 1/3rd of the line joining the distal ends of anterior and posterior axillary folds.
2. The point is 1 cm distal to the elbow joint at the level of neck of radius. The point lies on the medial aspect of tendon of biceps brachii.

2 parallel lines joining the above points represents brachial artery.

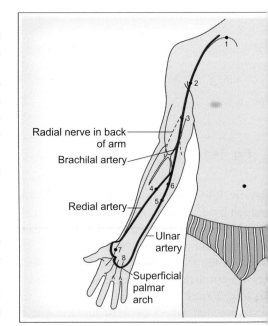

Fig. 14.3: Axillary art, brachial artery (in arm) ra artery, ulnar artery (in forearm) and superficial pal arch (in palm)

i. Brachial artery is compressed on the medial aspect of tendon of biceps during blood pressure recording

dial Artery in the Forearm (Fig. 14.3)

nts are:

A point 1 cm below the bent of elbow joint at the level of medial side of neck of the radius.

In front of the wrist between flexor carpi radialis and lower part of anterior border of radius, where pulsation is felt. It is the most important peripheral reflection of cardiac action.

Joint the 2 points by two = lines.

• It is the most important site of recording pulse.

lar Artery in Forearm (Fig. 14.3)

nts are:

The point is 1 cm distal to the elbow joint at the level of medial side of neck of the radius.

At the base of pisiform bone. It has a very superficial course in the forearm.

Join these 2 points with a lumen within.

perficial Palmar Arch (Figs 14.3 and 14.4)

nts are:

Lateral side of pisiform bone

Centre of thenar eminence

e points are joined by two curved line passing ough middle of palm. The summit of the line along the distal border of outstretched thumb.

Due to superficial and deep palmer arch the palm is more warmer than dorsum.

dial Nerve in the Back of the Arm (Fig. 14.3)

nts are:

At the termination of axillary artery, i.e. at the junction of anterior 2/3rd and posterior 1/3rd of the line joining the distal ends of anterior and posterior axillary folds.

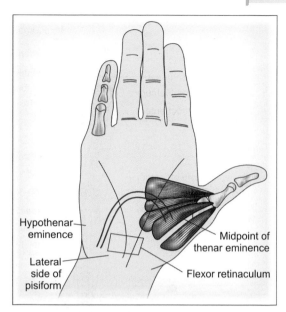

Fig. 14.4: Thenar and hypothenar eminences and superficial palmar arch

2. Junction of upper and middle third of the line joining insertion of deltoid to lateral epicondyle. Join the two points by a single line.

Ulnar Nerve in Forearm

Points at:
i. Behind medial epicondyle of humerus
ii. Lateral to pisiform bone.
   Join these 2 points with a single line.

INFERIOR EXTREMITY

Points (Fig. 14.5)

1. **Tip of Medial Malleolus**: Formed by lower projecting part of tibia.
2. **Tip of Lateral Malleolus**: Formed by lower end of fibula. It is half cm. lower than the medial malleolus.
3. **Tubercle of Navicular Bone**: 2 cm below the tip of medial malleolus and 2 cm in front of it.
4. **Adductor Tubercle**: Thigh is abducted and laterally rotated, hip and knee are slightly flexed.

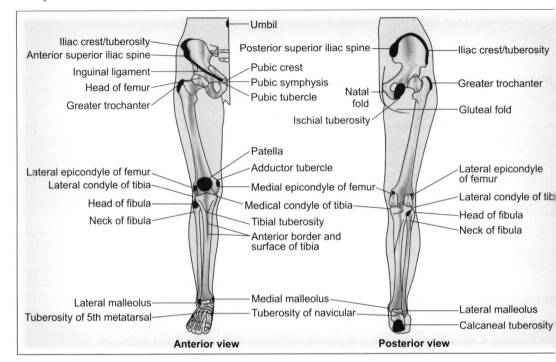

Anterior view   Posterior view

Fig. 14.5: Palpable features of inferior extremity

A small projection at the upper part of medial condyle of femur is palpated by tracing the tendon of adductor magnus from above.

- Importance:
  - Insertion of adductor magnus
  - Junction of epiphysis and diaphysis

Lines

1. **Popliteal Artery (Fig. 14.6)**

   Points at:

   i. 2.5 cm medial to the midpoint of the back of the thigh at the junction of middle and lower third of the thigh.

   ii. Middle of the back of the leg at the level of tibial tuberosity.

   2 parallel line joining the above points represent the popliteal artery.

2. **Posterior Tibial Artery**

   Points at:

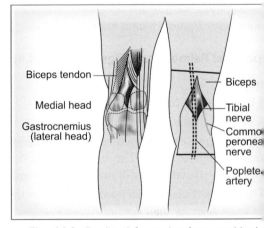

Fig. 14.6: Popliteal fossa (surface marking)

i. Middle of the back of the leg opposite tibial tuberosity.

ii. Midway between medial malleolus and tendocalcaneus.

2 parallel line joining the above points represent posterior tibial artery.

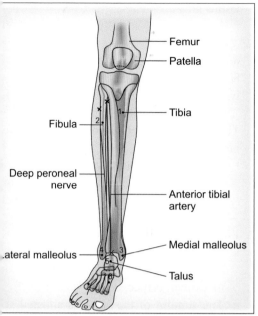

Fig. 14.7: Surface marking of leg (anterior tibial artery, deep peroneal nerve)

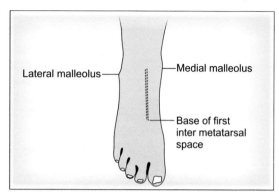

Fig. 14.8: Arteria dorsalis pedis (surface marking)

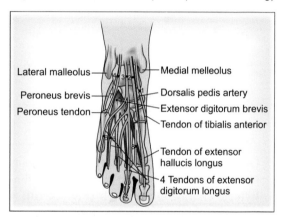

Fig. 14.9: Relation of arteria dorsalis pedis with long tendons of dorsum

Anterior Tibial Artery (Fig. 14.7)

Points at:

i. 2.5 cm below the medial side of the head of the fibula.

ii. Midpoint between medial and lateral malleolus 2 parallel line joining the above points represent anterior tibial artery.

Arteria Dorsalis Pedis (Figs 14.8 and 14.9)

Points at:

i. Midpoint between medial and lateral malleolus

ii. Point at the base of first intermetatarsal space
   • These (posteria tibial artery and dosarlis pedis artery are important for recording peripheral pulse

2 parallel lines joining the above points represents anterior tibial artery.

DOMEN

nes

Right and Left Lateral Planes (Fig. 14.10):

Plane passing through midclavicular point to nidinguinal point.

2. **Transpyloric Plane (Fig. 14.10):** Cuts the lower border of L1 vertebra. One hand breadth below the xiphisternal joint of the individual.on which the surface marking is done.
   • Pylorus of stomach, hila of kidneys, duodeno-jejunal flexure, neck of pancreas lies in this plane.

3. **Transtubercular Plane (Fig. 14.10):** Line joining the iliac tubercles represent this plane —(5 cm behind the anterior superior iliac spine.) This plane lies at the level of L4 vertebra. It lies slightly below the umbilicus.

Points

1. **Origin of Coeliac Artery:** Point 1.5 cm. above transpyloric plane in the midline.

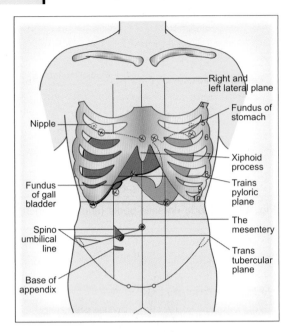

Fig. 14.10: Surface marking of abdomen

2. **Origin of Superior Mesenteric Artery**: A point just above the transpyloric plane in the midline.
3. **Pyloric Orifice of Stomach (Fig. 14.10)**: At the transpyloric plane 1.25 cm to the right of the midline.
4. **Tip of 9th Costal Cartilage (Fig. 14.10)**: At the junction of transpyloric planes and lateral border of rectus abdomininis (It is prominent in muscular body).
5. **Fundus of Gallbladder (Fig. 14.10)**: Tip of right 9th costal cartilage. It corresponds with an angle between right costal margin and line semi- lunaris (lateral border of rectus muscle).
6. **Base of the Appendix (Fig. 14.10)**: 2 cm below ileocecal orifice.
7. **Mc. Burney's Point**: At the junction between medial 2/3rd and lateral 1/3rd of spinoumbilical line (line joining umbilicus and anterior superior iliac spine).

Lines

1. **Inferior Border of Liver (Fig. 14.10):**

Points at:
i. Left 5th intercostals space 9 cm away fr the midline.
ii. At transpyloric plane in the midline
iii. Tip of 9th costal cartilage (right)
iv. 1.2 cm. below right costal margin, at the le of tip of 10th costal cartilage.
The above points are joined to represent infe border of liver.
- It is of great clinical value became live enlarged by a number of diseases. Norma in child upto 3 yrs. of age the lower bor exist below the costal margin.

2. **Fundus of Stomach (Fig. 14.10):**
i. One line is drawn directed upward backw and to the left starting from the left bor of cardiac orifice.
ii. The summit of the curve is situated at level of left 5th intercostals space just be the nipple.

3. **Lesser Curvature of Stomach (Fig. 14.1** Put a point at cardiac orifice and also in pyl orifice. The curvature is drawns starting fr the right margin of cardiac orifice upto the margin of pyloric orifice. Incisura angulari made in the mid line just below the transpyl plane.

4. **Root of the Mesentery**
Points are:
1st to draw transpyloric plane, transtuberc and right lateral plane.
i. 1 cm below the transpyloric plane, 2.5 to the left of the midline, it represe duodeno jejunal flexure.
ii. Junction of right lateral plane and transtu cular plane.
Join these two points by line with conve directed toward left.

5. **Kidney from the Back (Fig. 14.11):**
(Morris' parallelogram):
i. Two transverse lines at the level of thoracic and 3rd lumber spine.

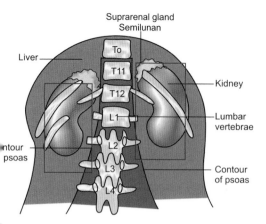

Fig. 14.11: Morris paralleogram (Dissection of kidney from back)

ii. Two vertical lines–2.5 cm away from the mid line and 10 cm away from the midline respectively.

Kidney is drawn–upper pole 3.8 cm away from dline, and lower pole 7.5 cm away from the dlines on the respective side (right or left).

ORAX

ints

Bifurcation of Trachea (Fig. 14.11): It is a point to the slightly right of midpoint of sternal angle.

Sternal Angle (Fig. 14.14): Junction of manubrium with the body of sternum.
. Importance of sternal angle
  • Counting of ribs
  • Junction of superior and inferior mediastinum.

Apex of the Heart (Fig. 14.14): In the left 5th intercostals space (ICS) 9 cm. away from midline (i.e. below and medial to left nipple).

es

Right Border of Heart (Fig. 14.14)
. Point at the upper border of right 3rd costal cartilage 1.25 cm from the lateral border of sternum.

ii. Point on the lower border of right 6th costal cartilage at the level of xiphisternal joint.
iii. Point on the right 4th space 3.8 cm from midline convex line Joining the above three points represent right border of Heart.
2. **Left Border of Heart (Fig. 14.14):**
   i. Point on lower border of left 2nd costal cartilage 1.2 cm from lateral margin of sternum.
   ii. Point in the left 5th intercostals space 9 cm away from the midline.(Where apexbeat in felt)
Line joining the above points convex upward and to the left represents the border of heart.
3. **Anterior Border of Left Lung (Fig. 14.12):**
   i. A point 2.5 cm above the midpoint of medial third of left clavicle.
   ii. A point on left sternoclavicular joint, a point at sternal angle slightly to the left of midline.
   iii. A point slightly to the left of the midline at the level of the 4th chondrosternal junction. From the 4th point the line passes laterally for 3.5 cm (from the midline), then downward and medially in a curved manner to the left 6th costal cartilage, about 4 cm. From the midline.

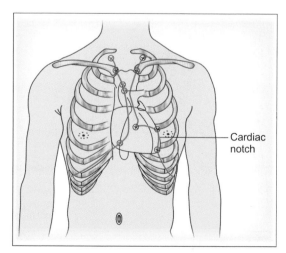

Fig. 14.12: Surface marking of (1) anterior border (2) Lower border of both lungs

4. **Right Costomediastinal Pieural Reflection**:
   Points at:
   i. Right sternoclavicular joint
   ii. Sternal angle in the midline
   iii. Level of right 4th sternochondral junction, in the midline
   iv. Xiphisternal joint—just to the right of the midline.
   (For costomediastinal reflection of pleura on the left side, 4th point is taken at the left extremely of the xiphisternal joint)

5. **Interior Border of Left Lung (Figs 14.12 and 14.13)**:
   Points at:
   i. Left 6th costal cartilage 4 cm. Away from midline
   ii. Left 8th rib in midaxillary line
   iii. Left 10th rib in scapular line
   iv. 2 cm to the left of 10th thoracic spine line joining the above points represent the inferior border of left lung.

6. **Arch of Aorta**
   Points at:
   i. Right end of sternal angle
   ii. Centre of manubrium sternum
   iii. Left end of sternal angle
   The line joining the points represents, the convex outer border of the arch of aorta.

7. **Superior Vena Cava (Fig. 14.12)**:
   Points at:
   i. Lower border of sternal and of right Ist cos cartilage
   ii. Upper border of the sternal end of the ri 3rd costal cartilage.
   Superior vena cava is repreented by 2 para lines 2 cm apart, coinciding with the abov points.

HEAD AND NECK

Points

1. **Isthmus of Thyroid Gland**
   Put a point at the center of the isthmus.
   Upper border: 1.2 cm below the lower bor of cricoid cartilage. Lower border 2 cm. be the upper border. Borders are 1.2 cm long lies over 1st end and 3rd tracheal ring.
   • Here tracheostomy is done by lifting isthmus.

2. **Anterior Arch of Cricoid Cartilage (Fig. 14.15)**:
   A point at the midline of anterior arch of cric most prominent part below the thyroid.

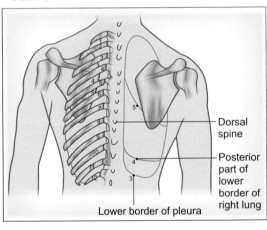

Fig. 14.13: Posterior chest wall: ribs, lungs and pleura

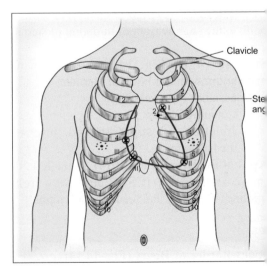

Fig. 14.14: Surface marking of heart (only give linear diagram) (1) Right border, (2) Left border Inferior border

Tip of Greater Cornu of Hyoid Bone (Fig. 14.15):

Most upper and lateral bony point from the body of the hyoid, can be palpated between thumb and the index finger.

Thyroid Eminence: Most prominent eminence in the mid line below the hyoid bone. More marked in male.

Nasion (Fig. 14.15): Overlies the frontonasal suture, marked by the depression at the root of the nose.

es

Right Lobe of Thyroid Gland

Points at:

i. 1.2 cm below the lateral end of isthmus, the line is drawn downward and taken laterally with a convexity downward for about 2 or 2.5 cm.

ii. On the anterior border of sternomastoid at the level of laryngeal prominence. The upper pole is joined with the lateral end upper border of isthmus

- Thyroid gland is frequently enlarged. In female it is darged in puberty. Non-cancering growth of thyroid is known as goiter.

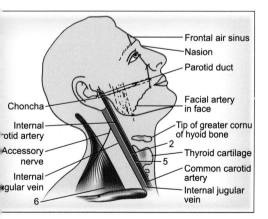

Fig. 14.15: Surface marking of head and neck

Labels: Frontal air sinus, Nasion, Parotid duct, Facial artery in face, Tip of greater cornu of hyoid bone, Thyroid cartilage, Common carotid artery, Internal jugular vein, Choncha, Internal otid artery, Accessory nerve, Internal jugular vein

2. **Duct of Parotid Gland (5 cm) (Fig. 14.15):**
   Points at:
   i. Lower border of concha
   ii. In between ala of the nose and red margin of the upper lip.
   Middle-third of the line joining these two points represents the parotid duct.
   - This is of clinical value as it can often felt by clinician to diagnose stone.

3. **Right Frontal Air Sinus (Fig. 14.15):**
   Points at:
   i. The nasion
   ii. 2.5 cm above the nasion
   iii. Junction of medial 1/3rd and lateral 2/3rd of supraorbital margin. The points are joined.
   - Frontal air sinuses are unequal is size, inflamed in sinusitis and point of tenderness is elicited in this region.

4. **Spinal Accessory Nerve**
   Points at:
   i. The lower and anterior point of tragus
   ii. Point opposite the tip of transverse process of atlas.
   iii. Junction of upper 1/4th and lower 3/4th of anterior border of sternomastoid.
   iv. Junction of upper 1/3rd and lower 2/3rd of posterior border of sternomastoid.
   v. Anterior margin of trapezius of the posterior trangle about 6 cm above the clavicle.

5. **Right Common Carotid Artery (Fig. 14.15)**
   Point at:
   i. Right sternoclavicular joint
   ii. Anterior margin of sternomastoid opposite the level of upper border of thyroid cartilage.
   It is represented by two parallel lines joining above two points.
   - Palpation of common carotid pulse is very important for cardiopulmonary resuscitation

6. **Right Internal Carotid Artery (Fig. 14.15):**
   Point at:
   i. Bifurcation of common carotid artery, i.e. a point at upper border of thyroid cartilage at

the level of anterior border of sternocleido-mastoid.

ii. Posterior border of mandibular condyle.

It is represented by two parallel lines joining above two points.

Bifurcation of Common Carotid Artery: A point at lower 1/3rd opposite upper border of thyroid cartilage at the anterior margin of sternocleido-mastoid.

7. **Facial Artery in Face (Fig. 14.15)**:

Points at:

i. The base of the mandible at the anterior border of masseter. (it is felt by pressing upper jaw with lower jaw).

ii. 1.25 cm lateral to the angle of mouth.

iii. Medial angle of the eye.

The first two points are joint by two zig. line. 2nd and 3rd point are connected by t straight line.

• This artery has got great clinical importan in plastic and cosmetic surgery.

Tip of Seventh Cervical Spine: A point at lov end of nuchal furrow, a prominent bony elevat in the midline felt when the head is bowed dov

8. **Internal Jugular Vein (Fig. 14.15)**:

Points at:

i. Louble of the ear.

ii. Medial end of the clavicle.

The points are joined by 2 parallel lines.

• Internal jugular vein is canulated frequen to measure the central venous pressure well as is dialysis of patient in kidney failu

Appendix

....	Good	Macro	Large
....	Out	Mast, masto	Breast
....	Exterior, External	Mega, megalo	Large
a	Outside of	Melano	Black
ro	Fiber	Meso	Middle
n	Shape	Micro	Small
act, galacto	Milk	Mono..............................	Singular
sso	Tongue	Morpho	Shape
co	Glucose	Oculo	Eye
th, gnatho	Jaw	Odonto	Tooth
nule	Grain like	Oligo	Few
ph	A recording instrument	Oo, oophoro	Ovary
e, gyneco, gyno	Woman	Orchi, orchio	Testis
nat, hemato...............	Blood	Osseo, osteo	Bone
i	One half	Ovi, ovo	Egg
at, hepato	Liver	Pachy..............................	Thick
io, histo	Tissue	Pan..................................	All
ro	Water	Patho, pathy	Disease
er..............................	Excessive	Penia	Deficiency
o	Beneath	Per..................................	Through
ter, hystero	Uterus	Peri..................................	Around
....	The ileum	Pexy	Fixation
a	Below	Phaco..............................	Lens (eye)
r	Between	Phase, phagia, phago	Eating
....	inflammation	Phleb, phlebo	Vein
a	Within	Phono	Sound
irido	The iris	Phos, photo	Light
yo..............................	Nucleus	Phren, phrenco	Diaphragm
at, kerato	Cornea	Plagia	Paralysis
esio	Motion	Pluri	More
t, lacto, lacti	Milk	Pneuma, pneumato.........	Air
to	Light or slender	Podo, podium	Foot
co..............................	White	Poly	Multiplicity
o	A stone	Pre, pro	Before

Procto	Anus
Psyche	Mind
Pylo	Pelvis
pyo	Suppuration
Re	Again
Recto	Rectum
Rhino	Nose
Sclero	Hardness
Scope	An instrument for viewing
Semi	One half
Sialo	Saliva
Somat, somato	Body
Spasmo	Spasm
Spermato, spermo	Semen spermatozoa
Splanchno	Viscera
Spleno	Spleen
Steno	Narrowness
Stoma, stomato	Mouth
Sub	Beneath
Super	In excess, in the upper p
Sym, syn	Together
Thel, thela	Nipple
Thermo	Heat
Thoraco	Chest
Thromb, thrombo	Blood clot
Tome, tomy	Cutting
Trans	Across
Trichi	Hair
Xanth, xantho	Yellow
Zym, zymo	Fermentation

MEDICAL PREFIXES, SUFFIXES, AND COMBINING USED IN ANATOMY

duct .... To move away from midline

scess .... Localised accumulation of pus and disintegrated tissue

etabulum .... Cup-like cavity

tin .... A contractile muscle protein

aptation .... Any change in structure or new environment

duct .... To move towards the midline of body

glutination .... Clumping

onist .... Muscle that bears the major responsibility for effecting a particular movement

ontois .... Embryonic membrane

eles .... Gene coding for same trait and found at the same locus on homologous chromosome

veolus .... Microscopic air sacs

algesia .... Reduced ability to feel pain

astomosis .... A union

eurysm .... Dilatation

giogram .... Diagnostic technique involving infusion of radiopaque substance into circulation for specific visualisation of blood vessel

us .... Distal end of GI tract

oneurosis .... Membranous sheet

achnoid .... Web-like

eola .... Circular pigmented area surrounding the nipple

rector pili .... Tiny smooth muscle attached to hair

thritis .... Inflammation of joint

eriole .... A minute artery

Aspiration .... The act of inhaling something into the lung

Ataxia .... Inaccurate movement

Atelectasis .... Lung collapse

Autoimmune .... Production of antibodies against own tissue response

Bolus .... A rounded mass of food

Bursa .... A fibrous sac with synovial membrane, containing synovial fluid

Calculus .... Stone

Callus....................... 1. Localised thickening of skin resulting from persisting friction

2. Repair tissue (fibrous or bony)

Calyx .... A cup-like extension

Canaliculus .... Extremely small tubular passage

Carcinogen .... Cancer causing agent

Carotene .... Yellow or orange pigment

Cataract .... Clouding of eye's lens

Cerebral palsy .... Neuromuscular disablity in which the voluntary muscles are poorly controlled or paralysed

Chemoreceptor .... Receptors sensitive to various chemicals

Chemotaxis .... Movement of a cell, organisms toward or away from a chemical substance

Cirrhosis .... Chronic disease of liver characterised by fibrosis

Cisternae .... Any cavity serving as reservoir

Cleavage .... An early embryonic phase consisting of rapid mitotic cell division

Clone .... Descendant of a single cell

Cochlea .... Snail-shaped chamber

Conjunctiva .... Thin protective mucous membrane lining the eyelids and covering the anterior surface of eye itself

Contraception .... Birth control

Contralateral .... Relating to opposite side

Corona radiata .... Crown-like arrangement

Cortex .... Outer surface layer of an organ

Deglutition .... Swallowing

Diaphragm .... Partition

Diaphysis .... Elongated shaft of a long bone

Dislocation .... Displacement from normal alignment

Dyskinesis .... Disorder of muscle tone and posture

Dysplasia .... A change in cell size and shape or arrangement

Dyspnea .... Difficult breathing

Edema .... Abnormal accumulation of fluid in tissues

Emesis .... Vomiting

Encephalopathy ...... Any disease of brain

Epitaxis .... Bleeding from nose

Extrinsic .... Of external origin

Exudate .... Any fluid that escapes from tissue containing pus

Fascicle .... Bundles of nerve or muscle fiber bound together by connective tissue

Fenestrated .... Pierced with one or more small opening

Fissure .... A groove

Fixator .... Muscle that immobilises one or more bones

Flexion .... Bending

Foramen .... Opening of a bone

Fossa .... A depression

Fovea .... A pit

Fracture .... A break in bone

Fundus .... Base of an organ

Gastrulation .... Developmental process t produces three primary ge layers

Gene .... One of the biological units heredity located in chromati

Genotype .... One's genetic make up

Gestation .... The period of pregnancy

Glomerulus .... Cluster of capilaries

Glottis .... Opening between vocal core

Gonad .... Primary reproductive organ

Hematoma .... Mass of clotted blood that for in an injured site

Hemostasis .... Stoppage of bleeding

Hepatitis .... Inflammation of liver

Hernia .... Abnormal protrusion of organ or a body part

Hilus .... The indented region of an org

Hirsutism .... Excessive hair growth

Histology .... Study of tissues

Homeostasis .... Stable internal environment the body

Hyperplasia .... Accelerated growth

Hypertrophy .... Increase in size

Hypothermia .... Low body temperature

In vitro .... In a test tube

In vivo .... In the living body

Incontinence .... Inability to control micturati volantarily

Infarct .... Region of dead tissue result from a lack of blood supply

Inflammation .... A nonspecific defensive r ponse of body to tissue inju

Infundibulum .... A stalk

Ischemia .... Local decrease in blood sup

Isometric .... Contraction in which the mus does not shorten contraction

Karyotype .... Chromosome character-istics an individual

Keratin .... Water-soluble protein found epidermis, hair and nails

Labia .... Lips, singual, labium

rimal .... Pertaining to tears

teal .... Special lymphatic capillaries of the small intestine that takes up lipid

unae .... A small space

nella .... A layer

ion .... Wound

ament .... Band of fibrous tissue that connects bone

bic system .... Functional brain system involved in emotional response

lignant .... Life threatening

ndible .... Lower jaw bone

stication .... Chewing

dial .... Toward the midline of the body

lanin .... Dark pigment formed by cell melanocyte

narche .... The first menstrual period

nopause .... Cessation of menstruation

crocephaly .... Formation of small brain tissue

dsagittal plane .... Specific sagittal plane that lies exactly in the midline (median) plane

ked nerve .... Nerve containing motor and sensory neurone

cus .... A sticky thick fluid

scle tone .... Sustained partial contraction of a muscle; keeps the muscle healthy and ready to act

ocardium .... Muscle coat of heart

ometrium .... Uterine musculature

opia .... Short sightedness

res .... Nostrils

crosis .... Dead tissue caused by disease or injury

onatal period .... The four-week period immediately after birth

oplasm .... An abnormal mass of proliferating cells, commonly known as tumors

ve impulse .... A self-propagating wave of depolarisation

Nociceptor .... Mechanism for the perception and transmission of painful or injurious stimuli

Nondisjunction .... Failure of one or more pairs of chromosome to separate at the mitotic stage of karyokinesis

Occlusion .... Closure

Olfaction .... Smell

Organelles .... Small cellular structure (like mitochondria, ribosome, etc.)

Osteomalacia .... Soft bone resulting from inadequate mineralisation

Osteophyte .... A bony outgrowth

Osteoporosis .... Gradual atrophy of skeletal tissue

Palate .... Roof of the mouth

Paresthesia .... An abnormal (burning or tingling) sensation

Parturation .... Give birth

Pectoral .... Pertaining to chest

Pedigree .... Ancestral history (family tree)

Petechae .... Minute hemorrhagic spot

Phagocytosis .... Engulfing

Pathology .... Study of changes in organs and tissues by disease

Phenotype .... To display (external feature)

Phlebitis .... Inflammation of a vein

Pinocytosis .... Engulfing of extracellular fluid

Polyps .... Benign mucosal tumor

Presbyopia .... Loss of near focusing ability

Prime mover .... Muscle that bears the major responsibility for a particular movement

Puberty .... Period of life when reproductive maturity is achieved

Radioactivity .... The process of spontaneous decay seen in some of the heavier isotopes

Ramus .... Branch

Referred pain .... Pain felt at a side other than the area of origin

Regeneration .... Replacement

Renal .... Pertaining to kidney

Renin .... Substance released by the kidney

Rennin .... Stomach secreted enzyme that acts on milk protein

Rhombencephalon .. Hind brain

Rugae .... Elevation or ridges as in stomach mucosa

Sebaceous gland ..... Oil secreted gland

Serosa .... Serous membrane (moist membrane)

Sinus .... Mucous membrane lined air filled, cavity

Somatic reflexes .... Reflexes that activate skeletal muscles

Somite .... A mesodermal segment of the body of embryo that forms skeletal muscles, vertebrae and dermis of skin

Splanchnic .... The vessel serving the digestive system circulation

Sprain .... Ligaments of a joint are stretched or torn

Stenosis .... Narrowing

Stimulus .... An extitant or irritant

Stroke .... Condition in which brain tissue is deprived of blood supply

Sudoriferous gland . Sweat producing gland

Sulcus .... A furrow

Surfactant .... Substance that reduces the surface tension, thus preventing the collapse of alveoli after each expiration

Synarthrosis .... Immovable joint

Synchondrosis .... A joint in which bones articulated by hyaline cartila

Synergist .... Stabilises joint to prev undesired movement

Systemic .... Pertaining to whole body

Tendon .... Cord of dense fibrous tis attaching muscle to bone

Tendonitis .... Inflammation of tendon shea typically caused by overuse

Thrombus .... A clot

Tract .... A collection of nerve fibers the central nervous system

Trophic hormone .... A hormone that regulates function of another gland

Tumor .... An abnormal growth of cells produces a swelling

Uvula .... Tissue tag hanging from s palate

Varicosities .... Dilatation and tortousity veins

Vas .... A duct

Ventral .... Anterior or in front

Venule .... A small vein

Vesicle .... A small liquid-filled sac

Villus .... A finger-like projection

Visceral .... Partaining to internal organ

Viscosity .... Sticky or thick

Vulva .... Female external genitalia

Xenograft .... Tissue graft taking from anot animal species

Zygote .... Fertilised egg

Index